Hand and Wrist Arthroscopy

Editors

CLARA WING-YEE WONG
PAK-CHEONG HO

HAND CLINICS

www.hand.theclinics.com

Consulting Editor
KEVIN C. CHUNG

November 2017 • Volume 33 • Number 4

ELSEVIER

1600 John F. Kennedy Boulevard • Suite 1800 • Philadelphia, Pennsylvania, 19103-2899

http://www.theclinics.com

HAND CLINICS Volume 33, Number 4
November 2017 ISSN 0749-0712, ISBN-13: 978-0-323-54881-6

Editor: Lauren Boyle
Developmental Editor: Kristen Helm

Hand Clinics (ISSN 0749-0712) is published quarterly by Elsevier Inc., 360 Park Avenue South, New York, NY 10010-1710. Months of publication are February, May, August, and November. Business and Editorial Offices: 1600 John F. Kennedy Blvd., Ste. 1800, Philadelphia, PA 19103-2899. Customer Service Office: 3251 Riverport Lane, Maryland Heights, MO 63043. Periodicals postage paid at New York, NY and at additional mailing offices. Subscription price is $398.00 per year (domestic individuals), $721.00 per year (domestic institutions), $100.00 per year (domestic students/residents), $454.00 per year (Canadian individuals), $839.00 per year (Canadian institutions), $541.00 per year (international individuals), $839.00 per year (international institutions), and $256.00 per year (international and Canadian students/residents). Foreign air speed delivery is included in all *Clinics* subscription prices. All prices are subject to change without notice. **POSTMASTER:** Send address changes to *Hand Clinics*, Elsevier Health Sciences Division, Subscription Customer Service, 3251 Riverport Lane, Maryland Heights, MO 63043. Customer Service (orders, claims, online, change of address): Elsevier Health Sciences Division, Subscription **Customer Service, 3251 Riverport Lane, Maryland Heights, MO 63043. Tel: 1-800-654-2452 (U.S. and Canada); 314-447-8871 (outside U.S. and Canada). Fax: 314-447-8029. E-mail: journalscustomerservice-usa@elsevier.com (for print support); journalsonlinesupport-usa@elsevier.com (for online support).**

Reprints. For copies of 100 or more of articles in this publication, please contact the Commercial Reprints Department, Elsevier Inc., 360 Park Avenue South, New York, New York 10010-1710. Tel.: 212-633-3874; Fax: 212-633-3820; E-mail: reprints@elsevier.com.

Hand Clinics is covered in *MEDLINE/PubMed (Index Medicus), Current Contents/Clinical Medicine, EMBASE/Excerpta Medica,* and *ISI/BIOMED.*

Contributors

CONSULTING EDITOR

KEVIN C. CHUNG, MD, MS
Chief of Hand Surgery, University of Michigan
Health System, Charles B.G. De Nancrede
Professor of Plastic Surgery and Orthopaedic
Surgery, Assistant Dean for Faculty Affairs,
Associate Director of Global REACH,
University of Michigan Medical School, Ann
Arbor, Michigan, USA

EDITORS

**CLARA WING-YEE WONG, MBChB, MRCS,
FRCSEd (Orth), FHKAM (Orth Surg),
FHKCOS**
Clinical Associate Professor (Honorary),
Division of Hand and Microsurgery,
Department of Orthopaedics and
Traumatology, Prince of Wales Hospital, The
Chinese University of Hong Kong, Shatin, NT,
Hong Kong SAR, China

**PAK-CHEONG HO, MBBS, FRCS (Edinburg),
FHKCOS, FHKAM (Orth Surg)**
Clinical Professor (Honorary), Consultant and
Chief, Division of Hand and Microsurgery,
Department of Orthopaedics and
Traumatology, Prince of Wales Hospital, The
Chinese University of Hong Kong, Shatin, NT,
Hong Kong SAR, China

AUTHORS

YUKIO ABE, MD, PhD
Director, Department of Orthopaedic Surgery,
Saiseikai Shimonoseki General Hospital,
Shimonoseki, Japan

ZAHAB S. AHSAN, MD
Resident Physician, Department of
Orthopaedics and Sports Medicine,
University of Washington, Seattle,
Washington, USA

**GREGORY I. BAIN, MBBS, FRACS,
FA, PhD**
Department of Orthopaedic Surgery, Flinders
University, Flinders Medical Centre, Adelaide,
South Australia, Australia

EVA-MARIA BAUR, MD
Senior Consultant, Practice for Plastic and
Hand Surgery, Murnau, Germany

SHAN-LIN CHEN, MD
Department of Hand Surgery, Beijing Jishuitan
Hospital, 4th Medical College of Peking
University, Beijing, China

**MICHAEL CHU-KAY MAK, MBChB, FRCS
(Edinburg), FHKCOS, FHKAM (Orth Surg)**
Division of Hand and Microsurgery,
Department of Orthopaedics and
Traumatology, Prince of Wales Hospital, The
Chinese University of Hong Kong, Shatin, NT,
Hong Kong SAR, China

KEVIN C. CHUNG, MD, MS
Chief of Hand Surgery, University of Michigan
Health System, Charles B.G. De Nancrede
Professor of Plastic Surgery and Orthopaedic
Surgery, Assistant Dean for Faculty Affairs,
Associate Director of Global REACH,
University of Michigan Medical School, Ann
Arbor, Michigan, USA

JAMES CLUNE, MD
Visiting Fellow, Section of Plastic Surgery, Yale School of Medicine, New Haven, Connecticut, USA

FERNANDO CORELLA, PhD
Orthopedic and Trauma Department, University Hospital Infanta Leonor, Hand Surgery Unit, Beata María Ana Hospital, Surgery Department, School of Medicine, Complutense University of Madrid, Madrid, Spain

RANDALL W. CULP, MD
Philadelphia Hand To Shoulder Center, Thomas Jefferson University, King of Prussia, Pennsylvania, USA

MIGUEL DEL CERRO, MD
Hand Surgery Unit, Beata María Ana Hospital, Madrid, Spain

FRANCISCO DEL PIÑAL, MD, PhD
Hand Surgeon, Private Practice, Madrid, Spain

JEFF ECKER, BMedSc (Hons), MBBS, FRACS
Director, Hand and Upper Limb Centre, Adjunct Professor, Curtin University of Technology, Hand and Wrist Surgeon, Western Orthopaedic Clinic, Perth, Western Australia, Australia

KENZO FUJII, MD
Department of Orthopaedic Surgery, Saiseikai Shimonoseki General Hospital, Shimonoseki, Japan

KEIJI FUJIO, MD
Chief Consultant of Hand Center and Medical Institute, Kansai Electric Power Hospital, Osaka City, Japan

MATHILDE GRAS, MD
Hand Surgeon, Institut de la Main, Clinique BIZET, Paris, France

DAVID G. HARGREAVES, MBBS, FRCS (Tr & Orth)
Orthopaedic Hand Surgeon, Department of Orthopaedics, University Hospital Southampton, Southampton, United Kingdom

JAN RAGNAR HAUGSTVEDT, MD, PhD
Senior Consultant, Hand Surgery, Department of Orthopedics, Østfold Hospital Trust, Graalum, Norway

RYAN P.C. HIGGIN, BM, BMedSci, MRCS (Eng)
Orthopaedic Registrar, Department of Orthopaedics, University Hospital Southampton, Southampton, United Kingdom

PAK-CHEONG HO, MBBS, FRCS (Edinburg), FHKCOS, FHKAM (Orth Surg)
Clinical Professor (Honorary), Consultant and Chief, Division of Hand and Microsurgery, Department of Orthopaedics and Traumatology, Prince of Wales Hospital, The Chinese University of Hong Kong, Shatin, NT, Hong Kong SAR, China

KARIM KANTAR, MBBS
Department of Orthopaedic Surgery, Flinders University, Flinders Medical Centre, Adelaide, South Australia, Australia

MASAAKI KOBAYASHI, MD, PhD
Department of Orthopaedic Surgery, Graduate School of Medical Sciences, Nagoya City University, Mizuho-ku, Nagoya, Japan

SIU-CHEONG JEFFREY JUSTIN KOO, MBBS, FRCS (Edinburgh), FHKCOS, FHKAM (Orth Surg), MHSM (New South Wales), MScSMHS (CUHK)
Department of Orthoapedic and Traumatology, Alice Ho Miu Ling Nethersole Hospital, Hong Kong SAR, China

RICARDO LARRAINZAR-GARIJO, PhD
Surgery Department, School of Medicine, Complutense University of Madrid, Chief of Orthopedic and Trauma, University Hospital Infanta Leonor, Madrid, Spain

DAVID M. LICHTMAN, MD
Uniformed Services University, Bethesda, Maryland, USA; Department of Orthopaedic Surgery, University of North Texas, Health Science Center, Fort Worth, Texas, USA

TOMMY LINDAU, MD, PhD (Hand Surgery)
Consultant Hand Surgeon, The Pulvertaft Hand Centre, Assistant Professor, University of Derby, Derby, United Kingdom

BO LIU, MD
Department of Hand Surgery, Beijing Jishuitan
Hospital, 4th Medical College of Peking
University, Beijing, China

**SIMON B.M. MACLEAN, MBChB, FRCSEd,
PGDipCE**
Department of Orthopaedic Surgery, Flinders
University, Flinders Medical Centre, Adelaide,
South Australia, Australia

CHRISTOPHE MATHOULIN, MD, FMH
Professor, Head of Department, Institut de la
Main, Clinique BIZET, Paris, France

BRETT F. MICHELOTTI, MD
Assistant Professor, Division of Plastic
Surgery, Department of Surgery, University of
Wisconsin Hospital and Clinics, Madison,
Wisconsin, USA

MONTSERRAT OCAMPOS, PhD
Orthopedic and Trauma Department,
University Hospital Infanta Leonor, Hand
Surgery Unit, Beata María Ana Hospital,
Madrid, Spain

HIDEKI OKAMOTO, MD, PhD
Department of Orthopaedic Surgery, Graduate
School of Medical Sciences, Nagoya City
University, Mizuho-ku, Nagoya, Japan

TAKANOBU OTSUKA, MD, PhD
Department of Orthopaedic Surgery, Graduate
School of Medical Sciences, Nagoya City
University, Mizuho-ku, Nagoya, Japan

MIN JONG PARK, MD
Department of Orthopaedic Surgery, Samsung
Medical Center, School of Medicine,
Sungkyunkwan University, Gangnam-gu,
Seoul, Korea

LORIS PEGOLI, MD
Hand and Reconstructive Microsurgery
Department, Humanitas San Pio X, Milan, Italy

ALESSANDRO POZZI, MD
Hand and Reconstructive Microsurgery
Department, Humanitas San Pio X, Milan, Italy

TAICHI SAITO, MD, PhD
International Research Fellow, Section of
Plastic Surgery, Department of Surgery,
University of Michigan Health System, Ann

Arbor, Michigan, USA; Department of
Orthopaedic Surgery, Okayama University
Graduate School of Medicine, Dentistry and
Pharmaceutical Sciences, Okayama, Japan

ISATO SEKIYA, MD, PhD
Department of Orthopaedic Surgery, Kainan
Hospital, The Aichi Prefectural Federation of
Agricultural Cooperative for Health & Welfare,
Yatomi, Aichi, Japan

JAE WOO SHIM, MD
Department of Orthopaedic Surgery, Samsung
Medical Center, School of Medicine,
Sungkyunkwan University, Gangnam-gu,
Seoul, Korea

CLARA SIMON DE BLAS, PhD
Computer Sciences and Statistics
Department, Rey Juan Carlos University,
Madrid, Spain

DAVID J. SLUTSKY, MD
Department of Orthopedics, Harbor-UCLA
Medical Center, The Hand and Wrist Institute,
Torrance, California, USA

JASON SOLOMON, MD
Department of Orthopedic Surgery, Arrowhead
Regional Medical Center, Colton, California,
USA

ENDRE SØREIDE, MD
Department of Orthopedic Surgery, Oslo
University Hospital, Ullevål, Oslo, Norway

JENNIFER M. STERBENZ, BS
Research Assistant, Section of Plastic
Surgery, Department of Surgery, University of
Michigan Health System, Ann Arbor, Michigan,
USA

GUANG-LEI TIAN, MD
Department of Hand Surgery, Beijing Jishuitan
Hospital, 4th Medical College of Peking
University, Beijing, China

**WING-LIM TSE, MBChB, MRCS, FRCSEd
(Orth), FHKAM (Orth Surg), FHKCOS**
Clinical Associate Professor (Honorary),
Associate Consultant, Division of Hand and
Microsurgery, Department of Orthopaedics
and Traumatology, Prince of Wales Hospital,
The Chinese University of Hong Kong, Shatin,
NT, Hong Kong SAR, China

CLARA WING-YEE WONG, MBChB, MRCS, FRCSEd (Orth), FHKAM (Orth Surg), FHKCOS
Clinical Associate Professor (Honorary), Division of Hand and Microsurgery, Department of Orthopaedics and Traumatology, Prince of Wales Hospital, The Chinese University of Hong Kong, Shatin, NT, Hong Kong SAR, China

JEFFREY YAO, MD
Associate Professor, Department of Orthopaedic Surgery, Robert A. Chase Hand & Upper Limb Center, Stanford University Medical Center, Palo Alto, California, USA

JIN ZHU, MD
Department of Hand Surgery, Beijing Jishuitan Hospital, 4th Medical College of Peking University, Beijing, China

Contents

The deep component of triangular fibrocartilage complex (TFCC) inserts onto the fovea of the ulnar head. This component is critical to provide distal radioulnar joint stability. The surgical techniques and results of transosseous inside-out TFCC foveal repair are discussed. The rewarding results encouraged the repair of TFCC to the fovea arthroscopically. Although the results are good, the factors of age (traumatic or degenerative) and quality of stump and TFCC proper, which relate to the results, should be considered in the future.

Injury of the triangular fibrocartilage complex (TFCC) is a common cause of ulnar-sided wrist pain. Volar and dorsal radioulnar ligaments and their foveal insertion are the most important stabilizing components of the TFCC. In irreparable tears, anatomic reconstruction of the TFCC aims to restore normal biomechanics and stability of the distal radioulnar joint. The authors proposed a novel arthroscopic-assisted technique using a palmaris longus tendon graft. Arthroscopic-assisted TFCC reconstruction is a safe and effective approach with outcomes comparable with those of conventional open reconstruction and may result in a better range of motion from minimizing soft tissue dissection and subsequent scarring.

Both ulnocarpal impaction syndrome and ulnar styloid impaction syndrome can produce ulnar wrist pain. The definition and clinical differentiation are explained. The relevant anatomy, biomechanics, causes, diagnosis, and arthroscopic treatments, as well as the surgical indications, techniques, and outcomes of these syndromes are discussed in detail.

The best outcome in distal radius fractures is achieved if anatomy is restored, in particular the intra-articular congruity. This is achieved partly with improved fixation, such as using volar locking plates, and partly by using an arthroscopy-assisted reduction and fixation technique. In addition to improving the intra-articular congruity, associated ligament and chondral injuries can be detected and treated. This article outlines various associated injuries with suggested management in a stepwise fashion. It is hoped that overall outcomes will be improved once patient-related and treatment-related factors have been evaluated and previously undetected associated ligament injuries have been found and treated.

Wrist arthroscopy is an efficient adjunct for intra-articular distal radius fracture fixation. However, performing wrist arthroscopy during the plate fixation is troublesome with the vertical traction applied and released. To facilitate the procedure, the authors developed a surgical technique, plate presetting arthroscopic reduction technique (PART), using a palmar locking plate. Since July 2005, they have performed PART for 248 intra-articular distal radius fractures with good and excellent results. Arthroscopic-assisted reduction of intra-articular fragments is superior to fluoroscopic assisted. PART also allows the detection of intra-articular migration of fracture fragments, screw protrusion, and associated soft tissue injuries.

Treatment of intra-articular malunion of the distal radius has evolved over the past 20 years, from open treatment to wet then dry arthroscopic techniques that provide excellent results with less morbidity than open approaches. Dry wrist arthroscopy provides a well-visualized surgical space in treating intra-articular malunion and results in less edema than wet techniques. The best results are attained in the first 3 months after injury. Alternative methods for avoiding total wrist arthrodesis in those who present later have been developed. The dry arthroscopic "inside-out" osteotomy technique for intra-articular malunions should be considered in patients with this condition.

There are times when clinical examinations, radiographs, and computed tomography scans do not provide sufficient information to know whether a scaphoid fracture or scaphoid bone graft has united, partially united, or not united. When this problem arises, arthroscopic examination of the scaphoid fracture or scaphoid bone graft provides additional information to solve the problem and plan further management in an evidence-based manner. The indications for the use of arthroscopy and surgical technique are described.

 Video content accompanies this article at http://www.hand.theclinics.com.

Arthroscopic scapholunate volar and dorsal ligament reconstruction achieves an anatomic reconstruction, avoids an open approach and capsular detachment, and provides a strong construct for early mobilization. Clinical results are discussed. Detailed "surgical tips" and technical modifications are provided.

The key to successful treatment of perilunate injuries is to achieve early anatomic reduction and maintain the carpal alignment. Open surgery may lead to capsular scarring and joint stiffness. Furthermore, there is an increased chance of damage of the already tenuous blood supply to scaphoid and the torn ligaments. Arthroscopic-assisted management of perilunate injuries has been suggested. This article describes the surgical technique and outcome of this minimally invasive approach for perilunate injuries.

The evidence behind management options for midcarpal instability (MCI) is scarce, relying solely on case series. Established treatments cause significant loss of wrist motion. As understanding of the condition has progressed, surgeons have been trying soft tissue techniques. The treatment option should be chosen for the appropriate type and grade of MCI. The Hargreaves grading system for palmar MCI aids treatment decision making. A possible role for arthroscopy in the treatment of MCI has been developed using arthroscopic thermal capsular shrinkage, appropriate for cases with dynamic instabilities. Static deformities require a soft tissue reconstruction or a partial wrist fusion.

Kienbock disease (KD) is a disease of uncertain etiology, leading to chondral and osseous change in the lunate and wrist. Traditionally, Lichtman's classification of KD, based on radiographic appearances, has been used to direct treatment. Diagnostic wrist arthroscopy allows direct assessment of the lunate and surrounding articulations. Wrist arthroscopy can also serve as a therapeutic tool for performing debridement, resection, or arthrodesis procedures. The new Lichtman-Bain algorithm takes into consideration the status of the lunate, the effect on the wrist, and surgical and patient factors to guide management.

 Video content accompanies this article at www.hand.theclinics.com.

Partial wrist arthrodesis (PWA) is a well-known procedure for treating degenerative or posttraumatic wrist conditions. Four-corner fusion (4CF) is mostly used for scapholunate advanced collapse and scaphoid nonunion advanced collapse. The author performed 39 procedures, including 4CFs, 2-corner fusions, 3-corner fusions, scaphoid-capitate/scaphoid-capitate-lunate fusions, scaphoid-trapezium-trapezoid arthrodeses, and radioscapholunate arthroscopic PWAs (A-PWAs). There were 8 revision cases, including 4 partial nonunions. All A-PWAs healed satisfactorily after revision surgery. This article discusses the surgical techniques and tips to avoid mistakes. The pros and cons for open versus arthroscopic techniques and for screws versus Kirschner wires are also discussed.

Focal chondral lesions are a common cause of chronic wrist pain, with no ideal treatment. The authors developed arthroscopic transplantation of osteochondral autograft from lateral femoral condyle to distal radius with satisfactory outcome in 4 consecutive patients between December 2006 and December 2010. In all cases, graft incorporation was completed by 3 to 4 months postoperation. All patients showed improvement in wrist function with no pain at follow-up at an average of 70.5 months (range 24–116 months). Second-look arthroscopy in 3 patients confirmed the preservation of normal articular cartilage. Patient satisfaction was high with no complications.

Dorsal and volar wrist ganglions are benign tumors; most of them are asymptomatic. They can disappear spontaneously. Arthroscopic resection can be performed for pain or cosmetic concern. Dorsal ganglion is more common (70%). The hypothesis of the origin is the result of mucoid dysplasia in association with intracapsular and extrasynovial ganglia that occur at the level of the dorsal scapholunate complex. Volar wrist ganglia are less common (20%) and occur mainly in the radiocarpal joint. They are due to capsular destruction at the volar insertion of the SL ligament and arise from the interval between radio scaphocapitate and long radiolunate ligament.

Rheumatoid arthritis (RA) is a systemic inflammatory disorder affecting multiple joints. Wrist involvement is common. Patients with persistent symptoms despite medical management are candidates for surgery. Synovectomy can provide pain relief and functional improvement for rheumatoid wrist. Arthroscopic synovectomy is a safe and reliable method, with minimal postoperative morbidity. This article reviews the role, technique, and results of arthroscopic synovectomy in the rheumatoid wrist.

Bennett fracture is the most common fracture of the thumb. Choosing the appropriate approach to fracture fixation requires a thorough knowledge of the anatomy surrounding the first carpometacarpal joint, which is necessary to prevent injury to local sensory nerves and tendons. Although no study has shown superior outcomes compared with open reduction internal fixation and fluoroscopically guided closed reduction and percutaneous pinning, arthroscopic-assisted fixation allows for debridement of the carpometacarpal joint and direct visualization of the articular surface during reduction and has minimal morbidity and associated complications.

 Video content accompanies this article at www.hand.theclinics.com.

The thumb carpometacarpal joint (CMCJ1) is born to have good freedom of motion. However, the excellent mobility at this joint also predisposes attenuation of capsuloligamentous structures, joint incongruity, instability, and osteoarthritis. The prevalence of radiographic CMCJ1 arthritis is high. There is no single ideal surgery for all stages of CMCJ1 arthritis, and for all kinds of patients. The arthroscopic approach seems to provide a better alternative with rewarding preliminary results. It includes arthroscopic synovectomy/debridement/thermal shrinkage, arthroscopic partial trapeziectomy and suture button suspensionplasty, and arthroscopic CMCJ1 excision/suture button suspensionplasty/K-wire fixation.

Scaphoid-trapezium-trapezoid (STT) joint arthritis is a common condition consisting of pain on the radial side of the wrist and base of the thumb, swelling, and tenderness over the STT joint. Common symptoms are loss of grip strength and thumb function. There are several treatments, from symptomatic conservative treatment to surgical solutions, such as arthrodesis, arthroplasties, and prosthesis implant. The role of arthroscopy has grown, and this procedure is probably the best treatment of this condition. Advantages of arthroscopic management of STT arthritis are faster recovery, better view of the joint during surgery, and possibility of creating less damage to the capsular and ligamentous structures.

This article describes the authors' experience with, and recent advancement in, the techniques that have allowed the development of many new arthroscopic procedures in the finger joints. It also describes the role and techniques of arthroscopy in small finger joints. Because the intra-articular anatomy of the first to the fifth metacarpophalangeal (MCP) joints is similar, this article discusses the hand MCP joints without distinguishing thumb from fingers.

Arthroscopy of the wrist continues to evolve and advance as a valuable clinical technique in hand surgery. This article addresses safety of wrist arthroscopy and provides an overview of the known iatrogenic complications. Ultimately, the likelihood of associated injuries during wrist arthroscopy is dependent on the surgeon's ability and understanding of the equipment. Case volume and duration of experience directly correlate with mitigating iatrogenic injury and optimizing patient outcomes.

HAND CLINICS

THE CLINICS ARE AVAILABLE ONLINE!
Access your subscription at:
www.theclinics.com

HAND CLINICS

Preface
Evolution and Inspiration from Hand and Wrist Arthroscopy

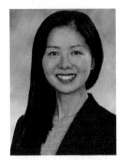

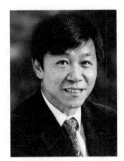

Clara Wing-yee Wong, MBChB, MRCS, FRCSEd (Orth),
FHKAM (Orth Surg), FHKCOS

Pak-cheong Ho, MBBS, FRCS (Edinburg), FHKCOS,
FHKAM (Orth Surg)

Editors

The clinical application of wrist arthroscopy is traced back to 1979 when Y.C. Chen reported the result of arthroscopic examination of the wrist and finger joints in 90 patients. The technique did not gain popularity until 1986 when a formal wrist arthroscopy workshop was organized in the United States by pioneers such as Gary Poehling, Terry Whipple, and James Roth. Since then, the technique and concept flourished through the impact of numerous international publications, training courses, and workshops throughout the world, and the establishment of major international bodies for the study of wrist disorders, including the International Wrist Investigator Workshop, European Wrist Arthroscopy Society, and lately, the Asia Pacific Wrist Association. Today, wrist arthroscopy has firmly established its value and reputation as an essential diagnostic and powerful therapeutic tool to evaluate and cure diseased wrists. It best illustrates how minimal invasive surgery can benefit patients most in concept and practice.

The diagnostic accuracy and specificity of wrist arthroscopy have been shown to be superior to arthrography, cineradiography, computed tomography, and MRI and have firmly established the standard. The therapeutic role has evolved with innovative techniques and customized surgical instruments, which have altered the management algorithm and opened up new horizons and standards for evaluation and treatment. More complex and precise new procedures can be performed with low complications. Anatomic structure repairing procedures, such as interosseous and capsular ligament repair, triangular fibrocartilage complex repair and reattachment, reduction and internal fixation of fracture dislocation, and chondroplasty for small chondral lesions, can be accomplished precisely under arthroscopic means. Functional reconstruction procedures give solutions on osseous, soft tissue, and cartilage problems. In osseous reconstruction, scaphoid nonunion and delay union can be treated by arthroscopic bone grafting and percutaneous fixation with high union rate. All forms of partial wrist fusion can be performed arthroscopically to maximize motion and enhance union. In soft tissue reconstruction, arthroscopic-assisted anatomic

Hand Clin 33 (2017) xv–xvi
http://dx.doi.org/10.1016/j.hcl.2017.08.001
0749-0712/17/© 2017 Published by Elsevier Inc.

reconstruction of the radioulnar ligaments can be performed to restore chronic distal radioulnar joint stability, and various forms of tendon graft reconstruction can be performed arthroscopically to restore the scapholunate gaps and stability with good long-term outcome. In cartilage reconstruction, arthroscopic osteochondral transplant can be done in chronic symptomatic posttraumatic osteochondral lesions. Arthroscopic solutions continue to evolve even in the smaller joints, such as thumb base, triscaphe, and finger joints. Portal site local anaesthesia has markedly diminished the risk and cost associated with arthroscopy and increased the acceptance of the surgery by both patients and surgeons. These new procedures are going to challenge the conventional ways. Further development in hand and wrist arthroscopy will probably be only limited by imagination and bioskill of the surgeons. We hope the 24 articles in this *Hand Clinics* are strong stimuli for you to practice more hand and wrist arthroscopies, and a rich source of inspiration for you to explore a much wider clinical application in the future.

Last, we would like to express our very sincere gratitude to all the contributors for sharing their wisdom and knowledge generously and for sacrificing their time and efforts to the birth of this issue.

Clara Wing-yee Wong, MBChB, MRCS, FRCSEd (Orth), FHKAM (Orth Surg), FHKCOS
Division of Hand and Microsurgery
Department of Orthopaedic and Traumatology
Prince of Wales Hospital
Chinese University of Hong Kong
16/F, The Club Lusitano
16 Ice House Street, Central
Hong Kong SAR

Pak-cheong Ho, MBBS, FRCS (Edinburg), FHKCOS, FHKAM (Orth Surg)
Division of Hand and Microsurgery
Department of Orthopaedic and Traumatology
Prince of Wales Hospital
Chinese University of Hong Kong
5F, Lui Che Woo Clinical Sciences Building
30-32 Ngan Shing Street
Shatin, NT
Hong Kong SAR

E-mail addresses:
clarawong@ort.cuhk.edu.hk (C.W.-y. Wong)
pcho@ort.cuhk.edu.hk (P.-c. Ho)

Diagnostic Wrist Arthroscopy

Brett F. Michelotti, MD[a],*, Kevin C. Chung, MD, MS[b]

KEYWORDS

- Wrist • Ligamentous injury • Diagnostic arthroscopy

KEY POINTS

- After a careful history and physical examination, wrist arthroscopy is the reference standard for identifying and characterizing intra-articular pathology.
- Wrist arthroscopy may be used to confirm the presence of articular wear, capsular and interosseous ligamentous pathology, and triangular fibrocartilage complex (TFCC) changes.
- Arthroscopy is a useful adjunct when determining whether or not a patient would benefit from soft tissue repair, reconstruction, or salvage procedure.
- Degenerative changes may be identified during arthroscopy that may or may not be contributing to a patient's complaints.
- Findings on wrist arthroscopy must be used in context of specific patient complaints and systematic physical examination findings to ensure that the correct treatment is selected.

INTRODUCTION

Although arthroscopically assisted treatments continue to be explored and analyzed for their effectiveness, the use of diagnostic wrist arthroscopy as an adjunct to a careful history and physical examination remains the reference standard in patients with pain thought to be originating from within the wrist.

When examined by an experienced hand surgeon, wrist problems in general and carpal instability are diagnosed approximately 75% of the time by history and physical alone.[1,2] Pertinent history regarding wrist pathology includes mechanism of injury, exacerbating hand and wrist maneuvers, pain-relieving hand and wrist positions/splints, prior corticosteroid injections that

had either a positive impact or no impact on symptoms, and prior surgical interventions.

Arthroscopy should be considered in the setting where a patient's pain has persisted despite nonoperative treatment with splinting and/or occupational therapy delivered by a certified hand therapist. A differential diagnosis should be established prior to arthroscopy to increase the probability of identifying a problem that is contributing to a patient's pain. A clinical scenario where this is best illustrated is a patient with dorsal wrist pain, exacerbated by loading and extension of the wrist. Physical examination, including provocative maneuvers, increase the probability that further diagnostic adjuncts will unveil a problem that can be acted on clinically. Using advanced imaging or arthroscopy as a screening tool may not have

Supported in part by the National Institute of Arthritis and Musculoskeletal and Skin Diseases (Midcareer Investigator Award in Patient-Oriented Research (2 K24-AR053120-06) (to Dr K.C. Chung).
Conflicts of Interest: The authors have no conflicts of interest.
Financial Disclosure: None.
[a] Department of Surgery, Division of Plastic Surgery, University of Wisconsin Hospital and Clinics, G5/358 – 600 Highland Avenue, Madison, WI 53792-3236, USA; [b] Section of Plastic Surgery, Department of Surgery, University of Michigan Medical School, 2130 Taubman Center, 1500 East Medical Center Drive, Ann Arbor, MI 48109-0340, USA
* Corresponding author.
E-mail address: michelotti@surgery.wisc.edu

hand.theclinics.com

the same clinical impact. Furthermore, although degenerative changes may be apparent on intra-articular examination, treatment may not improve a patient's symptoms. History and focused physical examination remain essential in determining whether or not a patient might predictably benefit from therapeutic intervention.

CLINICALLY RELEVANT ANATOMY

A systematic approach to evaluation of the wrist by arthroscopy starts with a thorough knowledge of the 3-D anatomy of the region. Traditionally, the workhorse arthroscopic portals are positioned over the dorsal wrist, avoiding the risk of injury to the neurovascular structures of the volar wrist. More recently, investigators have described volar arthroscopic portals that can be used to examine and repair dorsal soft tissue structures.[3–8]

The dorsal arthroscopic portals are named for their relation to the extensor compartments: 3-4, 4-5, 6 radial (R), 6 ulnar (U), radial midcarpal, and ulnar midcarpal portals. **Table 1** describes the anatomic structures that can be seen with each associated portal.

WRIST ARTHROSCOPY TECHNIQUE

The correct instrumentation and arthroscopy setup must be confirmed prior to initiating the delivery of anesthesia. Arthroscopy can be performed either with general anesthetic or regional anesthetic and sedation.

The patient is placed in the supine position with the shoulder abducted and elbow flexed at 90°. A tourniquet is placed above the elbow and the arm is padded in preparation for traction. The arm is secured to the hand table using a soft gauze wrap. Traction is applied through appropriately sized finger traps to gently distract the wrist. If the pulley system is positioned correctly, the fingers are directly collinear with the forearm.

The surgeon is seated on the side of the side of the hand table toward the feet of the patient. The arthroscopy viewing tower should be placed across from the surgeon. The assistant, important for stabilizing the forearm and wrist, can be seated on either side of the hand table (**Fig. 1**).

Standard equipment includes a 2.7-mm, 30° angled arthroscope; a 3-mm hook probe; and overhead traction. Instruments that are used in the treatment of intra-articular pathology include a radiofrequency ablation probe and a mechanical shaver. The shaver may be necessary to clear the wrist of synovitis or degenerative soft tissue changes to perform a comprehensive diagnostic evaluation of the wrist.

Traditionally, arthroscopy has been performed using fluid for articular distension and visualization, and wet arthroscopy has been considered reference standard. Recently, surgeons have challenged this paradigm and have elected to perform dry arthroscopy where no fluid is injected into the wrist. Proponents of the dry technique believe that fluid can disrupt normal tissue planes, making conversion to open surgery more difficult. Dry arthroscopy may also have a role in intra-articular fracture reduction and bone grafting.[9,10] This article focuses on wet arthroscopy.

DORSAL PORTALS: 3-4 PORTAL

The 3-4 portal is used to gain entry into the radiocarpal joint. Found at approximately 1 cm distal to the Lister tubercle, the 3-4 portal exists in the soft tissue concavity between the extensor pollicis longus tendon and the extensor digitorum communis tendons. After exsanguinating the extremity, the tourniquet is inflated to 100 mm Hg above the most recent systolic blood pressure (see **Fig. 1**).

An 18-gauge needle attached to a 10-mL saline-filled syringe is inserted into the 3-4 portal at approximately 10° of inclination toward the hand. This assumes that there is normal volar tilt of the radius (11°) (**Fig. 2**).

Careful inspection and palpation of the surface anatomy avoids inadvertent tendon injury. The bevel of the needle should be positioned parallel to the extensor tendons to reduce the risk of tendon laceration. If the needle does not enter the portal in perfect position, it may be difficult to place or manipulate the position of the arthroscope, resulting in poor visualization of wrist structures.

Entry into the joint is felt by a loss of resistance and a distinct pop through the dorsal capsule. The radiocarpal joint can be distended with 5 mL of saline to confirm needle placement. An 11-blade scalpel is then used to increase the size of the skin incision (**Fig. 3**). The blade should be placed along the needle, parallel to the extensor tendons, and used to cut skin only.

After removing the needle, a mosquito or narrow hemostat is directed along the same path into the radiocarpal joint. Gentle spreading of the mosquito will enlarge the capsular opening and permit entry of the arthroscope (**Fig. 4**). A blunt cannula is used to position the 2.7-mm arthroscope within the radiocarpal joint.

The arthroscope should be directed along the path that has been created by the mosquito. If slightly off, the trocar will not pass into the joint and may damage the articular surfaces of the distal radius, scaphoid, or lunate (**Fig. 5**).

4-5, 6U, AND 6R PORTALS

If wet arthroscopy is desired, gravity-driven inflow can be provided by the 6R or 6U portal or via the arthroscopic cannula. Outflow can be directed through the cannula or through the ulnar-sided portals, depending on the direction of inflow. Periodic irrigation and outflow of arthroscopic fluid clear debris, such as blood, clot, and loose cartilage bodies.

The 4-5 portal is accessed similar to the 3-4 portal. The point of entry is the interval between the extensor digitorum communis and extensor digiti minimi tendons, over the radiocarpal joint. Remembering that the normal inclination of the radius is approximately 22°, the entry point for the 4-5 portal is slightly more proximal than the 3-4 portal. Needle placement within the radiocarpal joint can be confirmed by direct arthroscopic visualization.

The 6R and 6U portals are designated by their relationship, R or U, to the extensor carpi ulnaris (ECU) tendon. The arthroscope can be used to triangulate and identify a safe entry point on either side of the tendon. Entry into the joint is again directly visualized.

SYSTEMATIC DORSAL RADIOCARPAL EVALUATION

When the arthroscope is placed correctly into the 3-4 portal, the surgeon should be able to view the proximal scaphoid, scapholunate (SL) ligament, lunate, and scaphoid fossa of the distal radius (**Fig. 6**). Evaluation should begin from radial to ulnar. If outflow is needed, a 6R portal can be placed via arthroscopic guidance.

The arthroscope is directed radially along the dorsal wrist capsule to view the radial styloid, proximal scaphoid articular cartilage, and scaphoid fossa. Volar soft tissue structures, from radial to ulnar, are radioscaphocapitate ligament (RSC), long radiolunate ligament (LRL), short radiolunate ligament, and the radio-SL ligament (RSL) or ligament of Testut (**Fig. 7**). Care should be taken to document articular wear, synovitis, and volar capsular injury or attrition.

The proximal membranous portion of the SL ligament, and the dorsal SL ligament can be visualized centrally, at the top of the arthroscopic image. Attenuation or hemorrhage represent at least a Geissler grade 1 injury. Geissler grade 2 injury represents gapping between bones of less than 1 mm. Grade 3 injury exists where gapping exceeds 1 mm. Geissler grade 4 injury is noted when the 2.7-mm arthroscope can be passed freely between bones, suggesting complete ligamentous disruption. Geissler grades 2–4 SL injury can be diagnosed via the midcarpal portals.

Moving ulnarly, the proximal articular cartilage of the lunate should be evaluated for wear. The lunate fossa can be appreciated on the distal radius. Staying within the joint but angling the scope toward the dorsal, ulnar wrist, the dorsal radiocarpal ligament can be inspected for injury. Volar radial and ulnar portals can be used to evaluate the full extent of the palmar intercarpal ligaments and the dorsal capsular structures, including the dorsal radiocarpal ligament.[5]

Advancing the scope ulnarly, the surgeon can appreciate the radial insertion of the TFCC, the central disk, ulnar attachments, the superficial palmar radioulnar ligament (PRUL) and dorsal radioulnar ligament (DRUL), the pisotriquetral orifice, and the prestyloid recess (**Fig. 8**). Small, controlled movements prevent inadvertent withdrawal of the scope from the joint and avoid trauma on scope reinsertion.

Any injury to the TFCC apparent via the 3-4 portal should be further investigated. A central perforation may be seen in the setting of ulnocarpal abutment (**Fig. 9**). A hook probe can be used via a 6R or 6U portal to examine the integrity of the TFCC (**Fig. 10**).[11,12] This cues the surgeon to detachment of the TFCC from the radius or, more commonly, the ulnar foveal attachments. Although a peripheral TFCC tear may be the source of ulnar-sided wrist pain, further evaluation may necessary to determine the cause of wrist instability, where present. Foveal attachments may appear intact by radiocarpal arthroscopy, where the deep fibers of the palmar and dorsal radiocarpal ligaments are not visualized.[13] When instability is present in the setting of intact superficial PRUL or DRUL foveal attachments, distal radioulnar joint (DRUJ) arthroscopy or arthrography may be warranted.

The 4-5 portal, entered similarly to the 3-4 portal and confirmed via direct visualization, can be used to confirm the presence of lunate fossa articular wear, changes of the proximal lunate, and injury/degeneration of the TFCC. Importantly, the 4-5 portal is used to better visualize the proximal membranous and dorsal lunotriquetral (LT) interosseous ligament. Hemorrhage or attrition cues the surgeon in to further evaluation from the midcarpal joint.

MIDCARPAL EVALUATION

Placement of the midcarpal portals should be performed after a thorough evaluation of all structures via the radiocarpal portal. Injuries to the SL or LT

Table 1
Anatomic structures by portal location

Portal	Location				
	Radial	Central	Volar	Dorsal/Distal	Ulnar
1–2 Portal	Scaphoid and lunate fossa, dorsal rim of radius	Proximal and radial scaphoid, proximal lunate	Oblique views of the RSC, LRL	Oblique views of the DRCL	TFCC poorly visualized
3–4 Portal	Scaphoid and lunate fossa, volar rim of radius	Proximal scaphoid and lunate, dorsal and membranous SLIL	RSC, RSL, LRL, ULL	Oblique views of DRCL insertion onto dorsal SLIL	TFCC radial insertion, central disk, ulnar attachment, PRUL, DRUL, PTO, PSR
4–5 Portal	Lunate fossa, volar rim of radius	Proximal lunate, triquetrum, dorsal and membranous LTIL	RSL, LRL, ULL	Poorly visualized	TFCC radial insertion, central disk, ulnar attachment, PRUL, DRUL, PTO, PSR
6-R Portal	Poorly visualized	Proximal lunate, triquetrum, dorsal and membranous LTIL	UL, ULT	Poorly visualized	TFCC radial insertion, central disk, ulnar attachment, PRUL, DRUL, PTO, PSR
6U Portal	Sigmoid notch	Proximal triquetrum, membranous LTIL	Oblique views of the UL, ULT	Oblique views of DRCL	TFCC oblique views of radial insertion, central disk, ulnar attachment, PRUL, DRUL
VR Portal	Scaphoid and lunate fossa, dorsal rim of radius	Scaphoid and lunate fossa, dorsal rim of radius	Palmar scaphoid and lunate, palmar SLIL	Oblique views of RSL, LRL, UL	Oblique views of radial insertion, central disk, ulnar attachment, PRUL, DRUL

Portal					
VU portal	Volar and palmar surfaces of the triquetrum and lunate	Palmar and proximal portions of the LT ligament	The volar TFCC	Ulnocarpal ligamentous complex	Ulnar wrist capsule
Volar midcarpal portal	Proximal capitate articular surface	Capitohamate articulation, capitohamate ligament	Palmar SL and LT ligaments	Dorsal radiocarpal, dorsal intercarpal ligaments	Triquetrohamate ligament, triquetrocapitate ligament, ulnar wrist capsule
Radial midcarpal portal	STT joint, distal scaphoid pole	SLIL, SL joint, distal scaphoid, distal lunate	Radial limb of RSL	Proximal capitate, CHIL, oblique views of proximal hamate	LTIL joint, partial triquetrum
Ulnar midcarpal portal	Distal articular surface of scaphoid	Distal lunate	Volar limb of RSC	Oblique views of proximal capitate, CHIL, proximal hamate	LTIL, LT joint, triquetrum
Dorsal DRUJ portal	Sigmoid notch, radial attachment of TFCC	Ulnar head	PRUL	Proximal surface of articular disk	Limited view of deep DRUL
Volar DRUJ portal	Sigmoid notch, radial attachment of TFCC	Ulnar head	DRUL	Proximal surface of articular disk	Foveal attachment of deep fibers of TFCC

Abbreviations: CHIL, capitohamate interosseous ligament; DRCL, dorsal radiocarpal ligament; LTIL, LT interosseous ligament; PSR, prestyloid recess; PTO, pisotriquetral orifice; UL, ulnolunate ligament; ULT, ulnotriquetral ligament.

Adapted from Slutsky DJ. Wrist arthroscopy portals. In: Slutsky DJ, Nagle DJ, editors. Techniques in hand and wrist arthroscopy. Philadelphia: Elsevier; 2006; with permission.

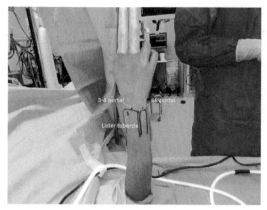

Fig. 1. Patient positioning.

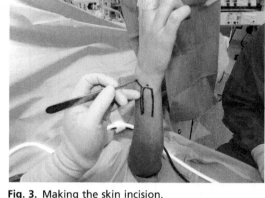

Fig. 3. Making the skin incision.

ligaments can be further classified via this approach. Midcarpal instability can be assessed and may be amenable to treatment by thermal capsular shrinkage.[14]

To enter the midcarpal joint, an 18-gauge needle, directed perpendicularly to the forearm axis, is inserted 1 cm distal to the 3-4 portal. The entry site should be just distal to the SL ligament and proximal to the capitate articular surface. The needle should be gently inserted into the joint to prevent injury to the scapholunate interosseous ligament (SLIL) or articular cartilage.

If there is return of arthroscopy fluid on entering the joint, this suggests disruption of the interosseous ligaments of the proximal carpal row where fluid is inappropriately communicating between the radiocarpal and midcarpal joints.

When the scope is oriented correctly, the surgeon should see the proximal capitate at the top of the image. The scaphocapitate joint and capitolunate joints can be seen radially and ulnarly. As the scope is directed radially, the surgeon can evaluate the

scaphotrapeziotrapezoid joint and the distal scaphoid pole for articular changes (**Figs. 11** and **12**).

Moving centrally and proximally, the SL articulation is assessed for ligamentous injury and instability. Gross instability can be estimated by the ability create a gap between the bones when directing the scope proximally toward the SL interval. If the scope does not easily pass between the bone (>2.7 mm gap, Geissler grade IV instability) then the distance between the 2 bones should be estimated by using the hook probe. Gapping less than a probe width (1 mm) or greater than a probe width signifies Geissler grade II and III instability, respectively (**Fig. 13**).

Volarly, the radial limb of the RSC ligament can be inspected for injury or attritional changes. Moving ulnarly, the proximal capitate, capitohamate articulation, and LT joint can be appreciated.

The ulnar midcarpal portal is entered in similar fashion, approximately 1 cm distal to the 4-5 portal. The articular surfaces of the distal scaphoid, lunate, triquetrum, proximal capitate, and hamate

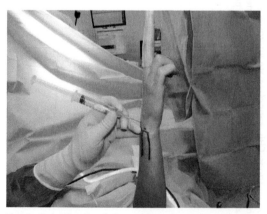

Fig. 2. Entering the 3-4 portal.

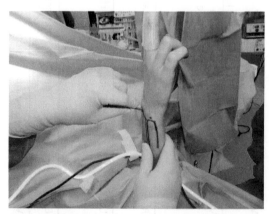

Fig. 4. Enlarging the skin incision.

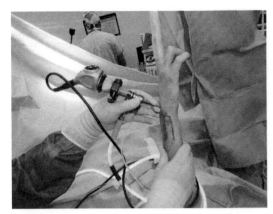

Fig. 5. Placing the arthroscope within the radiocarpal joint.

can again be inspected for articular wear (**Figs. 14** and **15**). Positioned directly distal to the LT interval, this portal can be used to estimate LT instability where distal to proximal pressure is applied via the scope while directly visualizing the joint for gapping.

ADVANCED ARTHROSCOPIC TECHNIQUES
Volar Radial, Ulnar, and Midcarpal Portals

Although the use of volar portals in wrist arthroscopy was described more than a decade ago, their application has not gained widespread acceptance.[7,15–17] Although technically unfamiliar, the volar radial and ulnar portals have a unique advantage over dorsal portals when visualizing the palmar component of interosseous ligaments, the dorsal wrist capsule, and associated extrinsic ligaments.[5–7]

The safety of the volar radial portal has been examined by Slutsky,[5] who used a combination of anatomic studies in which lead oxide and India ink preparations highlighted critical neurovascular anatomy. Important to placement of the volar radial portal is the ability to reproducibly locate and avoid the palmar cutaneous branch of the median nerve.

The volar radiocarpal portal is located at the level of the proximal wrist crease in the floor of the flexor carpi radialis (FCR) tendon sheath. After marking the proximal wrist crease on the skin, a 2-cm longitudinal incision over the FCR tendon is centered on the proximal wrist crease. The tendon sheath is incised and the FCR tendon is retracted ulnarly. A 22-gauge needle is directed perpendicular to the forearm axis at the intersection of the proximal wrist crease and midpoint of the FCR tendon sheath. This corresponds to the interval between the RSC and LRL. Injection of 5 mL of saline to distend the wrist can be used to confirm entry into the radiocarpal joint.

In his anatomic studies, Slutsky identified a safe zone of at least 3 mm around the volar radial portal trocar. Care should be taken to avoid imprecise placement of the trocar, which may result in injury to the palmar cutaneous branch of the median nerve or the palmar radiocarpal arch, which lie ulnar to the FCR tendon sheath and at the distal border to the pronator quadratus, respectively (**Figs. 16 and 17**).

The volar midcarpal portal can be identified and entered at approximately 11 mm (range 7–12 mm) distal to the volar radial portal.[5] The superficial palmar branch of the radial artery is avoided after direct visualization and protection.[18] From this portal, the surgeon may visualize the capitohamate ligament, which has been shown to minimize translational motion and stabilize the transverse carpal arch,[19,20] the palmar portion of the SL

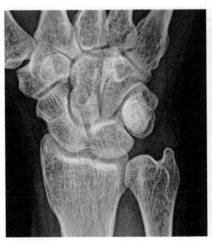

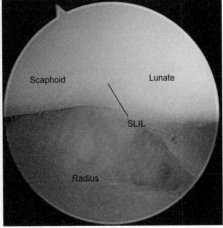

Fig. 6. Radiocarpal view via 3-4 portal.

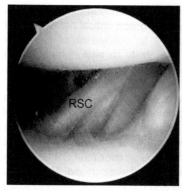
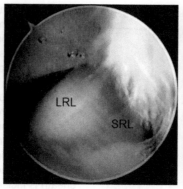
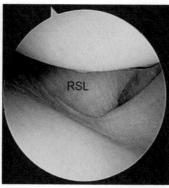

Fig. 7. Volar/radial extrinsic ligaments. SRL, short radiolunate ligament.

ligament, and the palmar aspects of the capitate and hamate for the presence of osteochondral fractures.

The volar ulnar portal may be used to evaluate and treat causes of ulnar-sided wrist pain, including LT ligament tears, DRUL, tears in the ECU subsheath and ulnar collateral ligamentous complex, and TFCC injuries. This portal is entered via a 2-cm longitudinal incision, beginning at the distal wrist crease and extending proximally along the ulnar border of the flexor digitorum superficialis tendons. After retracting the tendons radially, a 22-gauge needle is used to identify the radiocarpal joint. This may be confirmed with direct arthroscopic visualization or by injection of saline into the joint. Blunt dissection of the volar capsule should precede trocar placement. If the portal is positioned correctly, the trocar should enter the volar wrist through the ulnolunate ligament. The surgeon should visualize the palmar region of the LT ligament, distal and radial to the scope.

The volar ulnar portal permits the surgeon to directly visualize the palmar and proximal portions of the LT ligament, the volar TFCC, and volar and palmar surfaces of the triquetrum and lunate (**Fig. 18**).

In his anatomic study, Slutsky noted that the ulnar nerve and artery were more than 5 mm from the entry point of the trocar, although the palmar cutaneous branch of the ulnar nerve (nerve of Henle) was highly variable and at risk during portal placement.[5,6,21,22]

Distal Radioulnar Joint Arthroscopy

The integrity of the deep attachments of the TFCC establishes the stability of the DRUJ. Studies have shown that the DRUL confers stability both palmarly and dorsally.[23–25] Additionally, it is known that the ECU subsheath is an important stabilizer of the wrist and has been implicated as a pain generator in patients with ulnar-sided wrist pain.

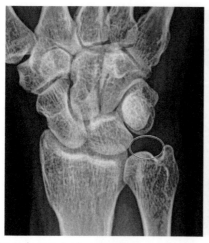
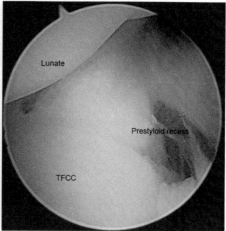

Fig. 8. TFCC and prestyloid recess.

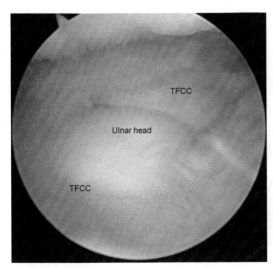

Fig. 9. Central perforation of the TFCC.

DRUJ arthroscopy permits a minimally invasive direct evaluation of the soft tissue stabilizers of the joint, articular cartilage of the sigmoid notch and ulnar head, and the proximal surface of the TFCC.

With respect to the articular cartilage of the sigmoid notch, arthroscopy can reliably detect shear injuries that may not be appreciated on CT or MRI.[25] These injuries are known to cause pain with rotation and compression of the wrist but may be clinically indistinguishable from other pain-generating pathology.

Synovitis of the DRUJ can be caused by a variety of disorders, including rheumatoid arthritis, gout, or pigmented villonodular synovitis. This can lead to swelling and pain over the ulnar head. DRUJ arthroscopy permits direct evaluation and/or débridement of the joint without disruption of the stabilizing ligamentous complex.

Perhaps the most important indication for DRUJ arthroscopy is the evaluation of the proximal attachments of the TFCC where there is concern for wrist instability. Arthrography of the radiocarpal joint does not detect deep palmar or DRUL disruption that could be responsible for DRUJ instability. By passing the arthroscope over the ulnar head via the DRUJ, the central disk and proximal radioulnar ligaments can be directly visualized and assessed for integrity.

Three diagnostic portals and a working portal have been described for DRUJ arthroscopy.[25] The proximal DRUJ portal is the point just proximal to the sigmoid notch, along the flare of the ulnar metaphysis. With the wrist in supination, the dorsal DRUJ capsule is relaxed, facilitating entry into the joint. An 18-gauge needle, directed slightly distally, is passed into the joint. Gentle blunt dissection is performed with a mosquito, following the path created by the needle. A blunt trocar, filled with arthroscopy fluid, is introduced after enlarging the dorsal capsulotomy (**Fig. 19**).

A systematic assessment of the DRUJ can be performed via the proximal DRUJ portal. The cartilage of the proximal ulnar head and sigmoid notch should be assessed for the presence of articular wear, shearing injuries, or loose bodies:

Relaxing the axial directed traction may permit easier view of the DRUJ as the space widens.
The wrist should be taken through a complete range of motion in pronation and supination to assess the entire joint surface.

The distal DRUJ portal is located between the fifth and sixth extensor compartments, just distal to the ulnar head. A 22-gauge needle can be directed into the DRUJ between the TFCC central

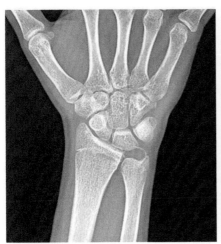

Fig. 10. Normal TFCC trampoline sign.

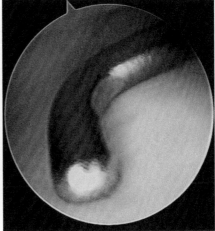

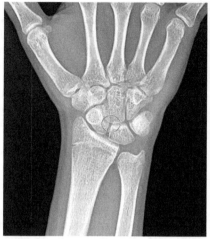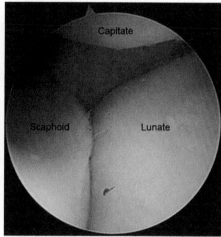

Fig. 11. Normal view of SL interval via midcarpal portal.

disk and cartilage of the ulnar head. Perfect placement is essential to avoid articular trauma upon scope placement. Entry into the distal DRUJ portal should be performed under direct arthroscopic visualization.

The arthroscope can be repositioned to the distal DRUJ portal once precise entry and position have been confirmed. This portal provides the best view of the proximal radioulnar ligamentous attachments into the base of the ulnar styloid.

A working portal, for a grasper or articular shaver, can be introduced 6 mm to 8 mm distal to the proximal DRUJ portal. This should be performed under direct visualization and care must be taken to avoid cartilage shearing on instrumentation.

The volar DRUJ portal, as described by Slutsky, may also be used to directly visualize the deep fibers of the radioulnar ligaments.[3] To access the DRUJ via a volar approach, a 2-cm longitudinal incision is designed along the ulnar border of the flexor digitorum superficialis tendons, centered over the proximal wrist crease. The finger flexor tendons are retracted radially and the ulnocarpal joint in entered with a 22-gauge needle. Entry into the DRUJ via the volar capsule is performed 5 mm to 10 mm proximal to the ulnocarpal joint. With flow of arthroscopy fluid, the joint space expands and permits passage of a 2.7-mm arthroscope. From this portal, the surgeon can directly visualize the foveal attachments of the radioulnar ligaments.

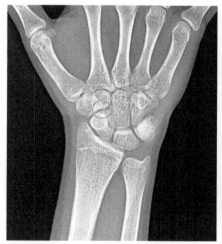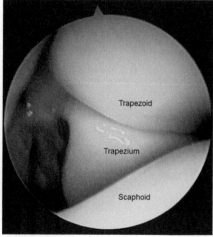

Fig. 12. Scaphotrapeziotrapezoid articulation.

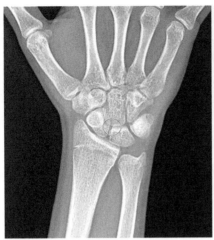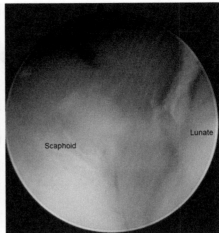

Fig. 13. Grade IV SL instability via midcarpal portal.

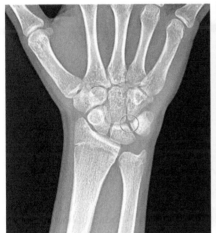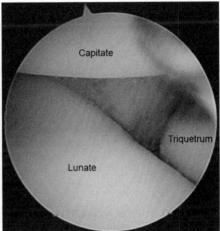

Fig. 14. LT interval via midcarpal portal.

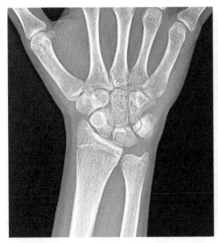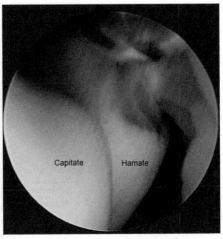

Fig. 15. Capitohamate interval via midcarpal portal.

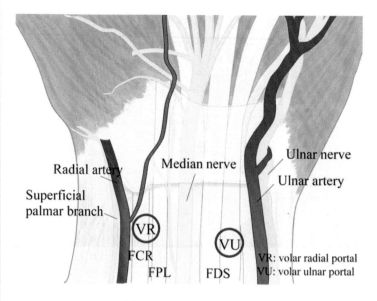

Fig. 16. Relative positions of the volar radial and volar ulnar portal. (*Courtesy of* N. Fujihara, MD, Nagoya, Aichi, Japan.)

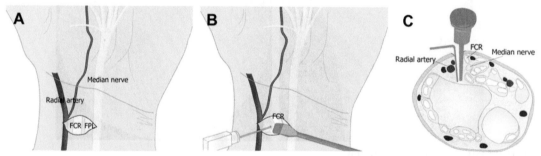

Fig. 17. Technique for volar radial portal placement. (*Courtesy of* N. Fujihara, MD, Nagoya, Aichi, Japan.)

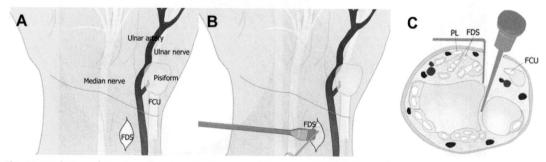

Fig. 18. Technique for volar ulnar portal placement. (*Courtesy of* N. Fujihara, MD, Nagoya, Aichi, Japan.)

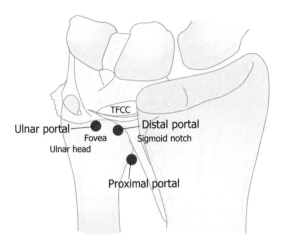

Fig. 19. Relative positions of dorsal DRUJ portals. (*Courtesy of* N. Fujihara, MD, Nagoya, Aichi, Japan.)

SUMMARY

Diagnostic arthroscopy is a useful adjunct in the diagnosis and treatment of intra-articular wrist pathology, after careful history and physical examination. A thorough understanding of the 3-D anatomy of the wrist is essential to optimize efficiency and to minimize complications associated with improper instrument placement.

Volar arthroscopic portal placement should be approached with caution. Cadaver dissection and trial portal placement may be necessary to prevent or minimize complications.

ACKNOWLEDGMENTS

The authors would like to acknowledge Nasa Fujihara for her work on the illustrations included in this article.

REFERENCES

1. Rhee PC, Sauve PS, Lindau T, et al. Examination of the wrist: ulnar-sided wrist pain due to ligamentous injury. J Hand Surg Am 2014;39(9):1859–62.
2. Sauve PS, Rhee PC, Shin AY, et al. Examination of the wrist: radial-sided wrist pain. J Hand Surg Am 2014;39(10):2089–92.
3. Slutsky DJ. Distal radioulnar joint arthroscopy and the volar ulnar portal. Tech Hand Up Extrem Surg 2007;11(1):38–44.
4. Slutsky DJ. The incidence of dorsal radiocarpal ligament tears in patients having diagnostic wrist arthroscopy for wrist pain. J Hand Surg Am 2008;33(3):332–4.
5. Slutsky DJ. Clinical applications of volar portals in wrist arthroscopy. Tech Hand Up Extrem Surg 2004;8(4):229–38.
6. Slutsky DJ. The use of a volar ulnar portal in wrist arthroscopy. Arthroscopy 2004;20(2):158–63.
7. Slutsky DJ. Wrist arthroscopy through a volar radial portal. Arthroscopy 2002;18(6):624–30.
8. Slutsky DJ, Nagle DJ. Wrist arthroscopy: current concepts. J Hand Surg Am 2008;33(7):1228–44.
9. Jones CM, Grasu BL, Murphy MS. Dry wrist arthroscopy. J Hand Surg Am 2015;40(2):388–90.
10. del Pinal F, Garcia-Bernal FJ, Pisani D, et al. Dry arthroscopy of the wrist: surgical technique. J Hand Surg Am 2007;32(1):119–23.
11. Ruch DS, Yang CC, Smith BP. Results of acute arthroscopically repaired triangular fibrocartilage complex injuries associated with intra-articular distal radius fractures. Arthroscopy 2003;19(5):511–6.
12. Atzei A, Rizzo A, Luchetti R, et al. Arthroscopic foveal repair of triangular fibrocartilage complex peripheral lesion with distal radioulnar joint instability. Tech Hand Up Extrem Surg 2008;12(4):226–35.
13. Slutsky DJ. Arthroscopic evaluation of the foveal attachment of the triangular fibrocartilage. Hand Clin 2011;27(3):255–61.
14. Mason WT, Hargreaves DG. Arthroscopic thermal capsulorrhaphy for palmar midcarpal instability. J Hand Surg Eur Vol 2007;32(4):411–6.
15. Levy HJ, Glickel SZ. Arthroscopic assisted internal fixation of volar intraarticular wrist fractures. Arthroscopy 1993;9(1):122–4.
16. Tham S, Coleman S, Gilpin D. An anterior portal for wrist arthroscopy. Anatomical study and case reports. J Hand Surg Br 1999;24(4):445–7.
17. Abe Y, Doi K, Hattori Y, et al. Arthroscopic assessment of the volar region of the scapholunate interosseous ligament through a volar portal. J Hand Surg Am 2003;28(1):69–73.
18. Omokawa S, Ryu J, Tang JB, et al. Vascular and neural anatomy of the thenar area of the hand: its surgical applications. Plast Reconstr Surg 1997;99(1):116–21.
19. Ritt MJ, Berger RA, Kauer JM. The gross and histologic anatomy of the ligaments of the capitohamate joint. J Hand Surg Am 1996;21(6):1022–8.
20. Garcia-Elias M, An KN, Cooney WP 3rd, et al. Stability of the transverse carpal arch: an experimental study. J Hand Surg Am 1989;14(2 Pt 1):277–82.
21. McCabe SJ, Kleinert JM. The nerve of Henle. J Hand Surg Am 1990;15(5):784–8.
22. Balogh B, Valencak J, Vesely M, et al. The nerve of Henle: an anatomic and immunohistochemical study. J Hand Surg Am 1999;24(5):1103–8.
23. Haugstvedt JR, Berger RA, Berglund LJ, et al. An analysis of the constraint properties of the distal radioulnar ligament attachments to the ulna. J Hand Surg Am 2002;27(1):61–7.
24. Taleisnik J. The ligaments of the wrist. J Hand Surg Am 1976;1(2):110–8.
25. Whipple TL. Arthroscopy of the distal radioulnar joint. Indications, portals, and anatomy. Hand Clin 1994;10(4):589–92.

Wrist Arthroscopy Under Portal Site Local Anesthesia Without Tourniquet and Sedation

Siu-cheong Jeffrey Justin Koo, MBBS, FRCS (Edinburgh), FHKCOS, FHKAM(Orth Surg), MHSM (New South Wales), MScSMHS (CUHK)[a],*, Pak-cheong Ho, MBBS, FRCS (Edinburgh), FHKCOS, FHKAM(Orth Surg)[b]

KEYWORDS

- Wrist arthroscopy • Portal site • Local anesthesia • Lidocaine

KEY POINTS

- In well-selected patients with adequate preparation and precaution, PSLA is a low-risk and comfortable procedure.
- The patient is neither sedated, nor under general or regional anaesthesia and tourniquet is not routinely used due to local hemostasis effect of anaesthetic mixture.
- 2% lidocaine with 1:200,000 epinephrine is injected through a 25G needle to portal sites, starting from joint capsule slowly back to the subcutaneous layer.
- The radiocarpal joint is then distended with saline injection and portal is created with transverse superficial skin incision followed by dilation by curved hemostat.
- Appropriate choice of the finger trap type, a proper application technique and adequate padding around the arm can enhance the comfort of patient.

INTRODUCTION

Historically, all joint arthroscopies are performed under general or regional anesthesia. Together with the aid of a tourniquet to achieve bloodless field, clear vision can be obtained during the procedure.

However, Rolf and colleagues[1,2] have successfully demonstrated the use of local injection of anesthetic agent to the portal sites in knee and ankle arthroscopy, bringing us to a new horizon because it can obviate the need for and risk of general anesthesia. We have transferred the successful experience of wide-awake local anesthesia into wrist arthroscopy and developed the technique of portal site local anesthesia (PSLA), which is now our major mode of anesthesia when we perform wrist arthroscopy.

In this article, we discuss the indications and contraindications, techniques to perform wrist arthroscopy under PSLA, and monitoring methods, as well as the potential risks in using PSLA.

INDICATIONS AND CONTRAINDICATIONS

The technique of PSLA for wrist arthroscopy has been used since 1998 in our center. All

Disclosure Statement: The authors have nothing to disclose.
[a] Department of Orthoapedic and Traumatology, Alice Ho Miu Ling Nethersole Hospital, 11 Chuen On Road, Tai Po, NT, Hong Kong SAR, China; [b] Division of Hand and Microsurgery, Department of Orthopaedic and Traumatology, Prince of Wales Hospital, Chinese University of Hong Kong, 5F, Lui Che Woo Clinical Sciences Building, 30-32 Ngan Shing Street, Shatin, NT, Hong Kong SAR, China
* Corresponding author.
E-mail address: jjsckoo@gmail.com

Hand Clin 33 (2017) 585–591
http://dx.doi.org/10.1016/j.hcl.2017.06.001

diagnostic arthroscopy and many therapeutic procedures including, soft tissue procedures such as synovectomy, thermal shrinkage for scapholunate interosseous ligament, ganglionectomy, and triangular fibrocartilage complex (TFCC) debridement and repair, as well as minor bone procedure in radial styloidectomy and wafer procedure are suitable cases for PSLA (**Box 1**). Before the surgery, the patient should be well-informed about the procedure and be able to conform to the instructions given by the surgeon.

Absolute contraindications for PSLA include known hypersensitivity to lidocaine and epinephrine. The presence of cardiac disease has been mentioned in the literature as a relative contraindication because this group of patients may be sensitive to epinephrine.[3] Procedures that require extensive bone work, such as proximal row carpectomy and scaphoidectomy with 4-corner fusion, may not be suitable. Patient factors such as young and immature patients, and patients with severe anxiety, mental retardation, uncontrolled psychiatric illness, or a low pain threshold are not appropriate candidates for this technique (see **Box 1**).

TECHNIQUE OF WRIST ARTHROSCOPY UNDER PORTAL SITE LOCAL ANESTHESIA

During the operation, no monitored anesthesia care or sedation is required. The patient is in the supine position and the operated arm is put on a hand table. The operated arm is prepared and draped from the hand to the upper arm level. It is important to maintain good comfort of the patient during the surgical procedure. We find that the appropriate choice of finger trap type, proper application technique, and adequate padding around the arm can patient enhance.

The affected hand is subjected to digital traction through the plastic finger traps by using a sterilizable Wrist Traction Tower (ConMed Linvatec Corp., Goleta, CA) with an adjustable tension spring to control the traction force. We prefer the use of plastic over metal trap because the latter is poorly tolerated by the patient when the operation is performed under PSLA. This protection is particularly important for patients with fragile skin, such as in rheumatoid arthritis. Three-finger traps are being used for the index, middle, and ring fingers for an even distribution of the traction force. The traps should reach the bases of the fingers at the web space level to ensure maximum skin contact (**Fig. 1**).

The patient's arm is placed on the metal base plate of the traction tower, when the shoulder is abducted, elbow flexed to 90°, forearm in neutral rotation, and the hand in an erected position. A broad self-adhesive Velcro band is used to wrap around the arm and the base plate at the level close to the bent elbow to provide countertraction.

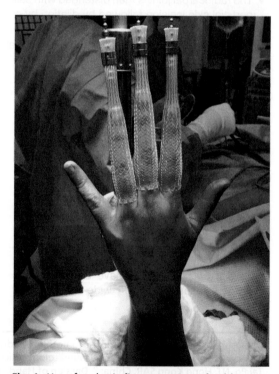

Fig. 1. Use of a plastic finger trap is preferable, especially in patients with fragile skin. Finger traps are used in index, middle, and ring fingers for even distribution of traction force and the traps should reach the base of finger at the web space level to ensure maximum skin contact.

Box 1
Wrist arthroscopy procedures indicated for portal site local anesthesia

Soft tissue procedure

Arthroscopic debridement

Removal of loose body

Synovectomy and biopsy

Ganglionectomy

Triangular fibrocartilage complex repair

Triangular fibrocartilage complex debridement

Thermal shrinkage for interosseous ligament

Release of wrist contracture

Bone procedure

Radial styloidectomy

Arthroscopic wafer procedure

Distal Scaphoidectomy

To improve the comfort level of the patient during the traction process, thick surgical towels are placed both underneath the arm and in between the Velcro band and the arm. Usually 10 to 12 pounds of traction force suffices for joint distraction and excessive traction should be avoided. With the wrist under traction, the various standard portals for wrist arthroscopy are then marked out on the skin through careful thumb tip palpation.

Two percent lidocaine with 1:200,000 epinephrine is injected through a 25-G needle to various portal sites, starting from joint capsule first and then withdrawn slowly to the subcutaneous layer. Intra-articular infiltration is not necessary under most circumstances, unless an extensive intra-articular procedure is anticipated, such as arthroscopic synovectomy in a rheumatoid wrist. Each portal site receives 1 to 2 mL of the solution. An aspiration test is performed before the injection to ensure no inadvertent injection into the systemic circulation. In contrast with another study that advocated delay of surgery for a minimum of 30 minutes after injection of the local anesthetic solution, we find that surgery can be started almost immediately after the injection (**Fig. 2**). The anesthetic mixture also provides effective local hemostasis in the joint capsule and synovium, and therefore obviates the routine use of a tourniquet.

During the surgery, further hemostasis could be achieved by various means, such as radiofrequency coagulation, increasing the height of saline bag suspension, or manual pumping of saline fluid. A sterile tourniquet can be applied to the arm if these measures fail. It is important to minimize the tourniquet time to avoid undue patient discomfort owing to muscle ischemia. If the surgeon prefers to put a tourniquet on the patient's arm as for a stand-by purpose, the tourniquet should be applied loosely to avoid a venous constriction effect that might cause more bleeding from the surgical site.

The radiocarpal joint is then distended by injecting 3 to 5 mL of saline at the 3/4 portal (**Fig. 3**). Transverse superficial skin incision along the skin crease is created over the portal site to have better scar healing and cosmetic outlook. Only the skin layer is incised to avoid inadvertent nerve, vessel, and extensor tendon injury. It is then followed by the gentle dilating of portal site with the tip of curved hemostat until the joint capsule is perforated, as perceived by the egress of saline fluid from the portal (**Fig. 4**).

An arthroscopic cannula with a blunt-ended trocar is gently placed through the portal. Extreme care is exercised to avoid inadvertent injury to the articular cartilage or ligamentous structures. A sharp-ended trocar is absolutely contraindicated. After removing the trocar, the cannula is then

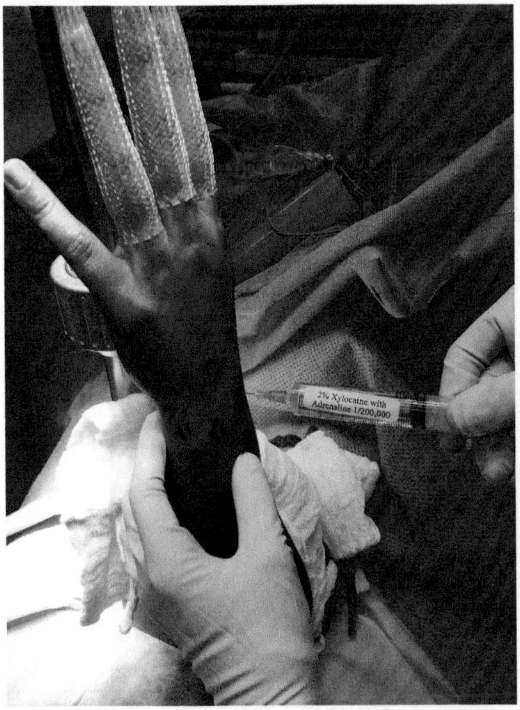

Fig. 2. Two percent lidocaine with 1:200,000 epinephrine is injected with a 25-G needle to various portal sites, starting from the joint capsule and then withdrawn slowly to the subcutaneous layer.

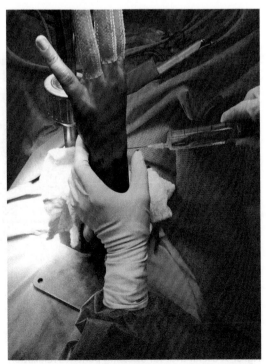

Fig. 3. The joint under examination is then distended by injecting 3 to 5 mL of saline through the 3/4 portal.

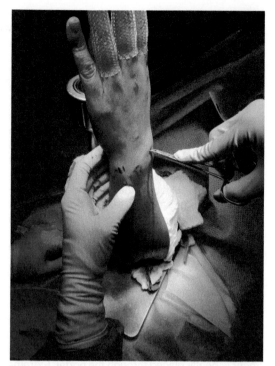

connected by long tubing to a 3-L saline bag hung at 1.5 m above the patient using a drip post or similar device. Continuous saline irrigation is provided with the aid of gravity to provide a clear view of the joint. An infusion pump is not necessarily and potentially harmful in causing extravasation of fluid and discomfort of the patient. Only when the joint and the cannula are completely filled with saline fluid, the 2.7-mm or 1.9-mm arthroscope is then inserted to avoid pushing the column of air inside the cannula into the joint.

TECHNICAL TIPS

The patient is neither sedated nor under general or regional anesthesia during the procedure, so the patient's understanding, cooperation, and relaxation are of paramount importance for the success of the surgery. When difficulty is being encountered during the portal establishment, it is generally due to the patient's anxiety and inadequate muscle relaxation of the forearm and hand, as well as from inadequate anesthesia. A useful trick is to look at the posture of the fingers of the patient. An anxious patient usually actively extends all fingers. In this way, the actively contracted forearm and hand muscle–tendinous units across the wrist would severely compromise the joint space of the wrist, rendering portal establishment impossible. It can be confirmed by observing an extended position of the thumb and little finger, which are not included in the finger traction normally (**Fig. 5**). Under such circumstances, the

Fig. 4. Only the skin layer is incised to avoid inadvertent nerve, vessel, or extensor tendon injury. It is then followed by the gentle dilating of portal site with the tip of a curved hemostat until the joint capsule is perforated, as perceived by the egress of saline fluid from the portal.

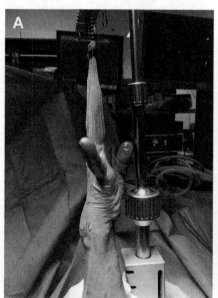
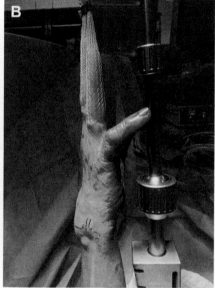

Fig. 5. A useful trick for assessing patient's relaxation state is to look at the posture of the fingers of the patient. (*A*) Patients who are not under a relaxed state will have the thumb and little finger extended, whereas (*B*) the thumb and little finger assume semirelaxed posture in a relaxed patient.

patient should be calmed, taught, and encouraged to relax until the thumb and little finger assume a semiflexed, relaxed posture.

During the surgery, manipulation of the volar wrist joint capsule and ligaments can produce sharp pain. This pain can be managed by local infiltration of the volar capsule and radiocarpal ligaments through the 4/5 working portal under direct arthroscopic vision (**Fig. 6**). Pain relief is usually immediate. The patient may also experience more pain during the use of radiofrequency apparatus for tissue ablation, because the wrist joint is more sensitive to temperature change than it is to mechanical manipulation. Limiting the radiofrequency application time and maintaining good fluid ventilation are effective measures to avoid undue pain.

ADVANTAGES OF PORTAL SITE LOCAL ANESTHESIA

We find that sedation is not necessary to achieve good results, in contrast with most published series on knee surgery. It is possible that voluntary muscle spasm is not so critical in case of wrist arthroscopy as compared with knee arthroscopy. Without sedation, the patient is able to watch the monitor, observe the operative procedure, and communicate with the operating surgeons and nursing staff throughout the procedure (**Fig. 7**). Interaction between patient and surgeon is beneficial to both. It enables the patient to have a better understanding of his or her own pathology, and participate in the decision making of the treatment and the subsequent rehabilitation program. The operating surgeon can closely monitor the status of the nerves around the wrist and the integrity of the extensor tendons during some procedures of

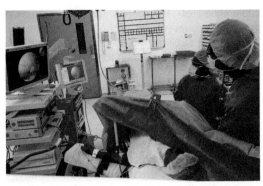

Fig. 7. Without sedation, the patient is able to watch the monitor, to observe the operative procedure, and to communicate with the operating surgeons and nursing staff throughout the procedure.

higher risk of iatrogenic injury,[4,5] such as thermal shrinkage of the ulnar extrinsic ligaments in palmar midcarpal instability and arthroscopic ganglionectomy in dorsal wrist ganglion. Complications can be avoided.

We also find that a clear arthroscopic view can be obtained with PSLA, even without the use of a tourniquet. From experience with knee arthroscopy, Karaoglu and colleagues[6] found that bleeding in arthroscopy mainly came from the portal site incision. With the use of a local anesthesia and epinephrine mixture injected into the portal site, a clear view can be obtained without significant hemodynamic changes.

PAIN CONTROL EFFICIENCY AND CLINICAL OUTCOME

In 2012, we performed a retrospective study to evaluate the effectiveness of PSLA in providing adequate pain control during wrist arthroscopic procedures in 111 patients performed between January 2007 and December 2009. The indications for wrist arthroscopy included 30 chronic wrist pain of unknown origin, 30 wrist ganglion, 27 posttraumatic arthritis, 11 TFCC injury, 5 rheumatoid arthritis, and 4 carpal instability. Therapeutic procedures were performed in all 111 cases, including 82 arthroscopic debridements, 30 ganglionectomies, 11 TFCC debridements, 6 arthroscopic synovectomies, 4 arthroscopic wafer procedures, 4 synovial biopsies, 3 TFCC repairs, 2 radial styloidectomies, and 2 thermal shrinkages. The average procedure time was 73 minutes (range, 20–255). All procedures did not require sedation. Only 6 of 111 cases needed to be converted to forearm intravenous regional anesthesia after diagnostic wrist arthroscopy owing to conversion to open surgery. None of the conversions were due to patient's

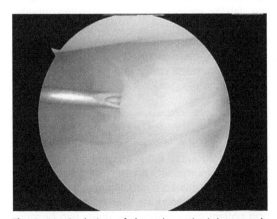

Fig. 6. Manipulation of the volar wrist joint capsule and ligaments can produce sharp pain. This can be managed by local infiltration of the volar capsule and radiocarpal ligaments through the 4/5 working portal under direct arthroscopic vision.

intolerance of PSLA. All procedures were completed uneventfully without complications. The average subjective pain visual analog scores at the worst moment during the operation and on average throughout the operation were 5.24 and 3.63, respectively (both with a range from 0 to 10). Overall, 51 patients reported sharp pain, 33 reported dull pain, 11 reported a mixed nature of pain, and 16 described no pain or discomfort at all. When they were asked about the most uncomfortable part of the surgery, 64 reported the intra-articular maneuver by the surgical instrument used during the operation, 6 reported the finger traction system, 18 reported the injection of local anesthetic solution, 7 described specifically during the introduction of the arthroscope into the joint, and 16 reported no discomfort at all. Their overall comment on the degree of comfort of the procedure was as follows: very comfortable (n = 6), comfortable (n = 29), tolerable (n = 64), and barely tolerable (n = 13). Fifty-eight patients reported a better understanding of the condition after watching the procedure intraoperatively. When they were asked about whether they would choose the same mode of anesthesia for another operation in the future, 88 patients (79%) had positive answer and 23 patients would opt for other methods.[7]

Hagert and colleagues[8] also reported their experience with wide-awake wrist surgery in 9 patients between June and August 2011. Their experience included 3 arthroscopic procedures and 2 combined arthroscopic–open surgeries in the series. For arthroscopic procedure, they used 20 mL of 1% lidocaine (10 mg/mL) with epinephrine (5 μg/mL) and 2 mL sodium bicarbonate (50 mg/mL) solution for dorsal infiltration with additional 5 mL of 1% lidocaine with epinephrine for intra-articular injection of the radiocarpal joint. No patient noticed pain during the procedure after the first poke of the needle and none required sedation or tourniquet. All of the patients would choose the same local anesthesia again. They recommended administration of the local anesthesia mixture at least 30 minutes before the surgery to allow time to acquire the desirable anesthetic level. In contrast, our experience showed that using lidocaine of higher concentration (2%) could achieve much faster onset and allow an almost immediate start of the operation.

POTENTIAL RISKS

Potential risks in PSLA include the effect of local anesthetic mixture leaking into systemic circulation, the vasoconstrictive effect of epinephrine, and the theoretical risk of permanent cartilage damage when lidocaine is accidentally injected into the joint. Different adverse effects of lidocaine and epinephrine when leaked into systemic circulation have been well-documented in the literature, including central nervous and cardiovascular toxicity.[9] Strict adherence to the practice of an aspiration test before injecting the local anesthetist mixture decreases the incidence of inadvertent injection into the systemic circulation. The addition of epinephrine to the lidocaine solution also renders the potential for systemic toxicity extremely remote.

Much concern on use of epinephrine in the hand comes from the belief that epinephrine causes finger necrosis by its vasoconstriction effect on the end artery. However, this concern has been dispelled by work from Lalonde and colleagues.[10,11]

The fear of causing permanent cartilage damage by lidocaine comes from the report on laboratory animal study by Dogan and colleagues[12] on the effect of injecting 0.5% bupivacaine into a rabbit knee joint. They showed more inflammatory changes in bupivacaine group. Anz and colleagues[13] reported that 0.5% bupivacaine reduced 100% cell viability in a canine cartilage in vitro model. There was a positive correlation on the reduction of bovine articular chondrocytes with the concentration and duration of exposure to lidocaine in a study by Miyazaki and colleagues.[14]

However, there was no direct causality between local anesthetic infusion and chondrolysis shown in clinical studies. Chondrolysis was observed only in patients undergoing shoulder and knee arthroscopy and receiving local anesthesia in a pain pump.[15–18] Ravnihar and colleagues[19] showed that a single intra-articular injection of lidocaine in knee arthroscopy did not influence the viability, morphology, and cultivation potential of chondrocytes in articular cartilage biopsy specimens for autologous chondrocyte implantation. Up to now, there is no study on the effect of lidocaine toward articular cartilage in wrist arthroscopy.

SUMMARY

The use of PSLA in wrist arthroscopy eliminates the need for and risks of general anesthesia. Without a tourniquet, a clear arthroscopic view can still be obtained by adding epinephrine in the local anesthetic mixture. The operating surgeon and patient can have better interaction because no sedation is necessary for the procedure. This enhances the patient's understanding of the disease, facilitates clinical decision making, and improves patient compliance with the rehabilitation program. In our review of 111 wrist arthroscopy procedures, pain control using PSLA achieved a satisfactory comfort level in 88% of patients during the procedure without any complication. We conclude that the PSLA technique without a tourniquet is a feasible and preferred mode of anesthesia for wrist arthroscopic surgery in the hands of experienced wrist arthroscopists. In well-selected patients with adequate preparation and precautions, it is a low-risk and surprisingly comfortable procedure.

REFERENCES

1. Rolf C. Knee arthroscopy under local anaesthesia. Hong Kong J Orthop Surg 1998;2(2):158–63.
2. Rolf C, Saro C, Engsträm B, et al. Ankle arthroscopy under local and general anaesthesia for diagnostic evaluation and treatment. Scand J Med Sci Sports 1996;6:255–8.
3. Lalonde DH. Reconstruction of the hand with wide awake surgery. Clin Plast Surg 2011;38(4):761–9.
4. del Piñal F, Herrero F, Cruz-Camara A, et al. Complete avulsion of the distal posterior interosseous nerve during wrist arthroscopy: a possible cause of persistent pain after arthroscopy. J Hand Surg 1999;24(2):240–2.
5. Fortems Y, Mawhinney I, Lawrence T, et al. Late rupture of extensor pollicis longus after a wrist arthroscopy. Arthroscopy 1995;11(3):322–3.
6. Karaoglu S, Dogru K, Kabak S, et al. Effects of epinephrine in local anesthetic mixtures on hemodynamics and view quality during knee arthroscopy. Knee Surg Sports Traumatol Arthrosc 2002;10(4);220–8.
7. Ong MT, Ho PC, Wong CW, et al. Wrist arthroscopy under portal site local anesthesia (PSLA) without tourniquet. J Wrist Surg 2012;1(02):149–52.
8. Hagert E, Lalonde DH. Wide-awake wrist arthroscopy and open TFCC repair. J Wrist Surg 2012;1(01):055–60.
9. Tucker GT, Mather LE. Clinical pharmacokinetics of local anaesthetics. Clin Pharmacokinet 1979;4(4):241–78.
10. Lalonde DH, Bell M, Benoit P, et al. A multicenter prospective study of 3,110 consecutive cases of elective epinephrine use in the fingers and hand: the Dalhousie Project clinical phase. J Hand Surg 2005;30(5):1061–7.
11. Thomson CJ, Lalonde DH, Denkler KA, et al. A critical look at the evidence for and against elective epinephrine use in the finger. Plast Reconstr Surg 2007;119(1):260–6.
12. Dogan N, Erdem AF, Erman Z, et al. The effects of bupivacaine and neostigmine on articular cartilage and synovium in the rabbit knee joint. J Int Med Res 2005;32(5):513–9.
13. Anz A, Smith MJ, Stoker A, et al. The effect of bupivacaine and morphine in a coculture model of diarthrodial joints. Arthroscopy 2009;25(3):225–31.
14. Miyazaki T, Kobayashi S, Takeno K, et al. Lidocaine cytotoxicity to the bovine articular chondrocytes in vitro: changes in cell viability and proteoglycan metabolism. Knee Surg Sports Traumatol Arthrosc 2001;19(7):1198–205.
15. Wiater BP, Neradilek MB, Polissar NL, et al. Risk factors for chondrolysis of the glenohumeral joint. J Bone Joint Surg Am 2011;93(7):615–25.
16. Hansen BP, Beck CL, Beck EP, et al. Postarthroscopic glenohumeral chondrolysis. Am J Sports Med 2007;35(10):1628–34.
17. Saltzman M, Mercer D, Bertelsen A, et al. Postsurgical chondrolysis of the shoulder. Orthopedics 2009;32(3):215.
18. Buohko JZ, Gurney-Dunlop I, Shin JJ. Knee chondrolysis by infusion of bupivacaine with epinephrine through an intra-articular pain pump catheter after arthroscopic ACL reconstruction. Am J Sports Med 2015;43(2):337–44.
19. Ravnihar K, Barlič A, Drobnič M. Effect of intra-articular local anesthesia on articular cartilage in the knee. Arthroscopy 2014;30(5):607–12.

REFERENCES

Chronologic and Geographic Trends of Triangular Fibrocartilage Complex Repair

Taichi Saito, MD, PhD[a,b,*], Jennifer M. Sterbenz, BS[c],
Kevin C. Chung, MD, MS[d]

KEYWORDS

- Wrist • Arthroscopy • TFCC repair • Chronologic trends • Geographic trends

KEY POINTS

- The repair methods for ulnar tears were noted as inside-out, outside-in, all-inside, and open repair, with the outside-in technique being the most common.
- Although the most reported method of TFCC repair is by attachment to the joint capsule, repair of ulnar-side tears by foveal attachment has been demonstrated recently.
- The effectiveness of the repair of radial-side tears was controversial and the methods of repair reported were inside-out, outside-in, all-inside, and open repair.

INTRODUCTION

The triangular fibrocartilage complex (TFCC) is an important stabilizer of the wrist joint, specifically the distal radioulnar joint (DRUJ). Disorders of the TFCC are one of the most common causes of ulnar-side wrist pain that interferes with daily activities, such as opening a door or shaking hands.[1]

The TFCC consists of four main components: (1) the triangular fibrocartilage proper (the fibrocartilage articular disk), (2) the distal radioulnar ligaments (volar and dorsal), (3) the meniscus homologue, and (4) the floor of the tendon sheath of the extensor carpi ulnaris (ECU) tendon. The articular disk rises from the hyaline cartilage of the sigmoid notch and the lunate facet of the distal radius. The disk becomes thicker along its ulnar attachment, and is wedge-shaped at the coronal section. The distal volar and dorsal radioulnar ligaments conjoin and insert into the base of the ulnar styloid. The meniscus homologue is a connective layer between the articular disk and the triquetrum. The floor of the sheath of the extensor tendon is incorporated into the TFCC on its dorsoulnar side. The ulnar aspect of the disk has two portions: one portion inserts into the ulnar styloid, and the other inserts at the fovea of the ulnar head (**Fig. 1**).[2,3] The deepest

Disclosure Statement: None.
[a] Section of Plastic Surgery, Department of Surgery, University of Michigan Health System, 2130 Taubman Center, SPC 5340, 1500 East Medical Center Drive, Ann Arbor, MI 48109-5340, USA; [b] Department of Orthopaedic Surgery, Okayama University Graduate School of Medicine, Dentistry and Pharmaceutical Sciences, 2-5-1 Shikata-cho, Kita-ku, Okayama 700-8558, Japan; [c] Section of Plastic Surgery, Department of Surgery, University of Michigan Health System, 2800 Plymouth Road, Building 14, G200, Ann Arbor, MI 48109, USA; [d] Section of Plastic Surgery, Department of Surgery, University of Michigan Medical School, University of Michigan Health System, 2130 Taubman Center, SPC 5340, 1500 East Medical Center Drive, Ann Arbor, MI 48109-5340, USA
* Corresponding author. Section of Plastic Surgery, University of Michigan Health System, 2130 Taubman Center, SPC 5340, 1500 East Medical Center Drive, Ann Arbor, MI 48109-5340.
E-mail address: taichis@med.umich.edu

Hand Clin 33 (2017) 593–605
http://dx.doi.org/10.1016/j.hcl.2017.07.010

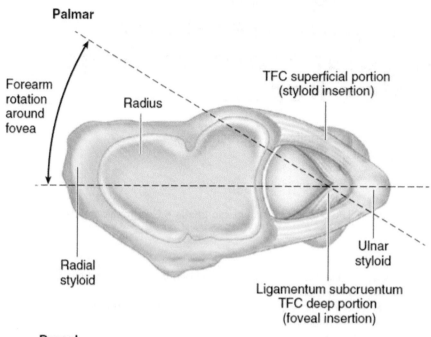

Fig. 1. Axial illustration of the TFCC. TFC, triangular fibrocartilage. (*From* Michelotti B, Brown M, Chung KC. Wrist arthroscopy. In: Chung KC, editor. Operative techniques: hand and wrist surgery. 3rd edition. Philadelphia: Elsevier; 2018. p. 170; with permission.)

portion has been called the ligamentum subcruentum.[4] The foveal attachment does more than the styloid insertion to stabilize the DRUJ because it has a closer relationship to the rotational axis of the forearm.[5] Therefore, a foveal detachment of the TFCC often results in DRUJ instability.[2,6]

The anatomy of the blood supply to the TFCC was revealed using latex injections.[7] There are three main arterial supplies to the TFCC: (1) the palmar and dorsal branches of the ulnar artery, (2) the dorsal branch of the anterior interosseous artery, and (3) the palmar branch of the anterior interosseous artery. Several studies have showed penetration of the vessels into about 10% to 20% of the peripheral articular disk using ink injections.[7,8] The peripheral palmar, ulnar, and dorsal areas have good healing ability because they have sufficient vascularization, whereas the central and radial areas typically need debridement in cases of injury because they have poor blood supply.

TFCC injuries are managed initially using nonsurgical measures, such as the immobilization of the wrist and forearm, activity modification, and analgesics, for the first 2 or 3 months. Moritomo and colleagues[9] reported that 46% of patients with avulsion of the TFCC from the fovea were

pain-free after conservative treatment. Operative treatment is considered in cases of persistent pain, DRUJ instability, and/or concomitant fractures. Operative treatment consists of open or arthroscopic debridement, and open or arthroscopic repair. These operative treatments are contraindicated for cases with severe ulnocarpal arthritis, or severe DRUJ arthritis associated with DRUJ instability.

This article reviews the classification of TFCC injuries and some repair methods based on the location of the tissue disruption. We also assess trends of TFCC repair organized by year and geographic area using literature published between 1990 and 2016 to provide current practice patterns of TFCC management around the world.

CLASSIFICATION

TFCC tears are categorized into two main classes by Palmer: class 1, traumatic lesions; and class 2, degenerative lesions (**Table 1**). These were further divided into subtypes.

Class 1 tears are identified based on the anatomic location of tissue disruption. Class 1A (central) tears are the most common type of traumatic TFCC tears and are debrided if

Table 1
Palmer classifications of TFCC tears

Class	Description
Class 1	Acute traumatic
1A	Central TFCC perforation
1B	Peripheral ulnar-side TFCC tear (with or without ulnar styloid fracture)
1C	Distal TFCC disruption (disruption from distal ulnocarpal ligaments)
1D	Radial TFCC disruption (with or without sigmoid notch fracture)
Class 2	Degenerative
2A	TFCC wear
2B	TFCC wear with lunate and/or ulnarchondromalacia
2C	TFCC perforation with lunate and/or ulnar chondromalacia
2D	TFCC perforation with lunate and/or ulnar chondromalacia with lunotriquetral ligament perforation
2E	2D + ulnocarpal arthritis

conservative treatment fails. Class 1B tears are peripheral tears in the vascular zone that are often the most appropriate to repair surgically because they often cause instability of the DRUJ. Class 1C tears are avulsions of the TFCC attachment to the ulnar carpus arising from the disruption of the volar ulnar extrinsic ligament complex. This ligamentous disruption often results in DRUJ instability. Class 1D tears are an avulsion of the TFCC from its radial attachment. This tear is often involved with marginal sigmoid notch fractures and the insertion sites of the dorsal and volar radioulnar ligaments that also cause instability of the DRUJ.

Class 2 tears are identified based on their point in the degenerative process. Degenerative tears are the result of chronic loading on the ulnar side of the wrist. These changes start with TFCC wear and chondromalacia of the ulnar lunate and ulnar head. TFCC perforation, lunotriquetral ligament perforation, and ulnocarpal arthritis develop sequentially.

LITERATURE REVIEW

We performed a literature search using the MEDLINE (PubMed) and EMBASE databases for articles that demonstrated a TFCC repair technique. The TFCC injury area and method of repair were extracted and categorized by geographic region and year. TFCC repair methods consist of arthroscopic inside-out, outside-in, all-inside, and open surgical repair. There are also two sites that the ulnar stump of the TFCC can be attached to after the injury: one is soft tissue, such as the joint capsule; and the other is the ulnar fovea. Therefore, we extracted the information about the area that the ulnar-side tears were attached to. If an article showed a technique that had been previously reported by the same author, the article was excluded.

We identified 41 articles written about the repair of ulnar TFCC tears and 10 articles written about the repair of radial TFCC tears. Conservative treatments were attempted for all cases reported in this review before undergoing TFCC repair. The mean time from the initial injury to operation was 8.9 months (range, 2–49; mean weighted value based on the number of patients). All patients underwent surgeries after failed conservative treatments and continuous wrist pain. It was reported that, before surgery, 9% of the patients complained of reduced grip strength, and that 15% of the patients had DRUJ instability, such as clicking or clunking. These symptoms were also indications for surgery. There were two studies that reported how many patients underwent open surgeries after failed conservative treatments.[9,10] Overall, 44% (52 of 119) of patients with a TFCC injury had surgeries after conservative treatments.

REPAIR OF THE ULNAR SIDE (PALMER 1B)
Trends in Chronologic Order

The annual number of articles that reported TFCC repairs increased gradually from 1991 to 2010 (**Fig. 2**). Although some authors began to report the repair of volar-side tears and dorsal-side tears more recently, articles that show the repair of ulnar TFCC tears have been the most frequent since 1991. These articles revealed that the ulnar side of the TFCC plays an important role in DRUJ stability.

Four surgical repair techniques have been reported: (1) inside-out, (2) outside-in, (3) all-inside (all-arthroscopic), and (4) open repair. To date, no direct-comparative study among these techniques has been published. The most described technique throughout the time period analyzed was outside-in (**Fig. 3**). The outside-in technique was first reported in the first half of the 1990s. For this technique, a 1.5-cm incision is initially made volar to the ECU tendon. A needle is then advanced through the ulnar capsule and into the torn TFCC (**Fig. 4**), after which a second needle is inserted adjacent to the first one. The suture end from the first needle is retrieved and brought

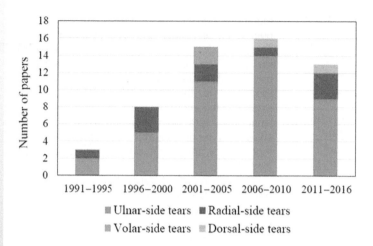

Fig. 2. Number of papers organized by year and the site of TFCC tears.

out via the second needle using a wire loop. The suture ends are then tied over the wrist capsule under tension.

The inside-out technique was originally reported by de Araujo and colleagues[11] in 1996. For this technique, a Tuohy needle is placed into the 3 to 4 or 1 to 2 portal to pass sutures in a radial to ulnar direction (**Fig. 5**). The needle is passed through the torn TFCC and advanced through a 1.5-cm longitudinal incision on the ulnar side of the wrist. A 2–0 PDS suture is then inserted through the needle and out the ulnar incision. A second pass through the TFCC tear is performed by moving the needle a few millimeters in the volar or dorsal direction. The second suture end is pulled through the needle, keeping the two suture ends free on the ulnar side of the wrist, and tied.

All-inside techniques, in which the entire repair is performed arthroscopically, were first demonstrated in the 2000s (see **Fig. 3**).[12–15] These techniques do not require an extra longitudinal incision and a subcutaneous suture knot. Yao

and colleagues[16,17] reported on this technique using the FasT-Fix system (Smith and Nephew Endoscopy, Andover, MA) with excellent results in 92% of their patients based on the Quick Disabilities of the Arm, Shoulder, and Hand (QuickDASH) and Patient-Rated Wrist Evaluation questionnaires. The system has two absorbable poly-L-lactate blocks that are prethreaded and pretied in a self-sliding knot. The two poly-L-lactate blocks are deployed through the capsule on either side of the TFCC tear and tightening the suture provides a reapproximation of the tear edge (**Fig. 6**).

Open repair techniques were the first established treatment method for TFCC tears.[18] Cooney and colleagues[18] demonstrated an open repair technique using a dorsal ulnar incision between the fourth and fifth extensor compartments. After inversion of the extensor retinaculum, the wrist capsule is incised parallel to the TFCC. Nakamura and colleagues[6] reported that open repair techniques are used if the fovea

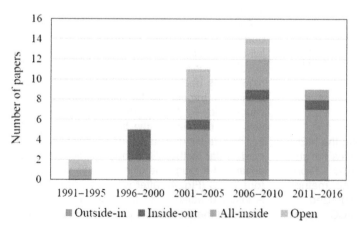

Fig. 3. Number of papers organized by year and suture technique for ulnar-side TFCC tears.

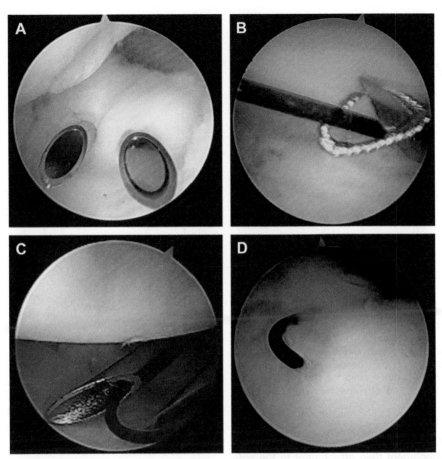

Fig. 4. Outside-in technique for ulnar-side TFCC tears. (*A*) A curved needle is penetrated through the capsule and the distal portion of the tear. A second needle is inserted parallel to the first. (*B*) A 2–0 or 3–0 PDS suture is passed through the needle and the suture is secured with the suture passer from the other needle. (*C*) The suture passer is withdrawn with the suture. (*D*) The needles are withdrawn and the suture ends are tied over the joint capsule.

and the DRUJ are poorly visualized from a DRUJ arthroscopic view, or if the TFCC is in poor condition such that arthroscopic repair may cause the sutures to cut through the TFCC. However, in the dorsal approach, the ECU tendon sheath floor and the superficial dorsal limb of the radioulnar ligament block the view of the fovea. Thus, Moritomo[19] recommended a palmar surgical approach for open TFCC repair and reported excellent results in 86% of their patients. In this palmar approach, a curvilinear or zig-zag incision is made along the medial side of the flexor carpi ulnaris tendon. The flexor carpi ulnaris tendon and the ulnar nerve are retracted to the radial side. The palmar capsule is then incised transversely from the palmar sigmoid notch of the radius to the base of the ulnar styloid.

With regard to the areas that ulnar-side TFCC tears were attached to, attachments to the soft tissue have been demonstrated since the 1990s

and are the most commonly reported (**Fig. 7**). In these conventional repair methods, peripheral TFCC tears are attached to the dorsal or ulnar joint capsule. A multicenter study revealed that 41 of 45 patients with an average follow-up of 37 months had good to excellent results by using a capsular repair of a peripheral TFCC tear.[20] However, TFCC tears originating at the fovea are not restored to the original site by this method, and instability of DRUJ may remain in some cases. Estrella and colleagues[21] demonstrated that results were poor in 14% of all patients who were treated by capsular repair, 40% of whom had persistent DRUJ instability.

Recently, the concept of the site where ulnar-side tears are attached during repair is changing. Reports on TFCC repair by attachment to the fovea have been increasing gradually since 2000. Between 2011 and 2016, more articles

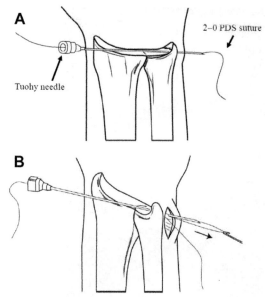

A

2–0 PDS suture

Tuohy needle

B

Fig. 5. Inside-out technique for ulnar-side TFCC tears. (*A*) The Tuohy needle is advanced to the ulnar wrist and a PDS suture is passed through the needle. (*B*) The needle is withdrawn and the second needle is penetrated through the triangular fibrocartilage at a point a few millimeters from the first. Both free suture ends are pulled out and tied over the ulnar capsule.

were published on the method of repair involving foveal reattachment than attachment to the soft tissue (see **Fig. 7**). This is likely because it was revealed that the foveal insertion of the TFCC plays a key role in the DRUJ stability.[22] Bain and colleagues[23] demonstrated that if the foveal footprint remains unattached, it becomes soaked in synovial fluid, leading to synovitis. Furthermore, they showed that this synovitis may inhibit healing of the foveal insertion, and lead to persistent DRUJ instability, wrist pain, and decreased grip strength.

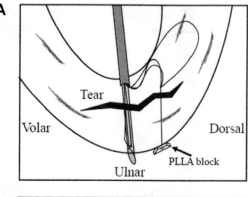

A

Tear

Volar   Dorsal

PLLA block

Ulnar

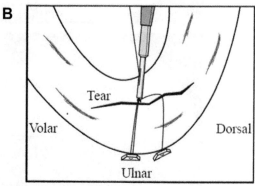

B

Tear

Volar   Dorsal

Ulnar

Fig. 6. All-inside technique for ulnar-side TFCC tears. (*A*) The first PLLA block is penetrated through the tear and advanced through the ulnar capsule. The needle introducer is then backed out to release the block outside the capsule. The second block is passed through the capsule and placed in the same manner. (*B*) The needle introducer is withdrawn, leaving the pretied suture. The suture is tightened, and the knot is cut by the knot pusher and cutter. PLLA, poly-ʟ-lactate.

Two methods of reattachment of the TFCC to the fovea are suture anchors and transosseous sutures.[6,24–26] Atzei and coworkers[25] reported results for the use of suture anchors for

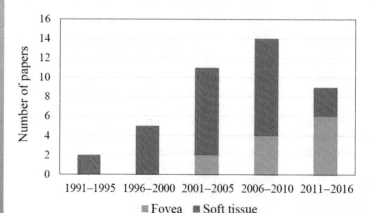

Fig. 7. Number of papers organized by attachment site and year for ulnar-side TFCC tears.

Table 2
Number of papers for each repair method for ulnar-side TFCC tears categorized by geographic region

Area	Country	No. of Paper	Attached Area		Suture Technique			
			Fovea	Soft Tissue	Outside-in	Inside-out	All-inside	Open
North America	United States	17	3	14	9	3	2	3
Asia	Japan	5	4	1	3	0	0	2
	Korea	5	3	2	4	0	1	0
	Taiwan	2	0	2	0	1	0	1
	China	1	0	1	1	0	0	0
	Hong Kong	1	1	0	0	1	0	0
	Philippines	1	0	1	1	0	0	0
Europe	Italy	3	1	2	1	0	2	0
	Belgium	3	0	3	3	0	0	0
	Austria	1	0	1	1	0	0	0
	Germany	1	0	1	0	0	1	0
	Norway	1	0	1	1	0	0	0
Total		41	12	29	24	5	6	6

reattachment. In this study, the mean pain score improved from 8.3 to 1.2, and the Modified Mayo Wrist Score was excellent or good in 94% of all patients. Nakamura and colleagues[6] showed the results of reattachment by a transosseous suture through a bone tunnel. The study revealed that 15 of 24 wrists resulted in no pain, and that the clinical outcome was excellent or good in 79% of patients.

Trends by Geographic Area

Articles that described TFCC repairs were mainly published in North America and Asia; fewer articles were reported in Europe (**Table 2** and **Fig. 8**). Similarly, methods of repair for ulnar TFCC tears were mainly shown in North America and Asia (**Fig. 9**). Outside-in techniques were most reported worldwide, and both open and inside-out repair were not reported in any publications from Europe.

Most articles from North America and Europe demonstrated the way that TFCC tears attach to soft tissue, such as a joint capsule (North America, 14 of 17 articles; Europe, 8 of 9 articles) (**Fig. 10**). However, more than half of the articles from Asia, mainly Japan and Korea, showed the way that ulnar-side TFCC tears attach to the fovea (Asia, 8 of 15 articles).

Recently, Atzei[27] proposed a new classification subgroup, type 1-B, in Europe. This classification was endorsed by the European Wrist Arthroscopy Society. Type 1-B is further divided into five classes that provide differentiation between distal

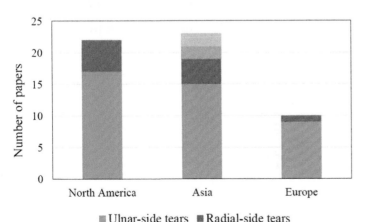

Fig. 8. Number of papers categorized by geographic region and the site of TFCC tear.

■ Ulnar-side tears ■ Radial-side tears
■ Volar-side tears ■ Dorsal-side tears

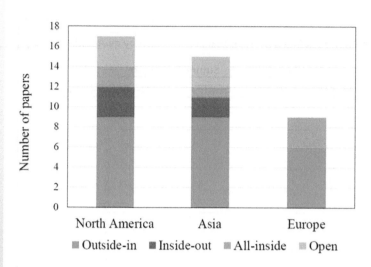

Fig. 9. Number of papers categorized by suture technique and geographic region for ulnar-side TFCC tears.

and proximal, and reparable and irreparable lesions (**Table 3**). Indications for treatment are also defined in this classification system. Foveal reattachments are required for complete and isolated proximal reparable tears (class 2 and 3) with DRUJ instability; conventional reattachments to the capsule are performed for isolated distal reparable tears (class 1). Considering that TFCC avulsion from the foveal insertion can cause DRUJ instability, these classifications and indications are rational. However, for an accurate diagnosis based on this classification, DRUJ arthroscopy is needed.

DRUJ arthroscopy was first reported by Whipple[28] in 1994. The procedure has rarely been performed because of its difficulty and the small size of the joint. Radiocarpal and midcarpal arthroscopies were often performed instead. Recently, several studies, mainly from Japan, have reported that DRUJ arthroscopies are important[29–33] because radiocarpal arthroscopies cannot visualize the foveal insertion of the deep fibers in the cases where the superficial portion of TFCC was not torn. The deep fibers are the main stabilizers of the TFCC so it is critical that they be visualized to make an accurate diagnosis; DRUJ arthroscopies are used to diagnose a rupture of the deep fibers. Nakamura and colleagues[30] reported that a DRUJ arthroscopy should be performed in any patients who have acute or chronic TFCC tears with DRUJ instability. Yamamoto and colleagues[31] demonstrated that pathologic findings of the proximal surface of the articular disk tended to relate to ulnar wrist pain,[29] and that, in 30% of all patients, DRUJ arthroscopies revealed pathologic findings that could not be identified with a radiocarpal arthroscopy.

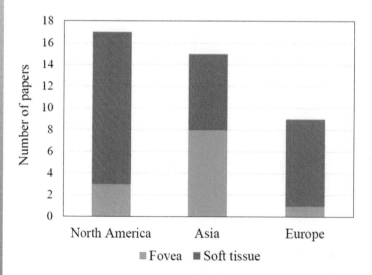

Fig. 10. Number of papers categorized by attachment site and geographic region for ulnar-side TFCC tears.

Table 3
Triangular fibrocartilage complex peripheral tear classification

	Clinical DRUJ Instability	Appearance of TFCC Distal Component	Status of TFCC Proximal Component	TFCC Healing Potential	Status of DRUJ Cartilage	Treatment
Class 1: repairable distal tear	None/slight	Torn	Intact	Good	Good	Repair: suture (ligament-to-capsule)
Class 2: repairable complete tear	Mild/severe	Torn	Torn	Good	Good	Repair: foveal refixation
Class 3: repairable proximal Tear		Intact	Torn	Good	Good	
Class 4: nonrepairable	Severe	Torn	Torn	Poor	Good	Reconstruction: tendon graft
Class 5: arthritic DRUJ	Mild/severe	Variable				Salvage: arthroplasty or joint replacement

REPAIR ON RADIAL SIDE (PALMER 1D)
Trends in Chronologic Order

We identified only 10 articles that reported on the repair of radial-side TFCC tears.[34–41] The repair of radial-side tears has been reported since the 1990s. However, the annual number of articles that reported the repair of radial-side tears did not increase over the time period covered in our literature search (see **Fig. 2**; **Fig. 11**). A radial-side tear is more uncommon and the repair methods are controversial. However, the repair of ulnar-side TFCC tears has better healing potential and results in good clinical outcomes. Some studies have reported that radial-side TFCC tears cannot heal because of a lack of blood supply.[7,8,42] However, other studies have showed good outcomes in healing radial-side tears.[35,37,39] Trumble and colleagues[43] reported that the repair of radial-side TFCC tears decreases pain significantly. Shih and colleagues[37] demonstrated that patients with radial-side TFCC tears had the same results as those with ulnar-side tears. They hypothesized that a combination of vascular ingrowth and synovial fluid can supply enough nutritional support to heal the tear. Therefore, TFCC repair may be performed for cases of radial-side tear with DRUJ instability.

Four repair methods were reported for radial-side tears: (1) outside-in, (2) inside-out, (3) all-inside, and (4) open repair techniques (see **Fig. 11**). The inside-out technique was most commonly used (6 of 10 articles).[34,35,37,41,44] The inside-out technique is performed by using transosseous sutures through the distal radius in ulnar to radial direction (**Fig. 12**). The suture is passed through the cannula, central rim of the TFCC, and bone tunnel, and then tied over the radius. The outside-in technique is also performed using transosseous sutures, but

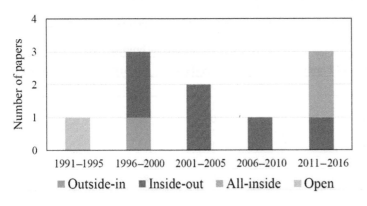

Fig. 11. Number of papers categorized by suture technique and year for radial-side TFCC tears.

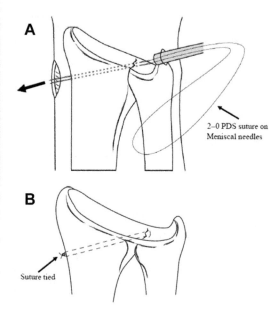

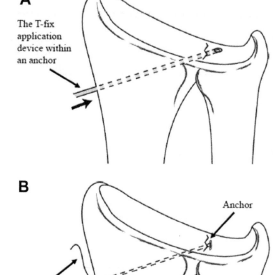

Fig. 12. Inside-out technique for radial-side TFCC tears. (*A*) A cannula is inserted into the joint. A meniscal needle is then passed through the triangular fibrocartilage and the radius after making a bone tunnel with a K-wire. (*B*) A second needle is advanced in the same manner. The suture is tied over the radius.

in the radial to ulnar direction (**Fig. 13**).[36,38] Recently, two all-inside repair techniques have been reported (see **Fig. 11**).[39,40] Trumble[39] first demonstrated one of them, an arthroscopic direct-repair technique, using an anchor to the radius in 2011. Cho and colleagues[40] noted another new all-inside technique using a small curved suture hook in 2012. In this technique, transosseous sutures are not necessary, and therefore, no extra skin incision is made to avoid the risk of irritating subcutaneous suture knot stacks over the radial side of the radius.

Fig. 13. Outside-in technique for radial-side TFCC tears. A special anchor system is used in this method. (*A*) The T-fix application device included an anchor is advanced until the triangular fibrocartilage is perforated after making a bone canal with a reamer. (*B*) The anchor is pushed out, unfolded, and retracted after removal of the application. The thread is tied periostally through a small incision.

Trends by Geographic Area

Table 4 and **Fig. 14** show the number of papers describing each suture technique for radial-side TFCC tears organized by geographic regions. The repair of radial-side TFCC tear was mainly reported in North America and Asia.[34,35,37–41,43] Only

Table 4						
Number of papers organized by repair method and geographic region for radial-side TFCC tears						
			Suture Technique			
Area	Country	No. of Paper	Outside-in	Inside-out	All-Arthroscopic	Open
North America	United States	5	0	3	1	1
Asia	Japan	1	0	1	0	0
	Korea	1	0	0	1	0
	Taiwan	1	0	1	0	0
	Hong Kong	1	0	1	0	0
Europe	Austria	1	1	0	0	0
Total		10	1	6	2	1

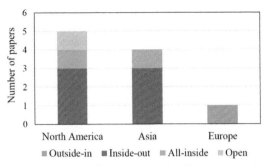

Fig. 14. Number of papers organized by suture technique and geographic region for radial-side tears.

one paper was from Europe, showing the outside-in technique.[36]

REPAIR IN OTHER AREAS

In regard to TFCC repair in other areas, we identified two articles that discussed volar TFCC tears (Palmer class 1C)[37,45] and two articles that demonstrated dorsal TFCC tears.[21,46] All four articles were published in Asia (see **Fig. 8**). The volar TFCC tears were repaired the same way as ulnar-side TFCC repairs (open or outside-in technique).[37,45] In both articles discussing dorsal tears, the outside-in technique was used.[21,46] Dorsal tears of the TFCC are not included in the original Palmer classification system. Dorsal tears were first discussed by Estrella and colleagues[21] in 2007; other authors have also reported the existence of dorsal TFCC tears.[46,47] Abe and colleagues[47] stated that a dorsal tear can entrap the ulnar head and cause restricted rotation of the forearm.

SUMMARY

This review shows the classification and repair methods of TFCC tears organized by tear area and in chronologic order. The outside-in technique for the ulnar-side repair was presented the most often. Although good results were revealed with each technique, the all-inside technique may be advantageous because this technique does not need a skin incision or a subcutaneous suture knot. Thus, the all-inside technique is a good option to decrease the risks of cutaneous nerve injury and irritation below the skin from the suture knot.

Soft tissue attachments were demonstrated most often in regards to the area that the stumps of ulnar-side TFCC tears were attached to. However, it has recently been recognized that the foveal attachment of the TFCC plays an important role in the DRUJ stability; reports of repair by attachment to the fovea have been gradually increasing. With soft tissue attachments, TFCC instability may remain in cases with torn proximal components. Therefore, surgeons should know the importance of foveal attachment methods. In cases with DRUJ instability but no TFCC tear findings after a radiocarpal arthroscopy, surgeons should consider performing DRUJ arthroscopies for a precise diagnosis because normal radiocarpal arthroscopies cannot detect a tear of the foveal attachment from the deep fibers. The Atzei classification is useful to determine a treatment strategy for peripheral TFCC tears.

Articles that showed methods of radial-side TFCC tear repair were scarce and were published mostly in North America and Asia. The outside-in technique for radial-side tear repair was demonstrated most frequently, whereas all-inside techniques have begun to emerge in recent years. Although the effectiveness of radial-side TFCC tear repair is controversial, radial-side repair may be indicated for the case with DRUJ instability.

With increasing globalization, the cultural diversity in local populations is bound to increase. Understanding differences in treatment methods or strategies provides physicians with the information they need to give their patients better options adapted to their cultural circumstances, such as health insurance and health infrastructure.

REFERENCES

1. Bain GI, Munt J, Turnor PC. New advances in wrist arthroscopy. Arthroscopy 2008;24(3):355–67.
2. Haugstvedt JR, Berger RA, Nakamura T, et al. Relative contributions of the ulnar attachments of the triangular fibrocartilage complex to the dynamic stability of the distal radioulnar joint. J Hand Surg Am 2006;31(3):445–51.
3. Nakamura T, Takayama S, Horiuchi Y, et al. Origins and insertions of the triangular fibrocartilage complex: a histological study. J Hand Surg Br 2001; 26(5):446–54.
4. Kleinman WB. Stability of the distal radioulna joint: biomechanics, pathophysiology, physical diagnosis, and restoration of function what we have learned in 25 years. J Hand Surg Am 2007;32A(7):1086–106.
5. Hagert CG. Distal radius fracture and the distal radioulnar joint: anatomical considerations. Handchir Mikr 1994;26(1):22–6.
6. Nakamura T, Sato K, Okazaki M, et al. Repair of foveal detachment of the triangular fibrocartilage complex: open and arthroscopic transosseous techniques. Hand Clin 2011;27(3):281–90.
7. Thiru RG, Ferlic DC, Clayton ML, et al. Arterial anatomy of the triangular fibrocartilage of the wrist and

its surgical significance. J Hand Surg Am 1986; 11(2):258–63.

8. Bednar MS, Arnoczky SP, Weiland AJ. The microvasculature of the triangular fibrocartilage complex: its clinical significance. J Hand Surg Am 1991;16(6): 1101–5.

9. Moritomo H, Masatomi T, Murase T, et al. Open repair of foveal avulsion of the triangular fibrocartilage complex and comparison by types of injury mechanism. J Hand Surg Am 2010;35(12):1955–63.

10. Park MJ, Jagadish A, Yao J. The rate of triangular fibrocartilage injuries requiring surgical intervention. Orthopedics 2010;33(11):806.

11. de Araujo W, Poehling GG, Kuzma GR. New Tuohy needle technique for triangular fibrocartilage complex repair: preliminary studies. Arthroscopy 1996; 12(6):699–703.

12. Bohringer G, Schadel-Hopfner M, Petermann J, et al. A method for all-inside arthroscopic repair of Palmer 1B triangular fibrocartilage complex tears. Arthroscopy 2002;18(2):211–3.

13. Conca M, Conca R, Dalla Pria A. Preliminary experience of fully arthroscopic repair of triangular fibrocartilage complex lesions. Arthroscopy 2004;20(7): e79–82.

14. Pederzini LA, Tosi M, Prandini M, et al. All-inside suture technique for Palmer class 1B triangular fibrocartilage repair. Arthroscopy 2007;23(10):1130. e1-4.

15. Yao J. All-arthroscopic triangular fibrocartilage complex repair: safety and biomechanical comparison with a traditional outside-in technique in cadavers. J Hand Surg Am 2009;34(4):671–6.

16. Yao J. All-arthroscopic repair of peripheral triangular fibrocartilage complex tears. Oper Tech Sports Med 2010;18(3):168–72.

17. Yao J, Lee AT. All-arthroscopic repair of Palmer 1B triangular fibrocartilage complex tears using the FasT-Fix device. J Hand Surg Am 2011;36(5): 836–42.

18. Cooney WP, Linscheid RL, Dobyns JH. Triangular fibrocartilage tears. J Hand Surg Am 1994;19(1): 143–54.

19. Moritomo H. Open repair of the triangular fibrocartilage complex from palmar aspect. J Wrist Surg 2015;4(1):2–8.

20. Corso SJ, Savoie FH, Geissler WB, et al. Arthroscopic repair of peripheral avulsions of the triangular fibrocartilage complex of the wrist: a multicenter study. Arthroscopy 1997;13(1):78–84.

21. Estrella EP, Hung LK, Ho PC, et al. Arthroscopic repair of triangular fibrocartilage complex tears. Arthroscopy 2007;23(7):729–37, 737.e1.

22. Moritomo H. Advantages of open repair of a foveal tear of the triangular fibrocartilage complex via a palmar surgical approach. Tech Hand Up Extrem Surg 2009;13(4):176–81.

23. Bain GI, McGuire D, Lee YC, et al. Anatomic foveal reconstruction of the triangular fibrocartilage complex with a tendon graft. Tech Hand Up Extrem Surg 2014;18(2):92–7.

24. Chou KH, Sarris IK, Sotereanos DG. Suture anchor repair of ulnar-sided triangular fibrocartilage complex tears. J Hand Surg Br 2003;28(6):546–50.

25. Atzei A, Rizzo A, Luchetti R, et al. Arthroscopic foveal repair of triangular fibrocartilage complex peripheral lesion with distal radioulnar joint instability. Tech Hand Up Extrem Surg 2008;12(4): 226–35.

26. Shinohara T, Tatebe M, Okui N, et al. Arthroscopically assisted repair of triangular fibrocartilage complex foveal tears. J Hand Surg Am 2013; 38(2):271–7.

27. Atzei A. New trends in arthroscopic management of type 1-B TFCC injuries with DRUJ instability. J Hand Surg Eur Vol 2009;34(5):582–91.

28. Whipple TL. Arthroscopy of the distal radioulnar joint. Indications, portals, and anatomy. Hand Clin 1994;10(4):589–92.

29. Yamamoto M, Koh S, Tatebe M, et al. Arthroscopic visualisation of the distal radioulnar joint. Hand Surg 2008;13(3):133–8.

30. Nakamura T, Matsumura N, Iwamoto T, et al. Arthroscopy of the distal radioulnar joint. Handchir Mikr 2014;46(5):295–9.

31. Yamamoto M, Koh S, Tatebe M, et al. Importance of distal radioulnar joint arthroscopy for evaluating the triangular fibrocartilage complex. J Orthop Sci 2010;15(2):210–5.

32. Abe Y, Tominaga Y. Ulnar-sided wrist pain due to isolated disk tear of triangular fibrocartilage complex within the distal radioulnar joint: two case reports. Hand Surg 2011;16(2):177–80.

33. Atzei A, Luchetti R, Braidotti F. Arthroscopic foveal repair of the triangular fibrocartilage complex. J Wrist Surg 2015;4(1):22–30.

34. Sagerman SD, Short W. Arthroscopic repair of radial-sided triangular fibrocartilage complex tears. Arthroscopy 1996;12(3):339–42.

35. Trumble TE, Gilbert M, Vedder N. Arthroscopic repair of the triangular fibrocartilage complex. Arthroscopy 1996;12(5):588–97.

36. Fellinger M, Peicha G, Seibert FJ, et al. Radial avulsion of the triangular fibrocartilage complex in acute wrist trauma: a new technique for arthroscopic repair. Arthroscopy 1997;13(3):370–4.

37. Shih JT, Lee HM, Tan CM. Early isolated triangular fibrocartilage complex tears: management by arthroscopic repair. J Trauma 2002;53(5):922–7.

38. Miwa H, Hashizume H, Fujiwara K, et al. Arthroscopic surgery for traumatic triangular fibrocartilage complex injury. J Orthop Sci 2004;9(4):354–9.

39. Trumble T. Radial side (1D) tears. Hand Clin 2011; 27(3):243.

40. Cho C-HL, Sin Y-K, Sin H-K. Arthroscopic direct repair for radial tear of the triangular fibrocartilage complex. Hand Surg 2012;17(3):429–32.

41. Tang CYK, Fung B, Rebecca C, et al. Another light in the dark: review of a new method for the arthroscopic repair of triangular fibrocartilage complex. J Hand Surg Am 2012;37(6):1263–8.

42. Chidgey LK. Histologic anatomy of the triangular fibrocartilage. Hand Clin 1991;7(2):249–62.

43. Trumble TE, Gilbert M, Vedder N. Isolated tears of the triangular fibrocartilage: management by early arthroscopic repair. J Hand Surg Am 1997;22(1):57–65.

44. McAdams TR, Swan J, Yao J. Arthroscopic treatment of triangular fibrocartilage wrist injuries in the athlete. Am J Sports Med 2009;37(2):291–7.

45. Chou CH, Lee TS. Peripheral tears of triangular fibrocartilage complex: results of primary repair. Int Orthop 2001;25(6):392–5.

46. Abe Y, Moriya A, Tominaga Y, et al. Dorsal tear of triangular fibrocartilage complex: clinical features and treatment. J Wrist Surg 2016;5(1):42–6.

47. Abe Y, Tominaga Y, Yoshida K. Various patterns of traumatic triangular fibrocartilage complex tear. Hand Surg 2012;17(2):191–8.

Arthroscopic Management of Triangular Fibrocartilage Complex Peripheral Injury

Jan Ragnar Haugstvedt, MD, PhD[a],*, Endre Søreide, MD[b]

KEYWORDS

- TFCC injury • TFCC repair • TFCC suture • Arthroscopic technique • Arthroscopic repair

KEY POINTS

- Triangular fibrocartilage complex (TFCC) is the most important stabilizer of the distal radioulnar joint.
- Injury of the TFCC may cause ulnar-sided wrist pain.
- The TFCC may be detached from the capsule or avulsed from the fovea.
- TFCC capsular reattachment could be performed with an arthroscopically assisted technique, providing good long-term results.

INTRODUCTION

As we gradually have come to understand more about the anatomy and biomechanics of the distal radioulnar joint (DRUJ), we have also learned the importance of preserving a well-functioning triangular fibrocartilage complex (TFCC). The stabilizing structures around the DRUJ include, among others, the dorsal and palmar distal radioulnar ligaments, the ulnocarpal ligaments, the joint capsule, and the subsheath of the extensor carpi ulnaris tendon.[1,2] The TFCC is the primary stabilizer of the DRUJ,[3,4] and is formed by the discus articularis proper, the ulnocarpal ligaments, the soft tissue, and the distal radioulnar ligaments that converge from separate origins on the radius to attach onto the ulna at the foveal region at the base of the ulnar styloid and along the ulnar styloid process itself[2,5] (**Fig. 1**). From a vascular injection study of the TFCC, we know that the peripheral margin of the TFCC is well-vascularized.[6]

According to Nakamura and colleagues,[1] the TFCC consists of 3 components, a hammock structure, with a distal, stable part suspending the ulnar carpus, the ulnotriquetral ligament, and the proximal part representing the true radioulnar ligaments. Palmer and Werner classified the disorders of the TFCC and divided the lesions into traumatic (class I) and degenerative (class II).[3,7] Degenerative changes of the TFCC develop with aging[8] and central defects of the TFCC are not considered repairable. However, for the traumatic lesions (class I), surgical repair has been performed. Repair of a meniscal tear in the knee is today considered a standard procedure with good outcomes, and over the last decades, several reports have also shown good results after

Declaration of Conflicting Interests: All named authors hereby declare that they have no conflicts of interest to disclose.
[a] Hand Surgery, Department of Orthopedics, Østfold Hospital Trust, Box 300, Graalum N-1714, Norway;
[b] Department of Orthopedic Surgery, Oslo University Hospital, Ullevål, Box 4956 Nydalen, Oslo N-0242, Norway
* Corresponding author. Olav Aukrurtvei 58C, Oslo 0785, Norway.
E-mail address: jrhaugstvedt@gmail.com

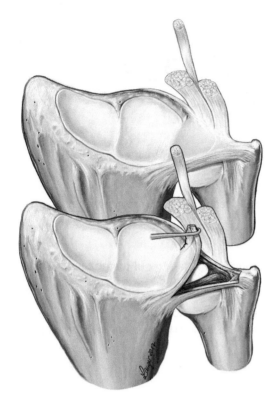

Fig. 1. The major stabilizer of the distal radioulnar joint is the triangular fibrocartilage complex (TFCC). The upper part of the figure displays a dorsal view of the TFCC with the distal radioulnar ligaments inserting into the styloid and the palmar distal radioulnar ligament in close relationship to the ulnocarpal ligaments. In the lower part of the figure, the discus articularis proper is elevated and the foveal insertion of the distal radioulnar ligaments, the ligamentum subcruentum, is shown. (*Courtesy of* J.R. Haugstvedt, MD, PhD, Graalum, Norway.)

open or arthroscopic repair of peripheral TFCC tears.[9–13]

CLASSIFICATION OF PALMER TYPE I-B TRIANGULAR FIBROCARTILAGE COMPLEX INJURIES

Biomechanical studies have suggested that the foveal insertion of the distal radioulnar ligaments is the most important of the 2 distal radioulnar ligament insertions for stability of the DRUJ.[14] This knowledge has helped us to understand that, although there is an intact distal part of TFCC, the DRUJ may still be unstable owing to rupture of the foveal ligament insertion. Based on this understanding a new classification of the Palmer type I-B injuries has been established.[15] The new classification considers injuries of the distal component of the TFCC as well as injuries of the

proximal component (**Fig. 2**). As an alternative to the hammock structure, it has been suggested to look at the TFCC as an iceberg: the emerging tip of the iceberg is the distal component of the TFCC and the submerged part is the proximal component of the TFCC.[16]

SYMPTOMS AND FINDINGS

In patients with an intra-articular distal radius fracture, an associated TFCC tear was found in 78% of cases.[17] Unless there is gross instability of the DRUJ, these patients suffer from pain from the distal radius fracture, and the TFCC injury is not diagnosed unless a diagnostic wrist arthroscopy is performed at the same time as a treatment of the distal radius fracture. If not diagnosed at the time of the injury, we have found that patients return with painful clicking of the wrist 6 months to 5 years after the trauma. Some also report ulnar-sided tenderness and a locking sensation; a few have reported instability of the DRUJ.[9,18]

A positive fovea sign—tenderness or pain with pressing the examiner's thumb distally and deep into the interval between the ulnar styloid process and flexor carpi ulnaris tendon, between the volar surface of the ulnar head and the pisiform—has been shown to indicate pathology of the TFCC and/or the ulnotriquetral ligament with a sensitivity of 95.2% and a specificity of 86.5%.[19] Stability of the DRUJ should be assessed in neutral, supinated, and pronated forearm rotation, and should always be compared with the contralateral forearm. Normal DRU ligaments will reveal a stable joint with a distinct endpoint; if no such endpoint is found, an avulsion of the foveal attachment of the DRU ligaments, the proximal component, should be suspected.

MRI may be helpful in the diagnosis of a peripheral tear of the TFCC and many patients bring the results of such an examination to the clinic. We do not, however, obtain MRI routinely in our preoperative planning, because we consider arthroscopy to be the gold standard for examination of the TFCC; an MRI that has been read as negative does not, in our experience, rule out a peripheral TFCC injury.

Although clinical examination and/or an MRI might arouse suspicion of a TFCC injury, an arthroscopic assessment is needed to confirm the diagnosis. If the patient suffers from an acute injury, we immobilize the patient in a cast for several weeks. If the patient has an older injury (several months) and suffers from ulnar-sided wrist pain and discomfort, we discuss treatment options with the patient. If the patient has a positive foveal sign, has long-lasting pain and symptoms that

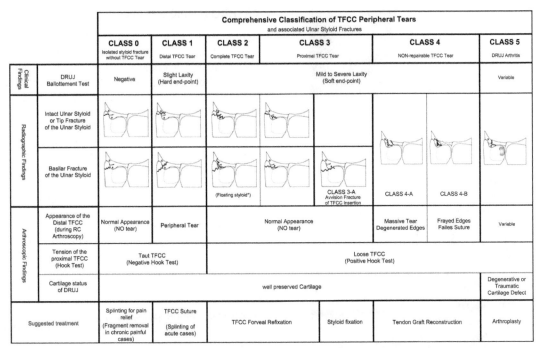

Fig. 2. Atzei's classification of type 1-B triangular fibrocartilage complex peripheral tears considering clinical, radiographic, and arthroscopic findings. DRUJ, distal radioulnar joint; RC, rotator cuff. (*From* Atzei A, Luchetti R. Foveal TFCC tear classification and treatment. Hand Clin 2011;27(3):270; with permission.)

impair quality of life, is informed about the possibilities of surgery and potential complications, then the patient should, in our opinion, be offered a diagnostic arthroscopy of the TFCC (in addition to the radiocarpal and midcarpal joints).

SURGICAL TECHNIQUES

With the patient in the supine position, the arm is draped and the hand is mounted in a vertical traction tower (**Fig. 3**). We apply traction, 10 to 15 pounds, to the fingers. The arthroscopic procedure can be performed under local, plexus, or general anesthesia. The surrounding skin and joint capsule of the portals used for the procedure should be properly anesthetized when using local anesthetics only. We prefer to use a tourniquet; however, the procedure could be performed without a tourniquet when local anesthesia is used.

We routinely start with a needle to localize the 3-4 portal. We make a small 1- to 2-mm transverse skin incision. We then use a small curved mosquito, with the curvature facing toward the radius, to spread out and open the soft tissue down to the capsule. After perforation of the joint capsule, we switch to a blunt trocar to enter the joint, with the trocar also pointing in a somewhat proximal direction. We then insert the arthroscope into the joint.

We prefer a 2.4-mm scope; however, we use a 1.9-mm scope in a small person. After verification of the arthroscope being in the radiocarpal joint, we establish an ulnar portal. Using a needle, we identify the correct position for the 6-R portal. The use of a needle ensures accurate positioning of the portal distal to the TFCC and the correct position for instrumentation. After correct positioning of the 6-R portal, we establish the portal making a small transverse skin incision as described. We perforate the capsule while viewing through the arthroscope. We typically use the 6-R portal for examination, for instrumentation, or for the placement of the arthroscope for a better view of the ulnar side of the wrist and the proximal row, and alternate between the different portals for the arthroscope, the probe, and the shaver.

In our opinion, dry arthroscopy, as described by del Pinal,[20] provides the best conditions for wrist arthroscopy. No inflow of water is established; however, the valve must be left open for inflow of air to the joint, and the possibility to irrigate the joint using a syringe with 5 to 10 mL of saline should be available. This necessitates a shaver connected to a suction device to drain out the joint after flushing.

After we have established the 3-4 and 6-R portals, cleaned the joint and secured a good view, we perform a diagnostic examination of the entire

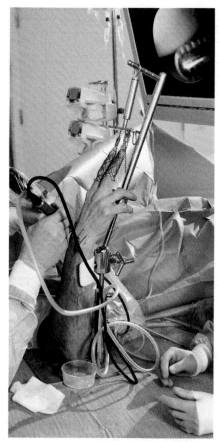

Fig. 3. The arm is mounted in a vertical tower allowing to flex the wrist. (*Courtesy of* P. Jørgsholm, MD, PhD, Vejle, Denmark.)

radiocarpal joint as well as the midcarpal joints, before any surgical procedure(s). Inspection of the TFCC may reveal a central or radial lesion; any presence of synovitis should be noted. The examination, however, is not completed by inspection only; thus, we insert a probe through the ulnar portal to evaluate the tension of the TFCC, often referred to as the trampoline test.[13] This test assesses the tautness of the TFCC by applying compressive force with a probe. The test is considered positive when the TFCC is soft and gives away. Another test, the hook test, has been described where traction is applied to the ulnar-most border of the TFCC with the probe inserted through an ulnar portal (6-R, 6-U, or a direct foveal portal).[15] The hook test is reported as positive when the TFCC can be pulled distally and radially toward the center of the radiocarpal joint. A positive hook test indicates a foveal detachment of the TFCC, a diagnosis that could be verified by arthroscopy of the DRUJ.

ARTHROSCOPIC REPAIR

Central and radial tears of the TFCC should be ruled out as the causes for reduced TFCC tautness, causing a positive trampoline test with a negative hook test. A central tear is not possible to repair, and a radial tear is usually not repaired, owing to the lack of vascularization of that area.[6] We evaluate the periphery of the TFCC and the capsular attachment. There is usually some synovitis at the region of a tear and we introduce a shaver from one of the ulnar portals to debride that area. When synovectomy is performed, a detachment of the TFCC from the capsule becomes visible (**Fig. 4**) and should be verified using a probe.

There are different techniques for performing an arthroscopically assisted repair of a peripheral TFCC injury. When we started, more than 20 years ago with an outside-in technique,[9] we used monofilament polyglyconate suture (Maxon, Convidin, Medtronic, Minneapolis, MN) making a loop at the end of the needle before this was introduced through the 6-R portal, perforating the capsule and the TFCC, and brought into the radiocarpal joint (**Fig. 5**). Using another suture loop, the first suture was brought to the outside through the 6-R portal (**Fig. 6**) and tied over the capsule. Additional sutures using the same technique, if needed, were placed to ensure restoration of the normal tautness of the TFCC.

This method has since been modified and, in our minds, simplified. We have had some patients needing removal of the sutures owing to symptomatic synovitis around the suture knot. Furthermore, we have experienced breakage of the suture while tying monofilament polyglyconate

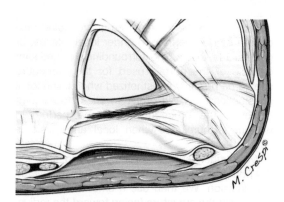

Fig. 4. The detachment of the triangular fibrocartilage complex from the capsule, a Palmer I-B lesion, or class I peripheral tear according to Atzei, becomes visible after debriding the synovitis that often covers the rupture. (*Courtesy of* C. Mathoulin, MD, FMH, Paris, France.)

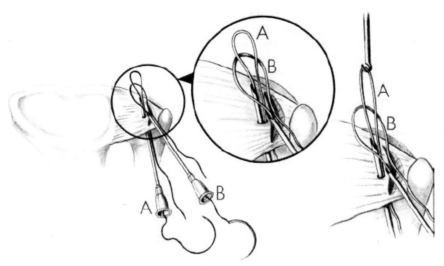

Fig. 5. An arthroscopically assisted technique to repair a peripheral triangular fibrocartilage complex (TFCC) tear. A suture loop was introduced through the TFCC into the radiocarpal joint while retrieving the loop with another suture loop. (*From* Haugstvedt JR, Husby T. Results of repair of peripheral tears in the triangular fibrocartilage complex using an arthroscopic suture technique. Scand J Plast Reconstr Surg Hand Surg 1999;33(4):444; with permission.)

sutures. Therefore, we prefer using a multistrand suture with a long chain ultra–high-molecular–weight polyethylene (FiberWire, Arthrex, Naples, FL), which in our experience has neither caused any synovitis or inflammation related to the knots, nor breakage of the suture. However, we are aware of other colleagues experiencing synovitis with the multistranded suture as we have experienced with the monofilament suture (Mayo Hand Club, personal communication, 2014).

After debridement of the area of the rupture, we use the 6-R portal to enter a multistranded suture

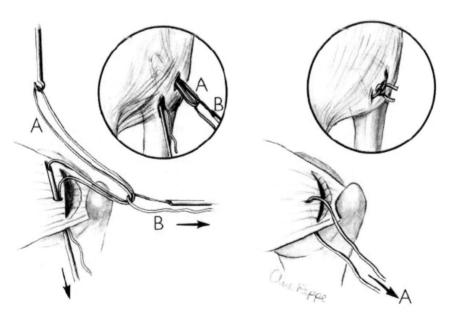

Fig. 6. With both ends of the suture outside the joint, a peripheral reattachment of the triangular fibrocartilage complex to the capsule was performed. (*From* Haugstvedt JR, Husby T. Results of repair of peripheral tears in the triangular fibrocartilage complex using an arthroscopic suture technique. Scand J Plast Reconstr Surg Hand Surg 1999;33(4):439–47; with permission.)

with polyethylene core (FiberWire 3-0) suture through a 21-G, 2″, 0.8 × 50-mm needle. The suture is entered from the tip of the needle. The needle (with the FiberWire suture inside) is advanced through the capsule from proximal of the TFCC with the needle directed in a distal direction; we want the suture to be placed through the TFCC 2 mm from the capsule, which can be verified visually through the arthroscope. The suture is left in this position while we introduce a mosquito, or a grasper, distal of the TFCC through the 6-R portal to retrieve the suture (**Fig. 7**). At the same time as the suture is pulled out, we withdraw the needle to avoid cutting the suture. We keep both ends of the suture clamped in a mosquito while we place a second suture using the same technique. With the 2 sutures in place, we pull the sutures to evaluate the tautness of the TFCC and the approximation of the TFCC to the capsule. Additional sutures are rarely needed to provide sufficient stability of the repair. We rotate the forearm to find the position for the best tautness; however, in most cases we do the repair in neutral forearm rotation. Before tying the sutures, we make a little wider incision around the 6-R portal, and debride the soft tissue down to the capsule to inspect the soft tissue to make sure that no nerves are entrapped by the suture. While tensioning the suture knots, the closure of the gap between the capsule and the TFCC is visualized through the arthroscope (**Fig. 8**). The suture ends are cut before we perform a trampoline

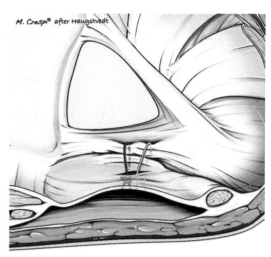

Fig. 8. We usually use 2 sutures to repair the rupture. The sutures will pull the triangular fibrocartilage complex (TFCC) in a peripheral direction to close the gap between the TFCC and the capsule. (*From* Haugstvedt JR. Secondary DRU joint problems instability, nonunion styloid, and ulnocarpal abutment. In: Hove LM, Lindau T, Hølmer P, editors. Distal radius fractures: current concepts. Heidelberg: Springer; 2014; with permission.)

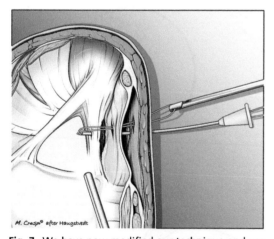

Fig. 7. We have now modified our technique and use a suture loop inside a needle, perforate the triangular fibrocartilage complex (TFCC), and bring the suture outside the joint using a mosquito or a grasper. We pass the suture through the 6-R portal proximal of the TFCC while the grasper is passed through the 6-R portal and perforates the capsule distal of the TFCC. (*Courtesy of* J.R. Haugstvedt, MD, PhD, Graalum, Norway.)

test for a final evaluation of this outside-in arthroscopically assisted TFCC repair. We use adhesive strips (Steri-Strips 3M, St. Paul, MN) to close the portals and apply local anesthesia around the portals for postoperative pain relief (if the surgery is performed under general anesthesia). We put on a dressing before putting on a cast.

This is our preferred method for a repair of a peripheral TFCC injury. There are, however, specifically designed kits for a repair; many companies have designed special kits with a variety of instruments, including suture retrievers, aiming to ease the surgical procedure. However, we consider the method described herein possible to perform for most surgeons in most cases; the equipment is inexpensive and available to everyone in an operating room.

Inserting the sutures in this manner increases the tautness of the TFCC because it is pulled in a peripheral direction. There are other ways of performing a repair where the suture is pulled in either a peripheral, or in a combination of a peripheral and a proximal direction. These methods are also described herein.

When we make an outside-in repair using horizontal loop sutures, we introduce a needle with a suture loop inside through the capsule proximal to the 6-R portal, with the tip of the needle distally directed and entering proximally to the TFCC. The loop suture is advanced into the joint, grasped with a grasper, and pulled from the radiocarpal joint to the outside through the 6-R portal (see **Fig. 7**). We then enter 1 more needle loaded with single suture to either side of the first suture loop, in the same direction as mentioned. The 2 ends of these 2 sutures are retrieved to the outside using a grasper (**Figs. 9** and **10**) and then passed through the loop in opposite directions before we pull the ends of the loop suture (the one in the middle; **Fig. 11**) to bring all 4 ends of the sutures outside the joint (**Fig. 12**). We evaluate the tautness of the TFCC, maintaining the sutures under tension throughout the evaluation. The sutures are tied under arthroscopic control after having ensured no entrapment of nerves in the sutures. A repair of the peripheral injury of the TFCC by 2 horizontal sutures will pull the TFCC in a peripheral and proximal direction (**Fig. 13**).

When possible, we sometimes use an inside-out technique for an ulnar-sided TFCC tear, a technique previously described by others.[18,21] We establish the 1-2 portal for insertion of an 18-G Tuohy (epidural) needle; however, the radiocarpal joint may sometimes be too tight to perform this type of suture technique, because it is difficult to cross the joint with the needle. The arthroscope should be placed in the 3-4 portal and we introduce the needle from the 1-2 portal and go across the joint to the ulnar side to the verified TFCC rupture with the needle (**Fig. 14**). While viewing the rupture and the tip of the needle through the arthroscope, we perforate the TFCC in an ulnar direction. We can see and feel the tip of the needle exiting close to the 6-U portal, but we always make an incision where the needle exits and debride down to the capsule to avoid any damage to any nerve before the needle is advanced out through the portal. When we pass the needle across the joint, we can either have a suture inside the Tuohy needle or we can introduce the suture from the outside (**Fig. 15**). We use a mosquito to hold onto the end of the suture being outside the 6-U portal as we withdraw the needle until the tip of the needle including the suture is viewed inside the joint (**Fig. 16**). We now redirect the needle and push it through the TFCC to bring the needle (and the suture) to the outside again (or we pass the needle through the capsule distal of the TFCC; **Fig. 17**). We then place another suture in a similar way, thus having performed 2 sutures to repair the peripheral ulnar TFCC injury.

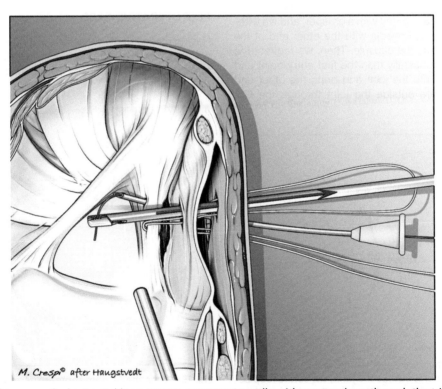

M. Crespi® after Haugstvedt

Fig. 9. When we make horizontal loop sutures, we enter 1 needle with a suture loop through the triangular fibrocartilage complex and bring the loop to the outside of the joint. Then we enter another needle with a suture inside and bring one end of this suture to the outside using a grasper. (*Courtesy of* J.R. Haugstvedt, MD, PhD, Graalum, Norway.)

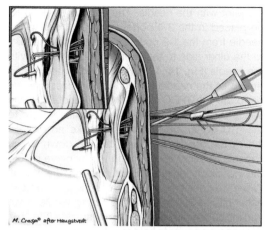

Fig. 10. A third needle is introduced and we bring 1 end of a suture inside this needle to the outside as well. (*Courtesy of* J.R. Haugstvedt, MD, PhD, Graalum, Norway.)

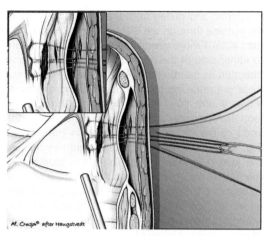

Fig. 12. Then we pull the loop to bring all the ends of the sutures outside of the joint proximal of the triangular fibrocartilage complex. (*Courtesy of* J.R. Haugstvedt, MD, PhD, Graalum, Norway.)

Still another technique is the all-inside technique, which has been described elsewhere.[22,23] As shown in **Fig. 18**, we place the arthroscope in the 3-4 portal and we insert a Tuohy needle with a suture inside from proximal of the TFCC through the meniscus to bring the suture inside the joint. We bring 1 end of the suture outside the joint through the 6-R portal with a grasper, and we withdraw the Tuohy needle with the other end of the suture outside the capsule. Then, we redirect the needle more distally than the first entry point and advance it into the joint and bring the other end of this suture outside the joint through the 6-R portal. We perform a gliding knot and use a knot pusher to finalize the repair.

In addition to these techniques, an arthroscopic knotless repair has been described.[24] However, we have no experience using this technique.

POSTOPERATIVE CARE

Having closed the wounds and put on a dressing, we apply a well-padded sugar-tong splint with the forearm in the neutral position that allows free

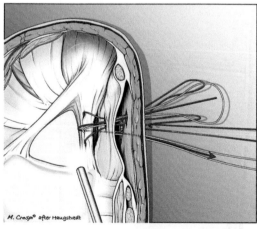

Fig. 11. When we have 1 loop and 2 ends from 2 different sutures outside the joint, the suture loop being in the middle, we bring the 2 ends from the 2 different sutures through the loop in opposite directions. (*Courtesy of* J.R. Haugstvedt, MD, PhD, Graalum, Norway.)

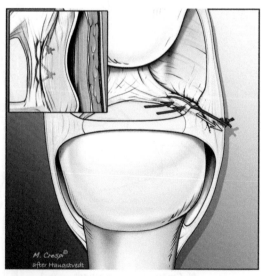

Fig. 13. When the 2 suture knots are performed, there will be traction in peripheral and proximal directions to close the capsular detachment of the triangular fibrocartilage complex. (*Courtesy of* J.R. Haugstvedt, MD, PhD, Graalum, Norway.)

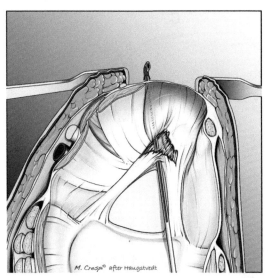

Fig. 14. For an inside-out technique, we use an 18-G Tuohy epidural needle that we pass from a radial portal across the joint to the ulnar side where the needle perforates the triangular fibrocartilage complex in a proximal direction to exit through a 6-U portal. When the needle is viewed, and palpated through the skin, we make an incision and debride the soft tissue to the capsule to ensure no nerve is injured. (*Courtesy of* J.R. Haugstvedt, MD, PhD, Graalum, Norway.)

flexion of the elbow, but no rotation of the forearm. We remove the splint after 2 weeks to control the wounds; however, we give the patient another splint or a cast to immobilize the forearm (rotation)

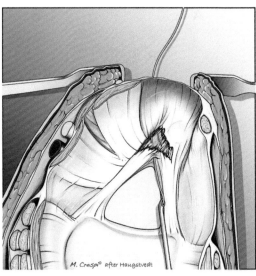

Fig. 16. With the suture inside the Tuohy needle, we withdraw the needle inside the joint until we see the needle and the suture through the arthroscope. (*Courtesy of* J.R. Haugstvedt, MD, PhD, Graalum, Norway.)

for 6 to 8 weeks. Some rehabilitation programs aim for earlier active range of motion exercises; however, many of our patients are referred from other parts of the country, making close follow-up difficult. We therefore recommend this long period of immobilization to prevent failure of the repair. After

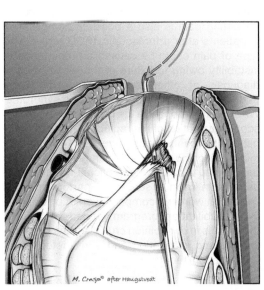

Fig. 15. After the needle is outside the joint through the 6-U portal, we can enter a suture into the needle from the tip of the needle. (*Courtesy of* J.R. Haugstvedt, MD, PhD, Graalum, Norway.)

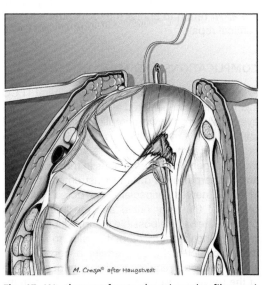

Fig. 17. We then perforate the triangular fibrocartilage complex and the capsule again with the needle, bringing the suture outside the joint again. Now we have the 2 ends of the suture outside the joint and a knot can be made. (*Courtesy of* J.R. Haugstvedt, MD, PhD, Graalum, Norway.)

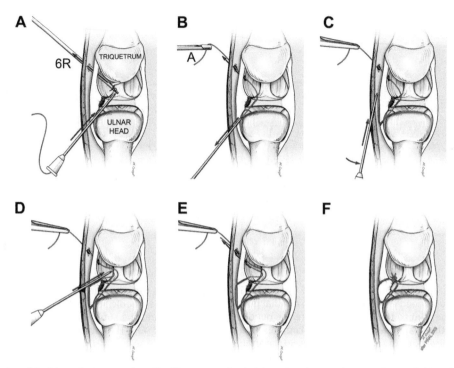

Fig. 18. The all-inside technique as described by Dr F. Del Piñal. For details, see the text. (*From* del Piñal F, García-Bernal FJ, Cagigal L, et al. A technique for arthroscopic all-inside suturing in the wrist. J Hand Surg Eur Vol 2010;35(6):476; with permission.)

removal of the cast, we refer the patients to a hand therapist for a rehabilitation program. We allow the patients to start with active exercises, then gradually they return to normal activities of daily living. We allow return to sports 5 to 6 months after the surgical repair.

COMPLICATIONS AND MANAGEMENT

Arthroscopic-assisted repair of a peripheral TFCC injury could be considered a safe procedure; however, there are known complications. As with all surgical interventions, there is the risk of infection or complications related to anesthesia. Aside from iatrogenic cartilage lesions in the radiocarpal and midcarpal joints owing to instrumentation, injuries to nerves, especially the dorsal sensible branch of the ulnar nerve and the interosseous posterior nerve, are possible complications. Nerve injuries range from a complete lesion to a dysesthesia; complete lesions require a nerve repair, and dysesthesia requires exploration for a release of the nerve to relieve the symptoms. Tendon injuries and damage of the extensor carpi ulnaris subsheath are also known complications, either as a laceration or entrapment. If clinical suspicion of such injuries is present, the structures should be surgically explored and repaired.

We emphasize careful debridement of the portals to prevent entrapment of the nerves, and/or tendons by the sutures used for TFCC repair. A more common complication, however, is synovitis owing to reaction to the sutures used. In these cases, we recommend removal of the sutures. Persisting pain is also a possible complication in patients after arthroscopic TFCC repair. This type of pain could be caused by recurrence of instability owing to failure of the repair, missed diagnosis of other radiocarpal or midcarpal pathologies, or chronic regional pain syndrome. We strongly emphasize the importance of arthroscopic evaluation of the radiocarpal and midcarpal joints, even though the TFCC pathology might be obvious at first glance. Long-lasting pain is also a possible complication that should be kept in mind if surgery is performed on a patient on workers' compensation. A postoperative rehabilitation program guided by a hand therapist is in our opinion crucial for the best outcomes, and prevention and early detection of possible complications.

OUTCOMES

We have published our results in patients undergoing arthroscopically assisted repair of peripheral

Table 1
Results from arthroscopically assisted peripheral triangular fibrocartilage complex repair

Authors	Result	No. of Patients/Total No. of Patients	Follow-up (mo)
Corso et al,[26] 1997	Satisfactory or better	42/45	37
Haugstvedt & Husby,[9] 1999	Good or excellent	14/20	23–59
Shih et al,[28] 2002	Good or excellent	34/37	26
Estrella et al,[18] 2007	Good or excellent	26/35	36
Reiter et al,[27] 2008	Good or excellent	29/46	11
Søreide et al,[12] 2016	Good or excellent	7/11	226–259

tears of the TFCC with a follow-up of 2 to 5 years.[9] We included 20 patients; 7 patients scored excellent, 7 good, 4 fair, and 2 poor, according to the Modified Mayo Wrist Score. In a recent follow-up assessing the long-term results for these patients, we found that the good results could remain 20 years after surgery.[12] This is, to our knowledge, the only long-term follow-up study that has been published, but there are many studies confirming these findings in short- and mid-term follow-ups[18,25–28] (**Table 1**). In a clinical comparison of 75 patients treated by open or arthroscopic repair of TFCC tears, the authors found no significant difference in outcomes after 3 to 4 years.[11] The authors found, however, an increase of postoperative superficial ulnar nerve pain in the open group compared with the arthroscopic group, although this difference was not statistically significant. They also reported that 15% to 20% of the patients required additional surgery for DRUJ instability, the reason for this is not stated in the paper. In our series, we found 1 patient with an excellent result at the first follow-up[9]; however, this patient had a poor result at the 20-year follow-up.[12] This patient had a positive trampoline test at the time of surgery, and a peripheral TFCC injury was diagnosed and repaired with an arthroscopically assisted outside-in technique. The DRUJ was stable at the first follow-up; however, at the time of the surgery, we did not pay attention to the proximal compartment of the TFCC,[15] and thus an additional foveal detachment (a complete tear of the proximal and distal component of the TFCC) might have been overlooked. The patient presented with a painful instability of the DRUJ at 20 years' follow-up; she had no endpoints when tested for instability, and she showed clinical and radiologic signs of degenerative changes in the DRUJ (she underwent a salvage procedure, and a semiconstrained prosthesis [Aptis] was inserted). This outcome emphasizes the importance of performing an adequate hook test to reveal complete tears of the peripheral TFCC.

SUMMARY

The TFCC is the most important stabilizer of the DRUJ and is a common concomitant injury to distal radius fractures. If the fracture is adequately treated, however, very few patients develop painful instability owing to the TFCC injury.[29] Pain, clicking, tenderness, and locking are typical presenting symptoms in patients with TFCC injuries; instability is an uncommon presenting symptom. If clinical examination raises suspicion of a TFCC lesion, we offer the patient diagnostic wrist arthroscopy for assessment of the TFCC, in addition to the radiocarpal and midcarpal joints. A peripheral TFCC lesion could be treated arthroscopically using an inside-out, an outside-in, or an all-inside technique. All of the techniques provide good to excellent results, which tends to persist over time, in 60% to 90% of cases.

REFERENCES

1. Nakamura T, Yabe Y, Horiuchi Y. Functional anatomy of the triangular fibrocartilage complex. J Hand Surg 1996;21(5):581–6.
2. Haugstvedt JR, Langer M, Berger RA. Distal radioulnar joint: functional anatomy, including pathomechanics. J Hand Surg Eur Vol 2017;42(4):338–45.
3. Palmer AK, Werner FW. The triangular fibrocartilage complex of the wrist–anatomy and function. J Hand Surg 1981;6(2):153–62.
4. Hagert E, Hagert CG. Understanding stability of the distal radioulnar joint through an understanding of its anatomy. Hand Clin 2010;26(4):459–66.
5. af Ekenstam F, Hagert CG. Anatomical studies on the geometry and stability of the distal radio ulnar joint. Scand J Plast Reconstr Surg 1985;19(1):17–25.
6. Thiru RG, Ferlic DC, Clayton ML, et al. Arterial anatomy of the triangular fibrocartilage of the wrist and its surgical significance. J Hand Surg 1986;11(2):258–63.
7. Palmer AK. Triangular fibrocartilage complex lesions: a classification. J Hand Surg 1989;14(4):594–606.

8. Mikic ZD. Age changes in the triangular fibrocartilage of the wrist joint. J Anat 1978;126(Pt 2):367–84.

9. Haugstvedt JR, Husby T. Results of repair of peripheral tears in the triangular fibrocartilage complex using an arthroscopic suture technique. Scand J Plast Reconstr Surg Hand Surg 1999;33(4):439–47.

10. Cooney WP, Linscheid RL, Dobyns JH. Triangular fibrocartilage tears. J Hand Surg 1994;19(1):143–54.

11. Anderson ML, Larson AN, Moran SL, et al. Clinical comparison of arthroscopic versus open repair of triangular fibrocartilage complex tears. J Hand Surg 2008;33(5):675–82.

12. Søreide E, Husby T, Haugstvedt JR. A long-term (20 years') follow-up after arthroscopically assisted repair of the TFCC. J Plast Surg Hand Surg 2016. [Epub ahead of print].

13. Hermansdorfer JD, Kleinman WB. Management of chronic peripheral tears of the triangular fibrocartilage complex. J Hand Surg 1991;16(2):340–6.

14. Haugstvedt JR, Berger RA, Nakamura T, et al. Relative contributions of the ulnar attachments of the triangular fibrocartilage complex to the dynamic stability of the distal radioulnar joint. J Hand Surg 2006; 31(3):445–51.

15. Atzei A. New trends in arthroscopic management of type 1-B TFCC injuries with DRUJ instability. J Hand Surg Eur Vol 2009;34(5):582–91.

16. Atzei A, Luchetti R. Foveal TFCC tear classification and treatment. Hand Clin 2011;27(3):263–72.

17. Lindau T, Arner M, Hagberg L. Intraarticular lesions in distal fractures of the radius in young adults. A descriptive arthroscopic study in 50 patients. J Hand Surg 1997;22(5):638–43.

18. Estrella EP, Hung LK, Ho PC, et al. Arthroscopic repair of triangular fibrocartilage complex tears. Arthroscopy 2007;23(7):729–37, 737.e1.

19. Tay SC, Tomita K, Berger RA. The "ulnar fovea sign" for defining ulnar wrist pain: an analysis of sensitivity and specificity. J Hand Surg 2007;32(4):438–44.

20. del Pinal F. Dry arthroscopy and its applications. Hand Clin 2011;27(3):335–45.

21. de Araujo W, Poehling GG, Kuzma GR. New Tuohy needle technique for triangular fibrocartilage complex repair: preliminary studies. Arthroscopy 1996; 12(6):699–703.

22. Lee CK, Cho HL, Jung KA, et al. Arthroscopic all-inside repair of Palmer type 1B triangular fibrocartilage complex tears: a technical note. Knee Surg Sports Traumatol Arthrosc 2008;16(1):94–7.

23. del Pinal F, Garcia-Bernal FJ, Cagigal L, et al. A technique for arthroscopic all-inside suturing in the wrist. J Hand Surg Eur Vol 2010;35(6):475–9.

24. Geissler WB. Arthroscopic knotless peripheral ulnar-sided TFCC repair. J wrist Surg 2015;4(2):143–7.

25. Trumble TE, Gilbert M, Vedder N. Isolated tears of the triangular fibrocartilage: management by early arthroscopic repair. J Hand Surg 1997;22(1):57–65.

26. Corso SJ, Savoie FH, Geissler WB, et al. Arthroscopic repair of peripheral avulsions of the triangular fibrocartilage complex of the wrist: a multicenter study. Arthroscopy 1997;13(1):78–84.

27. Reiter A, Wolf MB, Schmid U, et al. Arthroscopic repair of Palmer 1B triangular fibrocartilage complex tears. Arthroscopy 2008;24(11):1244–50.

28. Shih JT, Lee HM, Tan CM. Early isolated triangular fibrocartilage complex tears: management by arthroscopic repair. J Trauma 2002;53(5):922–7.

29. Mrkonjic A, Geijer M, Lindau T, et al. The natural course of traumatic triangular fibrocartilage complex tears in distal radial fractures: a 13-15 year follow-up of arthroscopically diagnosed but untreated injuries. J Hand Surg 2012;37(8):1555–60.

Arthroscopic Management of Triangular Fibrocartilage Complex Foveal Injury

Keiji Fujio, MD

KEYWORDS

- Inside-out • Arthroscopy • Fovea • TFCC

KEY POINTS

- It is important to make a precise diagnosis according to patient's history, meticulous physical findings, and MRI or arthrogram before operating.
- From the radiocarpal joint, the triangular fibrocartilage complex (TFCC) should be checked using the trampoline, hook, and floating sign. A distal radioulnar joint (DRUJ) scope may be introduced for a definitive diagnosis. The scope should be inserted from the radial DRUJ portal, checking the fovea using a probe or a 2.0-mm shaver.
- Enough debridement for the foveal side is important to reattach the TFCC. If the DRUJ scope can be used, shaving through the ulnar DRUJ portal is useful.
- 2-0 fiber wire is better used in the inside-out technique through the curved guide with the guide pin inserted in an oscillating manner.

INTRODUCTION: NATURE OF THE PROBLEM

The triangular fibrocartilage complex (TFCC) is an anatomically and biomechanically important 3-dimensional structure. The palmar and dorsal radioulnar ligaments of the TFCC have superficial and deep components.[1,2] The deep component inserts on the fovea of the ulnar head. Haugstvedt and colleagues[1] demonstrated that the deep component provides greater stability than the superficial component, according to their biomechanical study of the stabilizing effect of the TFCC on the distal radioulnar joint (DRUJ). To repair the deep component indicates effectiveness of transosseous repair for foveal detachment of the TFCC in stabilizing the DRUJ. There are various methods to repair the TFCC: inside-out,[3–12] outside-in,[13–17] and all-inside techniques.[18–25] In 2006, the author designed an inside-out repair technique[26] and found that it was also applicable for TFCC foveal repair. The inside-out technique for foveal injury is now introduced. The results of the arthroscopic reattachment of TFCC fovea are discussed.

INDICATIONS

The author's indications for transosseous inside-out TFCC foveal repair are as follows:

1. Pain or click during pronation and supination
2. Positive sign for instability, fovea sign, or ulnocarpal stress test
3. Confirm avulsion of TFCC at its ulnar insertion on MRI and DRUJ arthrography

CONTRAINDICATIONS

Transosseous inside-out technique is suitable for almost all cases of foveal tear except when the

Disclosure of Conflict of Interest: The author has nothing to declare for this study.
Kansai Electric Power Hospital, 2-1-7,Fukushima, Fukushima-ku, Osaka City, Japan
E-mail address: ykfujio@gmail.com

hand.theclinics.com

stump of the TFCC cannot be approximated to the fovea.

SURGICAL TECHNIQUE/PROCEDURE
Preoperative Planning

DRUJ stability is assessed with the fovea sign[27] and instability test. A positive ulnar fovea sign may indicate fovea disruption or ulnotriquetral ligament injury. DRUJ instability is assessed by passive anteroposterior translation of the distal ulna relative to distal radius in neutral rotation, supination, and pronation when the forearm muscles are fully relaxed. The degree of translation is compared with the contralateral side. Ulnar variance should be checked by radiograph. Coronal T2 short tau inversion recovery (STIR) MRI, which includes the helical view centering around the fovea (**Fig. 1**) and horizontal view paralleling the ulnar head diameter passing through ulnar styroid (**Fig. 2**), is useful for evaluation of the TFCC foveal insertion (**Fig. 3**).

Preparation and Patient Positioning

The operation is performed under general anesthesia or an upper arm block with the patient in the supine position. The arm is fixed to a hand table with the shoulder in 90° abduction. An upper-arm tourniquet is applied at 90 mm Hg above the systolic blood pressure. Finger traps are applied to the index and middle fingers. About 5 kg of traction is applied, or until dimples are seen on the dorsal metacarpophalangeal joints, with the Spider system (Smith & Nephew, London and Hull, United Kingdom) or Geissler traction system (ACUMED, Hillsboro, Oregon, USA). Created are 3-4 portal,

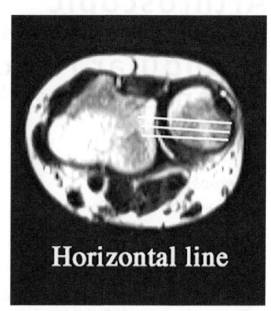

Fig. 2. MRI of horizontal view parallel to ulnar head diameter passing through the ulnar styloid.

4-5 portal, radial DRUJ portal (DRUJ-R), and ulnar DRUJ portal (DRUJ-U).

SURGICAL APPROACH
Diagnosis from Radiocarpal Joint and Distal Radioulnar Joint

Trampoline test, hook test, and floating sign from radiocarpal joint

A wrist arthroscope is inserted from the 3-4 portal for exploration to locate the TFCC tear. A probe is inserted via the 4-5 portal. The articular disc is then examined by the probe with the so-called

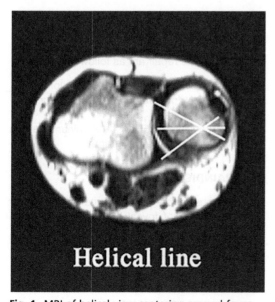

Fig. 1. MRI of helical view centering around fovea.

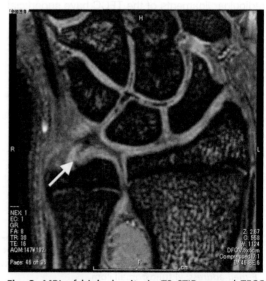

Fig. 3. MRI of high density in T2 STIR around TFCC foveal insertion. Arrow indicates foveal tear.

trampoline test[28] and the hook test.[29] In 1991, Hermansdorfer and Kleinman[28] showed that the trampoline effect may reveal diminished tension on the horizontal disc and is suggestive of an ulnar TFCC detachment. On the other hand, Iwasaki and colleagues[30] stated that by using this technique in the condition of foveal disruption, the normal trampoline effect is lost. However, it depends on personal experience in determining loss of tension and displacement of TFCC. In the author's opinion, the floating sign[31] (**Fig. 4**), in which TFCC around the fovea is floating during suction with a shaver, is usually helpful to make a decision on foveal detachment if there is no connection between radiocarpal joint (RCJ) and DRUJ, that is, no associated palmar 1A tear. Next, the torn TFCC is checked from the DRUJ scope directly. From the DRUJ-R portal, the scope is inserted, and probing is made from the DRUJ-U portal.

Foveal Debridement

Foveal debridement is an important procedure for subacute or chronic cases to promote bone to ligament reattachment. Debridement is performed from the DRUJ-U portal (**Fig. 5**).

If it is difficult to manage from the dorsal side, the shaver can be inserted from the volar fovea (**Fig. 6**). The TFCC remnant is slightly debrided to preserve the ligament tissue. For the foveal side, the remnant is debrided more aggressively to explore the foveal cortex.

Inside-Out Technique

A 2-cm longitudinal skin incision is made just volar to the ulnar styloid. The superficial ulnar nerve is

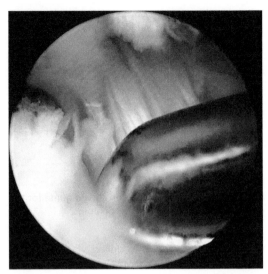

Fig. 5. The arthroscope is inserted through DRUJ-R portal, and debridement is done with a shaver inserted through the DRUJ-U portal.

retracted meticulously; the retinaculum is incised sharply, and the ulnar cortex is explored.

To repair an ulnar-sided TFCC tear, a single-lumen curved guide (**Fig. 7**) is inserted through the 4-5 portal, targeting the fovea. The curve at the tip of the guide makes targeting of the fovea accurate. In 1993, Bade and colleagues[32] reported the relationship between recess and fovea. An appropriate entry point for the isometric point would be just dorsal and radial to the recess as viewed from the RCJ (**Fig. 8**). At a neutral or slightly supinated position, the needle through the curved guide is easier to aim toward the center of fovea because the ulnar styloid moves in a volar direction (**Fig. 9**).

A stitcher needle (soft wire, sized 1.0 mm in diameter; Smith & Nephew), which has a hole at

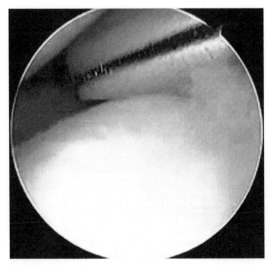

Fig. 4. TFCC is floating with the shaver suction on.

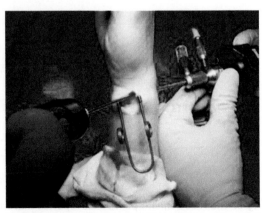

Fig. 6. The shaver is inserted through volar fovea if it is impossible to manage from dorsal side.

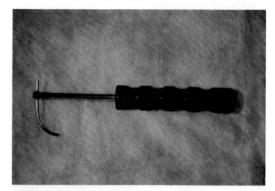

Fig. 7. The author's single-lumen curved guide for targeting toward the TFCC isometric point.

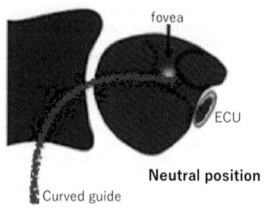

Fig. 9. Neutral or slightly supinated position is an easy position for placing the needle through the curved guide to the center of fovea because the ulnar styloid moves in the volar direction. ECU, extensor carpi ulnaris. (*Adapted from* Atzei A, Luchetti R. Repair of the foveal insertion of the TFCC through the DF portal. In: Slutsky DJ, editor. Principles and practice of wrist surgery. 1st edition. Philadelphia: Saunders, an imprint of Elsevier Inc; 2010. p. 564; with permission.)

the end of the needle, is drilled via the curved guide through the ulnar TFCC and distal ulna bone and comes out on the ulna aspect of distal ulna cortex. Then, a threaded 2-0 fiber wire is run through the hole, and the needle is pulled from the distal ulna or using a drive in an oscillating manner. This maneuver is repeated to pass the other end of the thread through the distal ulna bone.

Usually 2 knots are placed around the isometric point (**Fig. 10**).

After the traction is released, the 2 sutures are tied separately on the ulnar cortex.

COMPLICATIONS

Complications of the operation include injury to the superficial branch of ulnar nerve, breakage of the stitcher needle during insertion, and torn suture thread during passage. In order to avoid the above complications, careful dissection with

identification and retraction of the nerve is important. The curved guide should be held steady during drilling. The power drill should also be changed to an oscillating mode when passing the thread through the ulna bone.

POSTOPERATIVE CARE

- Immediate postoperative finger range-of-motion (ROM) exercise
- Long arm cast immobilization for 3 weeks
- Start wrist active ROM after the splint is removed

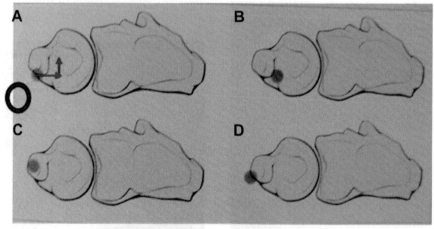

Fig. 8. The TFCC isometric point. Bade reported that type A is the most frequent type (A: 62%, B: 16%, C: 10%, D: 1.6%). (*From* Schmidt HM, Lanz U. Surgical anatomy of the hand. Stuttgart (Germany): Thieme; 2004. p. 59; with permission.)

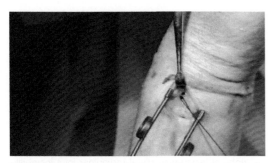

Fig. 10. Two sutures at the isometric point are made. Knots tied over the distal ulnar cortex.

- Start wrist passive ROM 6 weeks after surgery
- Achieve full rotation 3 months after surgery
- Avoid resisted twist motion within the postoperative 3 months

OUTCOMES

From October 2006 to December 2014, 150 patients, 92 men and 58 women (mean age 33.5 years old), underwent this operation and were reviewed. All patients were evaluated by the Mayo Modified Scoring System. Patients were evaluated at a mean follow-up time of 35.3 months. Except for 6 patients, all had complete relief of wrist pain and returned their previous work or sports. Grip strength averaged 94.1% of the contralateral side. Clinical score with modified Green and O'Brien Scoring System[33] averaged 93.1 points. There were 5 cases of superficial ulnar nerve irritation; symptoms resolved within 3 months, and 2 cases developed chronic regional pain syndrome.

SUMMARY

Surgical reattachment of TFCC to the fovea has been advocated to be important for stabilizing the DRUJ. The author has experienced hundreds of patients reattached for foveal TFCC avulsion with the arthroscopic inside-out technique since 1999. Because of the technical complexity especially for debridement, the arthroscopic procedure has been neglected. The current debridement technique and inside-out suture method can simplify the reattachment procedure.

REFERENCES

1. Haugstvedt JR, Berger RA, Nakamura T, et al. Relative contributions of the ulnar attachments of the triangular fibrocartilage complex to the dynamic stability of the distal radioulnar joint. J Hand Surg Am 2006;31:445–51.
2. Nakamura T, Takayama S, Horiuchi Y, et al. Origins and insertions of the triangular fibrocartilage complex: a histological study. J Hand Surg Br 2001;26(5):446–54.
3. Zachee B, De Smet L, Fabry G. Arthroscopic suturing of TFCC lesions. Arthroscopy 1993;9(2):242–3.
4. Corso SJ, Savoie FH, Geissler WB, et al. Arthroscopic repair of peripheral avulsions of the triangular fibrocartilage complex of the wrist: a multicenter study. Arthroscopy 1997;13(1):78–84.
5. Haugstvedt JR, Husby T. The results of repair of peripheral tears in the triangular fibrocartilage complex using an arthroscopic suture technique. Scand J Plast Reconstr Surg Hand Surg 1999;33(4):439–47.
6. Millants P, De Smet L, Van Ransbeeck H. Outcome study of arthroscopic suturing of ulnar avulsions of the triangular fibrocartilage complex of the wrist. Chir Main 2002;21(5):298–300.
7. Shih JT, Lee HM, Tan CM. Early isolated triangular fibrocartilage complex tears: management by arthroscopic repair. J Trauma 2002;53(5):922–7.
8. Ruch DS, Papadonikolakis A. Arthroscopically assisted repair of peripheral triangular fibrocartilage complex tears: factors affecting outcome. Arthroscopy 2005;21(9):1126–30.
9. Badia A, Khanchandani P. Suture welding for arthroscopic repair of peripheral triangular fibrocartilage complex tears. Tech Hand Up Extrem Surg 2007; 11(1):45–50.
10. Estrella EP, Hung LK, Ho PC, et al. Arthroscopic repair of triangular fibrocartilage complex tears. Arthroscopy 2007;23(7):729–37.
11. Mahajan RH, Kim SJ, Song DH, et al. Arthroscopic repair of the triangular fibrocartilage complex using a hypodermic needle: a technical note. J Orthop Surg (Hong Kong) 2009;17(2):231–3.
12. Wysocki RW, Ruch DS. Outside-in repair of peripheral triangular fibrocartilage complex tears. Oper Tech Sports Med 2010;18(3):163–7.
13. de Araujo W, Poehling GG, Kuzma GR. New Tuohy needle technique for triangular fibrocartilage complex repair: preliminary studies. Arthroscopy 1996; 12(6):699–703.
14. Trumble TE, Gilbert M, Vedder N. Arthroscopic repair of the triangular fibrocartilage complex. Arthroscopy 1996;12(5):588–97.
15. Skie MC, Mekhail AO, Deitrich DR, et al. Operative technique for inside-out repair of the triangular fibrocartilage complex. J Hand Surg Am 1997;22(5): 814–7.
16. Trumble TE, Gilbert M, Vedder N. Isolated tears of the triangular fibrocartilage: management by early arthroscopic repair. J Hand Surg 1997;22A(1):57–65.
17. Tang CYK, Fung B, Rebecca C, et al. Another light in the dark: review of a new method for the arthroscopic repair of triangular fibrocartilage complex. J Hand Surg 2012;37A:1263–8.
18. Bohringer G, Schadel-Hopfner M, Petermann J, et al. A method for all-inside arthroscopic repair of

Palmer 1B triangular fibrocartilage complex tears. Arthroscopy 2002;18(2):211–3.

19. Conca M, Conca R, DallaPria A. Preliminary experience 262 of fully arthroscopic repair of triangular fibrocartilage complex lesions. Arthroscopy 2004; 20(7):79–82.

20. Pederzini LA, Tosi M, Prandini M, et al. All-inside suture technique for Palmer class 1B triangular fibrocartilage repair. Arthroscopy 2007;23(10):1131–4.

21. Lee CK, Cho HL, Jung KA, et al. Arthroscopic all-inside repair of Palmer type 1B triangular fibrocartilage complex tears: a technical note. Knee Surg Sports Traumatol Arthrosc 2008;16(1):94–7.

22. Yao J. All-arthroscopic triangular fibrocartilage complex repair: safety and biomechanical comparison with a traditional outside-in technique in cadavers. J Hand Surg Am 2009;34(4):671–6.

23. del Pinal F, Garcia-Bernal FJ, Cagigal L, et al. A technique for arthroscopic all inside suturing in the wrist. J Hand Surg Br 2010;35(6):475–9.

24. Waterman SM, Slade D, Masini BD, et al. Safety analysis of all-inside arthroscopic repair of peripheral triangular fibrocartilage complex. Arthroscopy 2010;26(11):1474–7.

25. Yao J. All-arthroscopic repair of peripheral triangular fibrocartilage complex tears. Oper Tech Sports Med 2010;18(3):168–72.

26. Fujio K. Arthroscopic surgery for TFCC injury. Rinshoseikeigeka 2006;57(8):125–7.

27. Tay SC, Tomita K, Berger RA. The "ulnar fovea sign" for defining ulnar wrist pain: an analysis of sensitivity and specificity. J Hand Surg Am 2007;32(4):438–44.

28. Hermansdorfer JD, Kleinman WB. Management of chronic peripheral tears of the triangular fibrocartilage complex. J Hand Surg Am 1991;16:340–6.

29. Atzei A, Rizzo A, Luchetti R, et al. Arthroscopic foveal repair of triangular fibrocartilage complex peripheral lesion with distal radioulnar joint instability. Tech Hand Up Extrem Surg 2008;12(4):226–91.

30. Iwasaki N, Nishida K, Motomiya M, et al. Arthroscopic-assisted repair of avulsed triangular fibrocartilage complex to the fovea of the ulnar head: a 2- to 4-year follow-up study. Arthroscopy 2011;27(10): 1371–8.

31. Takeuchi H, Fujio K. Diagnosis for TFCC foveal tear – floating sign. J Jpn Soc Surg Hand 2014; 31(3):173–5 (in Japanese).

32. Bade H, Koebke J, Stangier R. Der Recessus ulnaris im Arthrogramm des proximalen Handgelenks. Handchir Mikrochir Plast Chir 1993;25:171–8 [in German].

33. Cooney WP, Bussey R, Dobyns JH, et al. Difficult wrist fractures. Perilunate fracture-dislocations of the wrist. Clin Orthop 1987;214:136–47.

Arthroscopic-Assisted Triangular Fibrocartilage Complex Reconstruction

Michael Chu-Kay Mak, MBChB, FRCS (Edinburg), FHKCOS, FHKAM (Orth Surg)*,
Pak-cheong Ho, MBBS, FRCS (Edinburg), FHKCOS, FHKAM (Orth Surg)

KEYWORDS

- Triangular fibrocartilage complex • Distal radioulnar joint • DRUJ instability • TFCC tear
- TFCC reconstruction • Wrist arthroscopy

KEY POINTS

- The triangular fibrocartilage complex (TFCC) is the primary stabilizer of the distal radioulnar joint, comprising the articular disc, the meniscus homologue, the volar and dorsal distal radioulnar ligaments, the subsheath of the extensor carpi ulnaris, the ulnar capsule, and the ulnolunate and ulnotriquetral ligaments.
- The volar and dorsal radioulnar ligaments have an important stabilizing effect in forearm rotation, with an isometric point of insertion in the fovea.
- In irreparable TFCC tears, anatomic TFCC reconstruction is the recommended treatment to restore stability of the distal radioulnar joint.
- The surgical technique of an arthroscopic-assisted approach in anatomic TFCC reconstruction is described. Soft tissue dissection is minimized and the joint capsule is not violated.
- Outcomes of this approach are comparable to the conventional open technique and may be superior in restoring range of motion.

RELEVANT ANATOMY AND BIOMECHANICS OF THE TRIANGULAR FIBROCARTILAGE COMPLEX

A solid understanding of the anatomy and biomechanics of the triangular fibrocartilage complex (TFCC) is crucial for undertaking its repair or reconstruction. The TFCC is a composite structure of ligamentous, fibrous, and fibrocartilaginous components that are blended as a homogeneous complex and function as a unit to stabilize the distal radioulnar joint (DRUJ), transmit load from the ulnar carpus to the ulna, and allow smooth wrist motion and forearm rotation.[1] Our current understanding of its functional anatomy is due largely to the work of Palmer and Werner in 1981[2] and the body of anatomic and biomechanical studies that followed. The TFCC is the primary intrinsic stabilizer of the DRUJ,[3] which is an inherently incongruent joint and relies mainly on soft tissue stabilizers. Division of the TFCC alone has been shown to result in dorsal DRUJ dislocation in neutral, pronation, and supination and volar dislocation in neutral and supination, in the presence of intact DRUJ capsule and pronator quadratus.[2] The TFCC consists of the articular disc, the meniscus homologue, the volar and dorsal distal radioulnar ligaments, the subsheath of the extensor carpi ulnaris, the ulnar capsule, and the ulnolunate and ulnotriquetral ligaments.[2,4] In particular, within the TFCC, the

Conflict of Interest: None.
Division of Hand and Microsurgery, Department of Orthopaedic and Traumatology, Prince of Wales Hospital, Chinese University of Hong Kong, 5F, Lui Che Woo Clinical Sciences Building, 30-32 Ngan Shing Street, Shatin, NT, Hong Kong SAR
* Corresponding author.
E-mail address: mmak@ort.cuhk.edu.hk

Hand Clin 33 (2017) 625–637
http://dx.doi.org/10.1016/j.hcl.2017.07.014

important stabilizing effect of the volar and dorsal radioulnar ligaments during forearm rotation have been demonstrated by multiple studies.[4–7] In pronation, the superficial dorsal and deep palmar fibers of the distal radioulnar ligaments become taut, whereas in supination, the superficial palmar and deep dorsal ligaments become taut.[5,8] On the other hand, the articular disc proper has a less important role in stabilizing the DRUJ and can be excised up to two-thirds without significant kinematic change.[9] The radioulnar ligaments are inserted into the fovea and the ulnar styloid, with the foveal insertion having the major effect on stability.[10] Nakamura and Yabe[11] described the distal portion of the TFCC as a hammocklike structure that supports the ulnar carpus, with a proximal portion being the radioulnar ligaments anchoring to the fovea. The hammock thus becomes unsteady once the anchor is broken.

The vascularity of the TFCC shows similarity to that of the meniscus of the knee. Thiru-Pathi and colleagues[12] showed that only the outer 15% to 20% of the articular disc is vascular, whereas Bednar and colleagues[13] reported that the vascularity of the TFCC is limited to the peripheral 10% to 40%. The feeding vessels are branches from the ulnar and anterior interosseous arteries. The radial and central portion of the TFCC receives nutritional support from synovial fluid. This pattern of vascularity dictates that only the periphery has predictable healing potential from surgical repair, whereas that of central tears is scarce.

EPIDEMIOLOGY AND PATHOMECHANISM OF TRIANGULAR FIBROCARTILAGE COMPLEX INJURY

Injury of the TFCC was cited as the most common cause of ulnar-sided wrist pain.[14,15] A systematic review reported a prevalence of TFCC abnormalities in symptomatic wrists ranging from 39% to 70% in patients between 50 and 69 years old.[16] Another study showed that up to 78% of distal radius fractures had associated TFCC injuries detected by arthroscopy in patients 20 to 60 years old.[17] The mechanism of injury commonly involves abrupt forceful rotation, or loading and distraction injury to the ulnar wrist and forearm.[17] Loading of the wrist in extreme extension and pronation or supination was the most common mechanism reported in a series and was verified in 2 cadavers by Coleman in 1960.[18,19] This frequently occurs in a fall on the outstretched upper extremity, particularly when falling to the side or backward. Patients with ulnar plus variance may also be more prone to injury due to the thinner TFCC.[20] Moritomo and colleagues[21] in 2010 also noted that wrist hyperextension with forearm rotation

was the most common injury mechanism. They further correlated the surgical findings of TFCC tear with mechanism of injury and suggested that forced wrist extension resulted in excessive traction of the ulnocapitate ligament, which in turn avulses the deep palmar radioulnar ligament from its foveal insertion. The second mechanism of injury was forceful rotation, in which hyperpronation was suggested to result in first an injury of the superficial dorsal radioulnar ligament and then the foveal insertion. Degenerative tears, which commonly result in attrition and perforation of the TFCC, were suggested to be caused by chronic repetitive loading of the wrist,[18] particularly in ulnar deviation and pronation.

CLINICAL ASSESSMENT OF TRIANGULAR FIBROCARTILAGE COMPLEX TEAR

The mechanism of injury, as described previously, is a useful clue to the diagnosis. There may be a "pop" sound with TFCC injury. Symptoms include ulnar wrist pain on rotation with or without loading, decreased range of motion, instability, weakness, and joint clunk. Chronicity and the presence of preexisting symptoms are noted. Physical signs are important to locate the site(s) of injury, help determine the type of lesion within the TFCC, and judge the extent of DRUJ instability. These include prominence of the ulnar head, and local tenderness corresponding to specific lesions. Common tender sites include the dorsal TFCC, the ulnar snuff box, or foveal area,[22] which is the interval between the ulnar head, triquetrum, flexor carpi ulnaris, and extensor carpi ulnaris tendons; the DRUJ dorsal capsule, lunate, triquetrum, and lunate triquetral ligament. Instability is elicited by provocative tests. Passive pronosupination of the forearm will be painful, which may limit the range of motion in peripheral TFCC tear. The DRUJ ballottement test is done in neutral, supination, and pronation. In the neutral position, there is normally up to 5 mm of dorso-volar translation of the DRUJ due to the inherent joint configuration. It is at the most stable locked position in maximal pronation and supination, and any translation should be regarded as abnormal. Furthermore, in full pronation, pain elicited by dorsal push of the ulnar head relative to the radius indicates tear of the deep palmar radioulnar ligament; whereas in full supination, pain elicited by volar push of the ulnar head indicates tear of the deep dorsal radioulnar ligament. The classic piano key sign may be positive in overt instability of the DRUJ.[23] The ulnocarpal ligament stress test is performed with the forearm in neutral rotation and the wrist in radial deviation, in which the ulnar head is balloted in the volar-dorsal direction similar to the DRUJ ballottement test. Normally in this position the DRUJ becomes more stable. Abnormal increase in translation indicates ulnocarpal ligament tear. Resisted supination and pronation, eliciting pain and weakness, is a sensitive but relatively nonspecific test for DRUJ instability. During resisted pronation, reduction in pain with a volar push on the dorsal ulnar head suggests peripheral TFCC tear. A radiograph of the wrist, in posteroanterior and lateral views with the forearm in neutral rotation, is part of routine assessment. Magnetic resonance arthrography is a useful modality to diagnose TFCC tears and concomitant injuries, and with wrist traction applied, has an accuracy of TFCC tear detection of 98%.[24]

MANAGEMENT AND INDICATION OF TRIANGULAR FIBROCARTILAGE COMPLEX RECONSTRUCTION

Initial management of suspected TFCC injury depends on the extent of instability, chronicity, and ulnar variance. In the acute injury, with dynamic or static reducible DRUJ instability, conservative treatment with a sugar-tong splint is given. Surgical intervention is indicated in the presence of persistent DRUJ instability after completing a course of splintage, history of acute on chronic ulnar wrist pain, and significant positive ulnar variance of 2 to 3 mm. Palmer[18] described a classification of different types of TFCC tears based on anatomic sites, in which a 1B tear is a peripheral traumatic tear on the ulnar aspect. More recently, Atzei and colleagues[25] proposed a subclassification of the Palmer 1B tear with corresponding surgical strategy, which, in addition to the anatomic site, incorporated degree of clinical instability, reparability of the tear, and cartilage condition of DRUJ. Arthroscopy is the gold standard in assessment of the TFCC and is essential in providing the previously described information. TFCC reconstruction with tendon graft is indicated in the irreparable TFCC with symptomatic DRUJ instability, which may happen with a neglected chronic injury, a massive tear in which the torn ends are under tension when opposed, or suboptimal healing after conservative treatment or surgical repair. This may result in torn ends that are sclerotic and degenerated, retracted, or frayed with thinned and friable scar tissue.

TRIANGULAR FIBROCARTILAGE COMPLEX RECONSTRUCTION

Various methods of TFCC reconstruction have been described in the literature, which fall into the categories of a direct extra-articular radioulnar tether,[26] an indirect stabilization via an ulnocarpal sling,[27,28] or reconstruction of the radioulnar ligaments.[29,30] The first 2 categories are largely historical in the context of restoring the function of TFCC as the normal axis of rotation is not restored and stability is insufficient. The reconstruction method of Scheker and colleagues[30] involves 2 separate tendon grafts to reconstruct the dorsal and volar distal radioulnar ligaments, requiring separate bone tunnels for each graft and substantial dissection on both sides. Adams and Berger[29] described an anatomic reconstruction that restores the radioulnar ligaments and their insertion into the fovea (see **Fig. 3**A), using a single graft that could be tensioned uniformly, and passes through the ulna at the foveal insertion site. This has since been widely used and reported by several investigators.[31,32] Based on this method of anatomic reconstruction, since 2000 we have used an arthroscopic-assisted technique, which we have reported previously.[33] The major advantage with an arthroscopic technique is its minimal invasiveness obviating the need of an open capsulotomy with a capsular flap of the original method. This minimizes soft tissue scarring, fibrosis, and stiffness. Under arthroscopic control, there can be a precise identification of the fovea for ulna tunnel preparation, and clear visualization allowing isometric placement of the graft at the fovea. It also allows thorough assessment of concomitant intra-articular pathologies, and earlier rehabilitation due to preservation of soft tissue integrity. In cases with substantial skeletal malalignment, such as in distal radius malunion and gross positive ulnar variance, corrective osteotomy should be performed in conjunction with TFCC reconstruction. If there is a basal ulnar styloid fracture nonunion, fixation has to be considered first if it contributes to loss of soft tissue stabilization. Contraindications include significant symptomatic DRUJ arthritis and forearm rotational instability due to insufficiency of the interosseous membrane. A diagnostic arthroscopy could be performed before definitive reconstruction to establish the reparability of the TFCC tear, or in one stage if diagnosis is certain. The surgical technique of arthroscopic-assisted TFCC reconstruction is presented.

SURGICAL TECHNIQUE
Setup and Instruments

The surgery is performed under general anesthesia or brachial plexus block. With the muscles relaxed, DRUJ stability is assessed with ballottement test comparing with the other side. The patient is positioned supine with longitudinal wrist traction of 10 to 15 lb. A tourniquet is applied over the arm. The following instruments are used:

1. 1.9-mm or 2.7-mm arthroscope
2. Motorized full-radius shaver (2.0/2.9 mm) and radiofrequency probe
3. Powered instrument including cannulated drills
4. 2-mm arthroscopic graspers and suction punch
5. Fluoroscopic image intensifier

Step 1: wrist arthroscopy and triangular fibrocartilage complex central opening preparation

The surgery starts with assessment of the radiocarpal joint with 3/4 viewing, 4/5 working, and 6U outflow portals. Associated chondral or ligamentous injuries are documented. The TFCC is assessed for loss of trampoline tension and detachment from foveal insertion with the hook test. Fibrous and excess synovial tissues are debrided with shaver and radiofrequency ablation. TFCC reconstruction is indicated when the foveal detachment is beyond repair. Chronic DRUJ instability is sometimes caused by suboptimal healing of the peripheral tear. Hook sign can be negative in the presence of a positive trampoline test. Because direct access to the fovea is essential for passage of the graft, a central perforation at the TFCC is desirable. If the central part of the TFCC is intact, a central perforation is created with an arthroscopic knife, shaver, or best with a radiofrequency ablation apparatus. If a central tear already exists, the tear is enlarged to 5 to 6 mm with an arthroscopic punch or radiofrequency ablation (**Fig. 1**). Any large floppy TFCC flap preventing direct access to the fovea is debrided until the edge of the TFCC perforation is smooth and the ulnar head is exposed. The torn ligamentous tissue or the ligamentum subcruentum should be readily identifiable.

Step 2: harvesting tendon graft

With the wrist taken off the traction tower and placed on a hand table, a 2-cm volar longitudinal incision is made midway between the palmaris longus (PL) tendon and radial border of the flexor carpi ulnaris (FCU) tendon at the level of the proximal wrist crease (**Fig. 2**A). The PL tendon is harvested in full length with a tendon-harvesting stripper.

With the flexor tendons and median nerve retracted radially and FCU, ulnar nerve, and artery retracted ulnarly, the volar surface of distal radius is reached. The distal border of the pronator

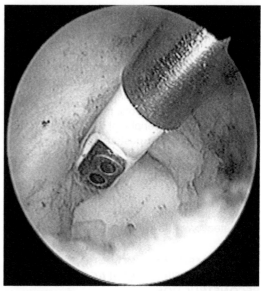

Fig. 1. The defect in the TFCC was enlarged with a radiofrequency probe until the fovea was exposed and torn edges are smooth.

quadratus serves as a landmark for the approximate level of the radial tunnel.

Step 3: radial tunnel preparation with passage of tendon graft

A 2-cm dorsal longitudinal incision is made extending proximally from the 4/5 portal (see **Fig. 2**B). The extensor retinaculum is divided over the fourth extensor compartment while preserving the distal and proximal fibers. The extensor tendons were retracted to the radial side to expose the distal radius at the ulnar edge of the lunate fossa adjacent to the sigmoid notch. A 1.1-mm guide pin is inserted on the dorsal surface of distal radius radial to the sigmoid notch. Under fluoroscopic guidance, the guide pin should be placed ideally at 5 mm proximal to the articular surface of lunate fossa and 5 mm radial to the sigmoid fossa with a volar tilt of 10° to 15° parallel to the surface of the lunate fossa (**Fig. 3**B). This is verified on fluoroscopy by anteroposterior and lateral views. A drill sleeve is used to prevent catching of soft tissue. Before the pin exits the opposite cortex, the tendons and neurovascular bundles on the volar side are gently retracted by an assistant to ensure that the guide pin exits at the ideal position, which is 5 mm radial to the sigmoid notch edge and just distal to the pronator quadratus. Only when the important soft tissue structures are out of harm's way and the assistant has direct visualization of the tip of the pin should it be advanced further (**Fig. 4**). With guide pin position confirmed by fluoroscopy, the tunnel is

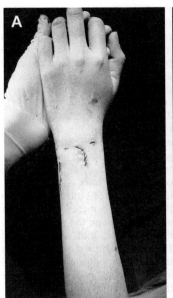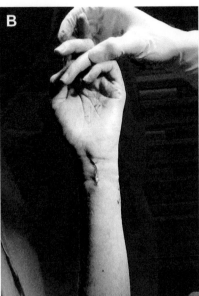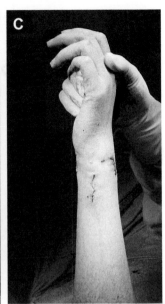

Fig. 2. (*A*) The dorsal incision is a 2-cm proximal extension of the 4/5 portal. (*B*) The 2-cm volar incision is placed between the PL and flexor carpi radialis tendons at the level of the proximal wrist crease. (*C*) A 3-cm longitudinal incision was made over the subcutaneous border of ulna starting 1 cm proximal to the tip of ulnar styloid.

enlarged to 2.2 to 2.5 mm depending on the caliber of the tendon graft, using cannulated drill bits and appropriate drill sleeves on both dorsal and volar sides to avoid iatrogenic injury to adjacent structures.

Step 4: ulnar tunnel preparation

With the wrist placed in a neutral position on the traction tower, a 3-cm longitudinal incision was made over the subcutaneous border of ulna starting 1 cm proximal to the tip of ulnar styloid (see **Fig. 2**C). The dorsal cutaneous branch of ulnar nerve should be identified and protected. After subperiosteal dissection, a 1.1-mm guide pin is inserted to the midpoint of the distal ulna at the level of 1.5 to 2.0 cm proximal to the tip of ulnar styloid at an acute angle targeting at the fovea of the ulnar head (see **Fig. 3**C). This can be facilitated by using the thumb to locate the position of the fovea at the base of the ulnar styloid to gauge position. The pin should be placed parallel to the shaft of the ulna. The intra-articular exit site of the guide pin is monitored under arthroscopy to ensure its central position at the fovea at the isometric point of insertion of the TFCC (**Fig. 5**). The ulnar bone tunnel is created with cannulated drills. Stepwise drilling to 2.9 mm or 3.2 mm under arthroscopic control is required because 2 limbs of the tendon graft will pass through this ulnar tunnel. The tip of the guide pin is held within the joint with a hemostat passing through the 4/5 portal to avoid iatrogenic damage of the articular cartilage of lunate and triquetrum by the drill bits.

Step 5: passing of the volar limb of tendon graft into joint and exteriorization through ulnar tunnel

After creation of the 2 bone tunnels, a 2-mm arthroscopic grasper is inserted into the radial bone tunnel from the dorsal to volar side. Once again, the volar structures are gently retracted to reveal the exit site of the grasper, ensuring no tendon or nerve entrapment by the graft during its passage. The PL tendon graft is grasped and passed through the tunnel from the volar to dorsal end (see **Fig. 3**D). The trocar of a 2.7-mm scope is introduced from the 4/5 portal and exits through the volar capsule at the interval between the ulnolunate ligament and short radiolunate ligament to create a volar capsular window (**Fig. 6**). The trocar is replaced by a 2-mm arthroscopic grasper introduced from the 4/5 portal to retrieve the volar limb of the PL graft into the joint through the interligament interval (see **Fig. 3**E; **Fig. 7**). Another grasper is introduced through the ulnar tunnel exiting the fovea and delivers the volar limb of the graft through this tunnel to the exterior (see **Fig. 3**F).

Step 6: passing of the dorsal limb of tendon graft into joint and exteriorization through ulnar tunnel

The tendon is first tied with a strong suture at its end. The graft with the suture on is then grasped and pushed into the joint through the 4/5 portal underneath the extensor tendons. In a similar fashion as passing the volar limb, the tendon end is pulled outside the ulnar tunnel using a grasper inserted

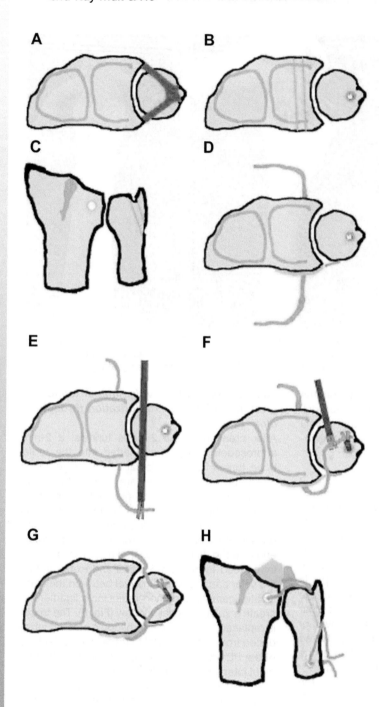

Fig. 3. (*A*) The anatomic reconstruction restores the volar and dorsal radioulnar ligaments and their insertion into the fovea. (*B*) A bone tunnel is created in the ulnar aspect of the distal radial metaphysis. (*C*) A second bone tunnel is created in the ulna from 1.5 to 2.0 cm proximal to the ulnar styloid to the center of the fovea, under arthroscopic verification. (*D*) A grasper is introduced into the radial tunnel and the tendon graft is passed into it from volar to dorsal. (*E*) A grasper is introduced from the 4/5 portal through a capsular window between the short radiolunate and ulnolunate ligaments. (*F*) The volar limb of the tendon graft is retrieved into the joint and passed into the ulnar tunnel to the exterior by a second grasper. (*G*) The dorsal limb is pushed into the joint through the 4/5 portal and passed into the ulnar tunnel. (*H*) A third transverse bone tunnel is made 1 cm proximal to the oblique tunnel in the ulna, and one limb of the graft is passed through it and tied to the other limb in a shoelace manner.

from the ulnar tunnel (see **Fig. 3**G; **Fig. 8**). The 2 limbs of tendon graft are secured with a hemostat.

Step 7: tensioning and tying around ulnar neck
At this junction, manual tightening of both limbs of the graft should result in a stable DRUJ upon ballottement. Another transverse bone tunnel is made approximately 1 cm proximal to the oblique tunnel at the distal ulna using a 2.5-mm drill bit. One of

the graft limbs is then inserted through the transverse tunnel in a figure-of-8 fashion (see **Fig. 3**H; **Fig. 9**). The graft is then tied to the other limb of the graft in a shoelace fashion, being maximally tightened with the forearm in neutral rotation. Ethibond suture is used to secure the tendon knot as well as to anchor the graft to the surrounding fascial structures. If the isometric point is attained as the graft position in the ulnar head, full range of

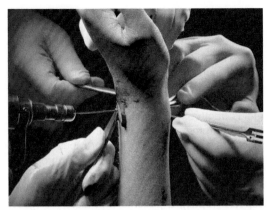

Fig. 4. The radial tunnel is created and enlarged while the volar structures are well protected and the exit site visualized.

passive pronosupination can be obtained without jeopardizing DRUJ stability. The wounds are then closed in layers.

REHABILITATION

The forearm is immobilized in a long arm cast with the forearm in neutral rotation for 3 weeks. This is changed to a removable above-elbow splint with elbow hinge to allow elbow flexion and extension for 3 weeks. Alternatively, a reversed sugar-tong splint with the forearm in neutral position serves a similar function without jeopardizing elbow motion. The patient is advised to perform active and passive rotational motion of forearm in its mid-range out of the splint under supervision by

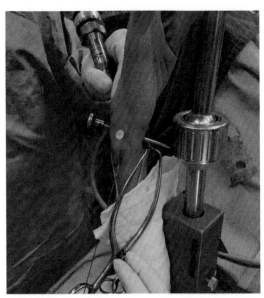

Fig. 6. A volar capsular window between the short radiolunate and ulnolunate ligaments is created by a trocar inserted from the 4/5 portal.

physiotherapist. By the seventh week after operation, free flexion-extension and pronosupination active exercise for the wrist is started. A below-elbow wrist splint is worn at rest for 3 more weeks and then worn only at night for another 3 weeks.

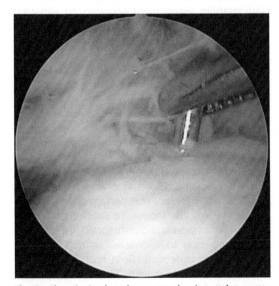

Fig. 5. The pin in the ulnar tunnel exits at the center of the fovea under direct arthroscopic view.

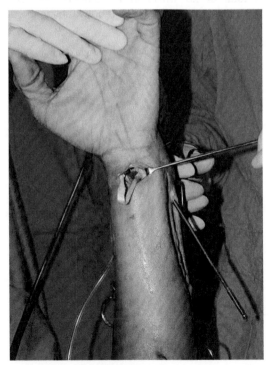

Fig. 7. The volar limb of the tendon graft is being passed into the joint by a grasper.

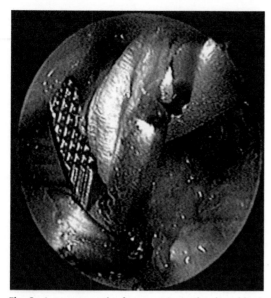

Fig. 8. A grasper at the fovea retrieves the dorsal limb of the tendon graft.

Passive range of motion exercise can be initiated by 6 to 8 weeks after the operation after restoration of stability of the DRUJ, followed by wrist and grip strengthening exercise.

OUTCOMES AND COMPLICATIONS

A total of 28 wrists in 28 patients received arthroscopic-assisted TFCC reconstruction in our

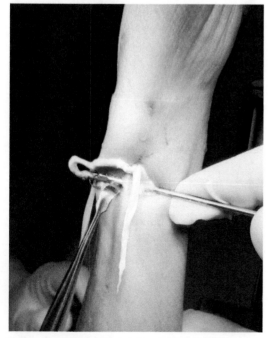

Fig. 9. One limb of the tendon graft is passed into the transverse ulnar bone tunnel.

center between 2000 and 2016 (**Table 1**). There were 15 male and 13 female individuals with an average age of 35 years at operation (ranging from 17 to 58). The average follow-up duration was 62 months (3–138). In all patients, there was a history of injury resulting in persistent ulnar wrist pain and weakness. Cases with previous distal radius fracture, DRUJ arthrosis, and ulna impaction syndrome were excluded. There were 16 recalcitrant patients who failed previous surgeries on their affected wrists (5 had arthroscopic debridement, 1 had open and 9 had arthroscopic TFCC repair, 1 had ulnar styloid fixation with capsular repair), 2 patients with history of gouty arthritis other than the wrist, and 2 patients with rheumatoid arthritis and systemic lupus erythematosus, respectively, at quiescent stage. Workers' compensation was involved in 13 patients.

Postoperatively, mean grip power increased from 58.6% to 71.6% of the contralateral nonaffected hand at the final assessment (**Table 2**). Compared with the preoperative range of motion, the mean pronosupination range improved from 84.6% of the normal side to 91.2% at the final postoperative assessment, and flexion-extension range improved from 77.1% to 83.71% (**Fig. 10**). The mean Mayo wrist score was 58 preoperatively and was 79 at the final assessment, with a 36% increase. The scores were excellent or good in 19 patients. The mean visual analog pain score decreased from 5.9 ± 1.5 preoperatively to 3.0 ± 2.5 postoperatively. In the 5 patients who were not able to return to their previous vocations, 4 were due to reasons unrelated to the wrist, which were back pain, disabling gouty arthritis, depression, and stroke with hemiplegia, respectively. Radiographic assessment revealed no widening of DRUJ or osteoarthritic changes on latest follow-up. There were consistently sclerotic changes at the radial and ulnar tunnels. Bony erosion over distal ulna was noted in one patient, likely related to the friction with the tendon knot. Tunnel sizes were static.

No fracture, or tendon injury occurred intraoperatively. There was one case of breakage of Kirschner-wire, which was removed from the joint. Ulnar nerve entrapment by the tendon graft occurred in one case, resulting in transient partial ulnar nerve palsy. Revision of the tendon graft and ulnar nerve release was performed, and the ulnar nerve palsy fully recovered subsequently. Two other patients developed neurapraxia of the ulnar nerve likely due to excessive retraction of the nerves during operation. Both had complete recovery within a few weeks. Three patients complained of discomfort over ulnar incision due to the graft knot or sensitive scar. No paraesthesia

Table 1
Demographics of patients who received arthroscopic-assisted TFCC reconstruction in our center between 2000 and 2016

Patient No.	Sex	Age	Injury side D: Dominant	Symptom Duration, mo	Previous Surgery	Arthroscopic Findings	Outcome	Complications
1	F	47	L	11	Arthroscopic TFCC repair	Massive dorsal tear	Unemployed	Nil
2	F	23	L (D)	22	Arthroscopic debridement	TFCC radial tear	RTW	Nil
3	M	42	L	17	Arthroscopic TFCC repair	TFCC volar central tear	RTW	Nil
4	M	34	L (D)	9	Ulna styloid fixation + soft tissue reconstruction	Ulna styloid nonunion	RTW	Nil
5	M	28	R (D)	21	Arthroscopic TFCC repair	Massive central tear	RTW	Nil
6	M	49	R (D)	24	Arthroscopic debridement	Massive tear with urate crystal, SNAC 2	Unemployed	Nil
7	M	23	L	12	No	Large fovea tear	RTW	Nil
8	M	17	R (D)	13	No	Massive dorsal tear	RTW	Nil
9	F	45	L	10	No	Massive central tear, villonodular synovitis	RTW	Nil
10	F	20	R (D)	8	No	Large fovea tear	RTW	Nil
11	F	22	R (D)	28	Arthroscopic debridement	Large fovea tear	RTW	Nil
12	F	41	L	23	Open TFCC repair	Massive central tear	RTW	Nil
13	M	28	R (D)	18	Arthroscopic TFCC repair	Large fovea tear	Unemployed	Dystonia
14	F	45	L	4	No	Radial tear	RTW	Graft rupture at 18 mo
15	F	36	L	14	No	Massive dorsal tear	RTW	Graft rupture at 14 mo
16	M	20	R (D)	132	No	Complete foveal tear, dorsal TFCC synovitis and scar	RTW	Nil
17	F	22	R (D)	28	Arthroscopic synovectomy	Complete foveal tear	RTW	Nil

(continued on next page)

Table 1
(continued)

Patient No.	Sex	Age	Injury side D: Dominant	Symptom Duration, mo	Previous Surgery	Arthroscopic Findings	Outcome	Complications
18	F	41	L	23	Arthroscopic foveal repair	Complete foveal tear	RTW	Graft rupture at 8 mo
19	F	52	R (D)	20	Diagnostic arthroscopy	Massive central to dorsal tear	RTW	Nil
20	M	20	R (D)	60	No	Central and complete foveal tear	RTW	Nil
21	M	32	R (D)	61	Arthroscopy and triquetral-hamate ligament thermal shrinkage for midcarpal instability, arthroscopic TFCC	Massive central to dorsal tear	RTW	Ulnar nerve entrapment by graft, neurolysis performed at 2 wk
22	M	19	R	7	Arthroscopic foveal repair	Complete foveal tear	RTW	Graft loosening at 4 wk (external to bone tunnel)
23	M	58	R (D)	38	Arthroscopic debridement of TFCC central tear and ulnar shortening osteotomy	Healed central tear with lax TFCC	RTW	Nil
24	F	48	L	19	Arthroscopic debridement of TFCC central tear	Massive central tear with dorsal fibrosis	Unemployed	Graft rupture at 12 mo
25	M	48	L	30	Arthroscopic foveal repair	Complete foveal tear	Unemployed	Nil
26	M	31	R (D)	27	Arthroscopic foveal repair	Complete foveal tear	RTW	Nil
27	F	36	L	156	No	Complete foveal tear	Housewife	Nil
28	M	51	R (D)	21	Diagnostic arthroscopy	Complete foveal tear, massive central tear	RTW	Nil

Abbreviations: RTW, return to work; TFCC, triangular fibrocartilage complex.

Table 2
Outcomes of patients who received arthroscopic-assisted TFCC reconstruction in our center between 2000 and 2016

	Preoperation		Latest Follow-up	
	Average and SD	Range	Average and SD	Range
Pronation	67.9 ± 22	6–94	76.3 ± 9.7	55–90
Supination	74.5 ± 25.8	0–95	81.5 ± 17.8	40–115
Pronation, %	82.8 ± 26.4	10–124	92.3 ± 12	68.7–114.3
Supination, %	85.1 ± 27.1	0–105	95.1 ± 34.6	40–242.8
Pronation + supination, %	84.7 ± 21.8	10–114	91.1 ± 16	52.7–126
Extension + flexion, %	77.1 ± 25.4	7–126.3	83.7 ± 28	42–131.6
Radial + ulnar deviation, %	71.4 ± 25.2	18–132.5	83.5 ± 21.9	50–119
Grip strength, %	58.6 ± 29.1	6.6–114	71.6 ± 26.2	16.7–106
Mayo wrist score	57.6 ± 15	15–90	79.3 ± 13.1	25–100
VAS pain score	5.9 ± 1.5	2–9	3 ± 2.5	0–7

Abbreviations: TFCC, triangular fibrocartilage complex; VAS, visual analog scale.

was noted over the territory of dorsal cutaneous branch of ulnar nerve.

There were 4 cases of graft rupture that presented at 10, 12, 14, and 18 months. Two of these occurred after new injuries of their wrists after the operation, and 2 occurred without reinjury. Arthroscopic debridement of the torn tendon graft edges was performed. Revision surgery with tendon grafting was performed for 2 cases. One patient fully recovered, but the second patient continued to be symptomatic. In one patient, loosening of

the graft external to the ulnar bone tunnel occurred at 4 weeks postoperatively and revision with graft retightening was performed. Subsequent recovery was smooth and he became a league handball player.

Adams and Berger[29] reported their outcome of open TFCC reconstruction in 2002. Pain relief was achieved in 12 of 14 patients and there were 2 recurrences. The postoperative grip strength reached 85% of the opposite hand and the range of pronation and supination was 90% and 87%

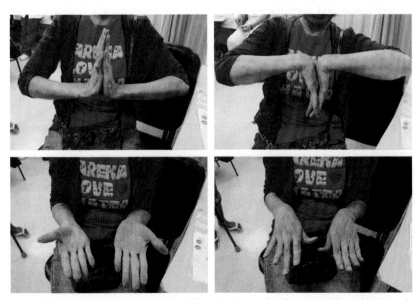

Fig. 10. A patient with TFCC reconstruction on the right side 7 months after operation, showing almost full range of motion.

compared with the preoperative range. Our results with a less invasive technique were at least comparable with the established open reconstruction, with a possible advantage in restoring range of motion. In our series, the range of pronation was 112% and supination was 109% compared with the preoperative values in our series. This could be attributed to the less invasive nature of the technique obviating the need for creation of a dorsal DRUJ capsular flap. As a result, motion is started earlier in our rehabilitation protocol at the fourth week, whereas in the series of Adams and Berger,[29] a long-arm cast was kept for 6 weeks. An extensive capsulotomy could also result in fibrosis and scarring with reduced range of motion.

SUMMARY

Reconstruction of the TFCC with autologous tendon graft is indicated in irreparable TFCC tears to restore DRUJ stability. The current recommended standard is anatomic reconstruction of the distal radioulnar ligaments to their foveal insertion by the method described by Adams and Berger.[29] Based on this reconstruction design, an arthroscopic-assisted technique is a less invasive alternative that offers several advantages. Arthroscopy offers a clear visualization of the TFCC tear and assessment of reparability. Under a direct and magnified view, one can ensure the creation of bone tunnel and placement of graft at the isometric foveal insertion point. Our results show that arthroscopic anatomic TFCC reconstruction is a safe and effective option with results comparable to the conventional open technique, and may achieve better range of motion through preservation of soft tissue and capsular integrity and accelerated rehabilitation.

REFERENCES

1. Nakamura T, Yabe Y, Horiuchi Y, et al. In vivo motion analysis of forearm rotation utilizing magnetic resonance imaging. Clin Biomech (Bristol, Avon) 1999; 14:315–20.
2. Palmer AK, Werner FW. The triangular fibrocartilage complex of the wrist— anatomy and function. J Hand Surg 1981;6:153.
3. Moritomo H. The distal interosseous membrane: current concepts in wrist anatomy and biomechanics. J Hand Surg 2012;37(7):1501–7.
4. Ishii S, Palmer AK, Werner FW, et al. An anatomic study of the ligamentous structure of the triangular fibrocartilage complex. J Hand Surg 1998;23(6): 977–85.
5. Ekenstam FA, Hagert CG. Anatomical studies on the geometry and stability of the distal radio ulnar joint. Scand J Plast Reconstr Surg 1985;19(1):17–25.
6. Schuind F, An KN, Berglund L, et al. The distal radioulnar ligaments: a biomechanical study. J Hand Surg 1991;16(6):1106–14.
7. Ward LD, Ambrose CG, Masson MV, et al. The role of the distal radioulnar ligaments, interosseous membrane, and joint capsule in distal radioulnar joint stability. J Hand Surg 2000;25(2): 341–51.
8. Xu J, Tang JB. In vivo changes in lengths of the ligaments stabilizing the distal radioulnar joint. J Hand Surg 2009;34(1):40–5.
9. Adams BD. Partial excision of the triangular fibrocartilage complex articular disk: a biomechanical study. J Hand Surg 1993;18(2):334–40.
10. Haugstvedt JR, Berger RA, Nakamura T, et al. Relative contributions of the ulnar attachments of the triangular fibrocartilage complex to the dynamic stability of the distal radioulnar joint. J Hand Surg 2006; 31(3):445–51.
11. Nakamura T, Yabe Y. Histological anatomy of the triangular fibrocartilage complex of the human wrist. Ann Anat 2000;182(6):567–72.
12. Thiru-Pathi R, Ferlic DC, Clayton ML. Arterial anatomy of the triangular fibrocartilage of the wrist and its surgical significance. J Hand Surg (Am) 1986; 11:258–63.
13. Bednar MS, Arnoczky SP, Weiland AJ. The microvasculature of the triangular fibrocartilage complex: its clinical significance. J Hand Surg (Am) 1991;16: 1101–5.
14. Pidgeon TS, Waryasz G, Carnevale J, et al. Triangular fibrocartilage complex. JBJS Rev 2015; 3(1):e1.
15. Sachar K. Ulnar-sided wrist pain: evaluation and treatment of triangular fibrocartilage complex tears, ulnocarpal impaction syndrome, and lunotriquetral ligament tears. J Hand Surg 2008;33(9): 1669–79.
16. Chan JJ, Teunis T, Ring D. Prevalence of triangular fibrocartilage complex abnormalities regardless of symptoms rise with age: systematic review and pooled analysis. Clin Orthop Relat Res 2014; 472(12):3987–94.
17. Lindau T, Arner M, Hagberg L. Intraarticular lesions in distal fractures of the radius in young adults. A descriptive arthroscopic study in 50 patients. J Hand Surg Br 1997;22(5):638–43.
18. Palmer AK. Triangular fibrocartilage complex lesions: a classification. J Hand Surg Am 1989;14: 594–606.
19. Coleman HM. Injuries of the articular disc at the wrist. J Bone Joint Surg Br 1960;42:552–9.
20. Palmer AK, Glisson RR, Werner FW. Ulnar variance determination. J Hand Surg (Am) 1982;7: 376–9.
21. Moritomo H, Masatomi T, Murase T, et al. Open repair of foveal avulsion of the triangular

fibrocartilage complex and comparison by types of injury mechanism. J Hand Surg 2010;35A:1955–63.

22. Tay SC, Tomita K, Berger RA. The "ulnar fovea sign" for defining ulnar wrist pain: an analysis of sensitivity and specificity. J Hand Surg Am 2007; 32:438–44.

23. Morrissey RT, Nalebuff EA. Dislocation of the distal radioulnar joint: anatomy and clues to prompt diagnosis. Clin Orthop 1979;144:154–8.

24. Lee RK, Griffith JF, Ng AW, et al. Wrist traction during MR arthrography improves detection of triangular fibrocartilage complex and intrinsic ligament tears and visibility of articular cartilage. Am J Roentgenol 2016;206(1):155–61.

25. Atzei A, Luchetti R, Garagnani L. Classification of ulnar triangular fibrocartilage complex tears. A treatment algorithm for Palmer type IB tears. J Hand Surg Eur Vol 2017;42(4):405–14.

26. Fulkerson JP, Watson HK. Congenital anterior subluxation of the distal ulna. A case report. Clin Orthop 1978;131:179–82.

27. Breen TF, Jupiter J. Tenodesis of the chronically unstable distal ulna. Hand Clin 1991;7(2):355–63.

28. Tsai TM, Stilwell JH. Repair of chronic subluxation of the distal radioulnar joint (ulnar dorsal) using flexor carpi ulnaris tendon. J Hand Surg Br 1984;9(3):289–94.

29. Adams BD, Berger RA. An anatomic reconstruction of the distal radioulnar ligaments for posttraumatic distal radioulnar joint instability. J Hand Surg Am 2002;27(2):243–51.

30. Scheker LR, Belliappa PP, Acosta R, et al. Reconstruction of the dorsal ligament of the triangular fibrocartilage complex. J Hand Surg Br 1994;19(3): 310–8.

31. Shih JT, Lee HM. Functional results post-triangular fibrocartilage complex reconstruction with extensor carpi ulnaris with or without ulnar shortening in chronic distal radioulnar joint instability. Hand Surg 2005;10:169–76.

32. Teoh LC, Yam AK. Anatomic reconstruction of the distal radioulnar ligaments: long-term results. J Hand Surg Br 2005;30:185–93.

33. Tse WL, Lau SW, Wong WY, et al. Arthroscopic reconstruction of triangular fibrocartilage complex (TFCC) with tendon graft for chronic DRUJ instability. Injury 2013;44(3):386–90.

Arthroscopic Management of Ulnocarpal Impaction Syndrome and Ulnar Styloid Impaction Syndrome

David J. Slutsky, MD[a,b],*

KEYWORDS

- Ulnar impaction • Wrist arthroscopy • Ulnar styloid • Management

KEY POINTS

- Ulnocarpal impaction syndrome consists of the triad of a triangular fibrocartilage complex (TFCC) tear, a lunotriquetral ligament tear, and an ulnar positive variance. There is often chondromalacia of the proximal ulnar aspect of the lunate and chondromalacia of the ulnar head.
- Wrist arthroscopy and an ulnar shortening procedure is indicated in the patient with a neutral to positive ulnar variance and persistent ulnar-sided wrist pain despite conservative treatment, aiming to unload the ulnocarpal joint.
- Ulnar styloid impaction syndrome is characterized by the impaction of the triquetrum against the ulnar styloid, causing chondromalacia, synovitis, and ulnar-sided wrist pain. In the presence of a long styloid, an excision of the ulnar styloid suffices. When it is the result of a combination of factors, surgical treatment varies and a simple excision of the ulnar styloid is no longer the only procedure necessary.
- Symptomatic nonunions of the ulnar styloid are uncommon and may occur in isolation or be associated with a TFCC tear. If the deep foveal ligaments are intact, a simple excision will suffice. If there is distal radioulnar joint instability or a TFCC tear, an arthroscopic or open TFCC repair may be necessary.

ULNOCARPAL IMPACTION SYNDROME
Relevant Anatomy and Biomechanics

Ulnar impaction can produce ulnar-sided wrist pain and can be related to ulnocarpal impaction (UCI) due to an ulnar positive variance (**Fig. 1**). Palmer and colleagues[1] demonstrated that there was an inverse relationship between the thickness of the triangular fibrocartilage and the ulnar variance. The more positive the ulnar variance, the thinner the triangular fibrocartilage. Hara and colleagues[2] found that the force-transmission ratio was 50% through the scaphoid fossa, 35% through the lunate fossa, and 15% through the triangular fibrocartilage in the neutral position. Werner and colleagues[3] demonstrated that lengthening the ulna by 2.5 mm increased the force borne by the ulna from 18.4% to 41.9% of the total axial load. Shortening of the ulna by 2.5 mm decreased the axial load borne by the ulna to 4.3%. Removal of the articular disc portion of the triangular fibrocartilage complex (TFCC) decreased the load on the intact ulna from 18.4% to 6.2%. The peak pressure at the ulnolunate articulation increased from

The author has no conflicts or disclosures.

[a] Department of Orthopedics, Harbor UCLA Medical Center, Torrance, CA 90503, USA; [b] The Hand and Wrist Institute, 2808 Columbia Street, Torrance, CA 90503, USA

* The Hand and Wrist Institute, 2808 Columbia Street, Torrance, CA 90503.

E-mail address: d-slutsky@msn.com

Hand Clin 33 (2017) 639–650
http://dx.doi.org/10.1016/j.hcl.2017.07.002

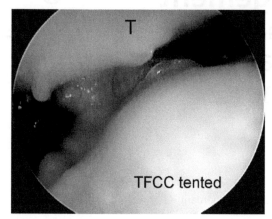

Fig. 1. Arthroscopic view of tenting up of the triangular fibrocartilage complex (TFCC) in a patient with an ulnar positive variance. T, triquetrum. (© 2017 David J. Slutsky)

1.4 N/mm^2 for the unaltered wrist to 3.3 N/mm^2 when the ulna was lengthened by 2.5 mm.

Degenerative central tears of the articular disk occur more frequently with advancing age. In a cadaver study of 180 wrist joints, Mikic[4] noted an incidence of 53% in those older than age 60 years compared with 7% in the third decade. Clinical experience has shown, however, that not all of these tears are symptomatic. Most symptomatic degenerative tears of the TFCC are related to chronic overloading of the ulnocarpal joint. Primary ulnar impaction is related to an increased ulnar variance. Viegas and Ballantyne[5] dissected 100 cadaver wrists and found a 73% incidence of TFCC tears in specimens with an ulnar positive variance versus 17% when there was a negative ulnar variance. Acquired ulna positive deformities can occur with distal radius fractures that heal with radial shortening, distal radial growth arrest, and Essex-Lopresti and Galeazzi fractures. This can also occur following a radial head excision; with congenital causes of ulnar positive variance, such as Madelung deformity or a premature closure of the distal radius growth plate; and following a wrist fusion. Ulnar impaction may also be dynamic and even occur in patients with an ulna neutral or negative variance during power grip in the pronated position.[6] This is because of the approximate 1.95 cm of radial shortening that occurs as the radius rotates across the ulna during pronation, which leads to a dynamic impingement.[7] UCI syndrome consists of the triad of a TFCC tear, a lunotriquetral (LT) ligament tear, and an ulnar positive variance. There is often chondromalacia of the proximal ulnar aspect of the lunate, a so-called kissing lesion, and there may be chondromalacia of the ulnar head (**Fig. 2**).

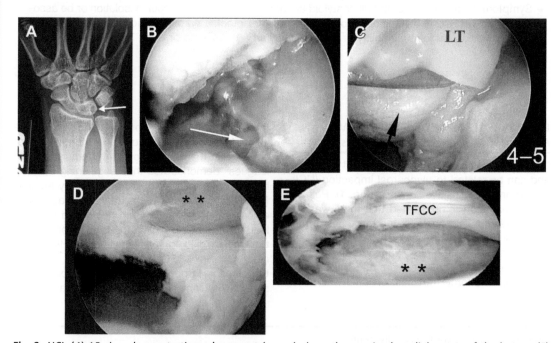

Fig. 2. UCI. (*A*) AP view demonstrating a bone cyst (*arrow*) along the proximal medial aspect of the lunate. (*B*) View from the 4 to 5 portal of a central TFCC tear with exposure of the ulnar head (*arrow*). (*C*) Elevator is placed underneath a LT ligament tear. Note the fibrillated cartilage on the proximal lunate (*arrow*). (*D*) View from the 4 to 5 portal of an area of exposed subchondral bone (*asterisks*) with a full-thickness cartilage tear long the proximal aspect of the lunate. (*E*) Debrided TFCC tear exposing an area of chondromalacia (*asterisks*) on the ulnar head. (© 2017 David J. Slutsky)

Classification

In Palmer's classification, degenerative TFCC tears are subdivided into 5 categories: type IIA, wearing of the TFCC without perforation or chondromalacia; type IIB, wearing of the TFCC with chondromalacia of the lunate or ulna; type IIC, true perforation of the TFCC with lunate chondromalacia; type IID, TFCC perforation plus lunate and/or ulnar chondromalacia and LT interosseous ligament (LTIL) tears without carpal instability; and type IIE, TFCC perforation with an LTIL tear and ulnocarpal arthritis.

Diagnosis

Patients with UCI syndrome present with chronic ulnar-sided wrist pain that may be increased by power grip, ulnar wrist deviation, and/or forearm rotation. They may complain of intermittent clicking localized to the ulnar carpus, as well as swelling after activity, decreased strength, and a loss of wrist and forearm motion. There may be tenderness over the fovea and possibly the triquetrum and ulnar head. Passive and active ulnar deviation produces pain. The ulnocarpal stress test is performed by applying axial stress to a maximally ulnar-deviated wrist during pronation and supination. Ulnar styloid triquetral impingement (USTI) occurs in supination and may be confused with UCI (see later discussion). Extensor carpi ulnaris (ECU) tendonitis may mimic USTI or UCI. The ECU synergy test was found to be highly specific, exploiting an isometric contraction of the ECU during resisted radial abduction of the thumb with the wrist in neutral position and the forearm supinated. Re-creation of pain along the dorsal ulnar aspect of the wrist is considered to be a positive test. Diagnostic local anesthetic injections may also help identify the pain generator.

Standard wrist radiographs are obtained to assess for arthritis involving the carpus and distal radioulnar joint (DRUJ) and to measure the ulnar variance. When evaluating ulnar-sided wrist pathologic states, a zero rotation posteroanterior (PA) view is essential. This is performed with the shoulder abducted 90°, the elbow flexed 90°, and the wrist in neutral. Because ulnar variance is dynamic, stress PA views can help. A pronated grip view[6] may reproduce a dynamic increase[6] in the ulnar variance. Osteoarthritis changes, such as joint space narrowing, sclerosis, and cystic changes or osteophytes can be seen along the ulnocarpal joint.

MRI is helpful to diagnose UCI syndrome.[8] Degenerative tears of the TFCC may be seen, as well as focal cartilage defects. MRI with intravenous contrast is better for visualizing bone marrow pathologic states. Marrow edema typically affects the ulnar aspect of the lunate, with or without involvement of the radial aspect of the triquetrum and ulnar head. Subchondral cystic changes appear as low-signal intensity on T1-weighted images and high-signal intensity on T2-weighted images (**Fig. 3**).[9] If sclerosis is present, low-signal intensity on both T1-weighted and T2-weighted images will be seen. A measurement of the ulnar variance using MRI is, however, not accurate because it is difficult to obtain a true anatomic position in the magnet gantry. Magnetic resonance arthrography can be performed by injecting gadolinium in the DRUJ to detect TFCC tears. A dedicated 23 mm wrist coil and 3 T magnet can improve the accuracy. One study found that the presence of MRI signs of UCI is a predictor of a good outcome following an arthroscopic wafer resection.[10]

ARTHROSCOPIC WAFER RESECTION

Wnorowski and colleagues[11] examined the biomechanical effects of an arthroscopic wafer resection in 9 ulnar positive cadaver forearms. Each specimen was evaluated biomechanically using axial load cells and pressure-sensitive film to evaluate the effect of serial resection of the TFCC and distal ulna on axial load and ulnar carpal pressures. There was a statistically significant unloading of the ulnar aspect of the wrist after excision of the centrum of the TFCC and resection of the radial two-thirds width of the ulnar head, to a depth of subchondral bone resection.

Indications

Wrist arthroscopy and an ulnar shortening procedure is indicated in the patient with a neutral to

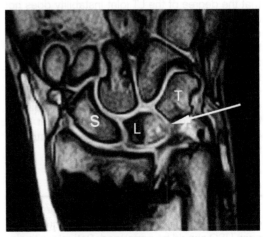

Fig. 3. T2-weighted MRI showing an area of increased signal intensity of the proximal medial pole of the lunate (*arrow*). L, lunate; S, scaphoid; T, triquetrum. (© 2017 David J. Slutsky)

positive ulnar variance and persistent ulnar-sided wrist pain despite conservative treatment with splints, nonsteroidal anti-inflammatory drugs (NSAIDs) with or without selected cortisone injections. The aim is to unload the ulnocarpal joint either through an ulnar shortening osteotomy (USO) or wafer resection of the ulnar head. In a biomechanical study, excision of 3 mm of subchondral bone decreased the force transmitted across the ulnar head by 50%; further bone resection did little to decrease this force.[11] The goal is to resect sufficient ulna to produce a 2 mm negative ulnar variance. An arthroscopically assisted ulnar shortening has the advantage of being less invasive and is not associated with complications such as nonunion or the need for subsequent plate removal.

Symptomatic incomplete TFCC tears (Palmer type IIA, IIB) are treated with debridement. The role of an ulnar shortening procedure in this group is unsettled. Osterman and Seidman[12] have recommended an ulnar shortening procedure in these patients. Tomaino and Elfar,[13] on the other hand, have reported good results by creating a central defect in the intact articular disc and then proceeding with an arthroscopic wafer resection. A wafer resection through the DRUJ portals is another option. Patients with a complete TFCC tear (Palmer type IIC, IID) and a dynamic or static ulnar positive variance are treated with arthroscopic debridement and an ulnar shortening procedure. Any associated LTIL tears are debrided if the LT joint is stable. If the LT joint is unstable, it can be pinned for 6 to 8 weeks. Some investigators recommend USO because this has been shown to tighten the ulnocarpal ligaments in a cadaver model,[14] which may stabilize the LT joint. Iwatsuki and colleagues,[15] however, showed that the degree of the LT joint instability does not appear to affect the clinical outcomes. In a study on USO, a second-look arthroscopy was performed in 25 subjects with an LTIL tear (group A) and compared with 25 subjects without a tear (group B). In group B, 11 wrists improved based on the Geissler grade, 9 wrists showed no changes, and 2 wrists became worse. Clinically, the subjects demonstrated improvement after USO regardless of the degree of degenerative LT ligament changes.

Contraindications

The limit for an arthroscopic wafer is 4 mm.[16] If greater than 4 mm of shortening is required, an open USO should be performed. Patients with significant ulnocarpal and/or DRUJ osteoarthritis (Palmer type IIE) are better suited for an excisional arthroplasty or ulnar head implant. DRUJ instability must be treated before an arthroscopic ulnar shortening procedure because this does not address any LT or ulnocarpal ligament instability.

Surgical technique: arthroscopic wafer resection

After an initial arthroscopic radiocarpal and midcarpal survey, the scope is placed in the 4 to 5 portal. The 6R and 6U portals are used for instrumentation, although it is useful to assess the completeness of ulnar head resection with the scope in the 6U portal. The 6U portal may also be used for viewing while the burr is placed in the 4 to 5 or 6R dorsal portals because this increases the space for triangulation of the instruments. Rapid irrigation is needed to clear the debris. The edges of the TFCC tear are debrided back to stable margins. A 2.9 mm burr is then used in a back-and-forth motion to resect 2 to 3 mm of the ulnar head (**Fig. 4**). The diameter of the burr can be used as a gauge of the amount of bony resection, but this should also be checked fluoroscopically. The forearm must be pronated and supinated to avoid leaving a shelf of bone. Care must be taken to avoid injury to the deep foveal insertion of the TFCC, as well as the sigmoid notch. The LTIL is evaluated from the 6R portal and any tears are debrided. Midcarpal arthroscopy is used to assess the degree of LT joint instability. A Geissler grade III instability can be treated with LT joint pinning for 6 weeks, although this approach has been recently challenged.[15] Any small areas of chondromalacia on the proximal lunate or triquetrum are observed. If there is a full-thickness cartilage defect of 1 cm or more; however, microfracture with a 0.045 mm K-wire can be performed in an attempt to stimulate fibrocartilage formation.

A wafer resection can also be performed through the DRUJ portals[17] when the TFCC is still intact (Palmer IIA, IIB). When performed with a TFCC tear (Palmer IIC), this allows for a more conservative TFCC debridement because the ulnar head resection is performed underneath the TFCC tear and not through it. The DRUJ wafer resection also facilitates preservation of the volar and dorsal radioulnar ligaments, as well as the foveal attachment of the deep radioulnar ligament. Postoperatively, the patient is placed in a below-elbow splint for 4 weeks and started on protected range of motion, including pronation and supination.

Alternative procedures: arthroscopic distal metaphyseal ulnar shortening osteotomy Yin and colleagues[18] published a technique for an arthroscopic distal metaphyseal USO for ulnar impaction. This is based on the open technique

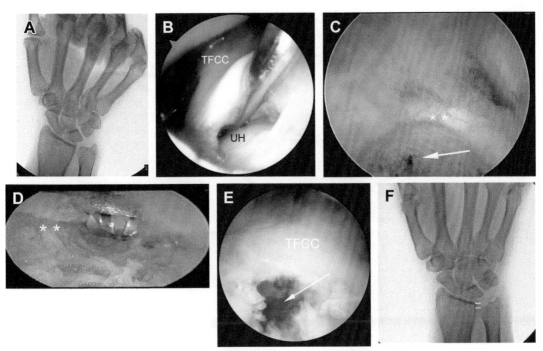

Fig. 4. (*A*) AP view of a patient with UCI and an ulnar positive variance. (*B*) View from the 4 to 5 portal of a central TFCC tear with exposure of the ulnar head (UH). (*C*) After a partial ulnar head resection, demonstrating exposed bleeding subchondral bone (*arrow*) and a rim of articular cartilage (*asterisks*). (*D*) View from the volar DRUJ portal with the burr removing a shelf of bone (*asterisks*) from the medial aspect of the ulnar head. (*E*) The TFCC tear is decompressed following the wafer resection (*arrow*). (*F*) AP radiograph view demonstrating an ulnar minus variance. (© 2017 David J. Slutsky)

for an osteochondral shortening osteotomy of the distal ulna as described by Slade and Gillon.[19] A triangle ABC is drawn on the dorsal skin over the ulnar head, which depicts the osteotomy (**Fig. 5**). Line AB is 3 mm proximal to the ulnar dome. Point A is just 1 mm from the ulnar cortex. The arrow (see **Fig. 5A**) indicates the amount to be shortened, which can be calculated by the angle CAB. Generally, if the angle is 15°, the amount will be about 4 mm. Three K-wires are inserted percutaneously into the ulna according to the triangle that marks the borders of the osteotomy under fluoroscopic control. The arthroscope is then placed in the proximal DRUJ portal and the K-wires are identified. A 1.9-mm motorized burr inserted via the distal DRUJ portal is used to remove the bone between the 2 K-wires while keeping the ulnar part of the cortex intact. The 3 K-wires are removed and the greenstick osteotomy is then closed by pressing on the dome of the ulnar head with a mosquito forceps in the distal DRUJ portal. A 1.2-mm screw introducer wire is drilled via the DRUJ distal portal, which is proximal to the TFCC, to fix the dome directed at a palmar and proximal direction. Therefore, the TFCC is not perforated. A cannulated headless compression screw is used to maintain compression. The distal aspect of the screw engages but does not perforate the ulnar cortex. An above-elbow cast is applied for 4 weeks followed by mobilization.

Outcomes

Meftah and colleagues[10] reviewed 26 subjects (mean age of 38.5) with arthroscopic wafer resection done from 1998 to 2005 who failed nonoperative treatments. The subjects' age, history of previous wrist fracture, presence of MRI signs, and ulnar variance were recorded as variables. Of these, 22 subjects (84.6%) had either good or excellent pain relief (median 4, range 1–4). Significant correlation was found between MRI signs of UCI and postoperative pain relief. History of previous distal radius fractures was negatively correlated with pain relief. No correlation was found between postoperative strength and any of the variables.

The debate about whether to perform an arthroscopic wafer versus an open USO rages on. In a study by Bernstein and colleagues[20] on UCI syndrome, subjects treated with arthroscopic TFCC debridement and wafer resections were compared with 16 subjects who were treated with

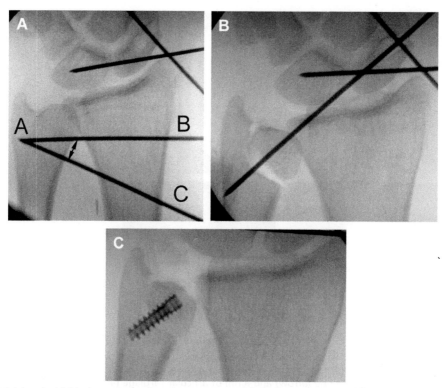

Fig. 5. (*A*) A triangle ABC is drawn to outline the osteotomy. (*B*) The bone is removed from between lines A and B and the osteotomy is closed. (*C*) The osteotomy site is held with a headless cannulated screw. Note the negative ulnar variance. (© 2017 David J. Slutsky)

arthroscopic TFCC debridement and an open USO. At mean follow-up times of 21 and 15 months, respectively, 9 out of 11 subjects showed good to excellent results after arthroscopic treatment compared with 11 out of 16 following an USO. The investigators concluded that a combined arthroscopic TFCC debridement and wafer procedure provides similar pain relief and restoration of function with fewer secondary procedures when compared with an open shortening. Vandenberghe and colleagues[21] had similar conclusions. They reviewed the outcomes in 28 subjects who underwent a USO compared with 12 subjects who underwent an arthroscopic wafer resection. At a mean follow-up of 29 months (range, 7–60 months) the mean Disability of the Arm, Shoulder, and Hand (DASH) score in the USO group improved from 40 to 26 (SD 18.3; *P*<.01). The Modified Mayo Wrist Score (MMWS) was 11 excellent, 10 good, 6 fair, and 1 poor. The mean visual analog scale (VAS) was 4.4 (SD 1.9). In the wafer group, the mean DASH score was 34 (SD 19.4; *P*<.01); with a MMWS of 4 excellent, 4 good, and 5 fair; and a mean VAS of 4.6 (SD 2.65). Of significance was that 27 secondary procedures were required in 21 subjects in the USO group and there were 3

nonunions. The time off work was 7 months (range, 0.5–30 months) in the USO and 6.1 months (range, 0–26 months) in the wafer group (*P*<.001).

ULNAR STYLOID IMPACTION SYNDROME
Relevant Anatomy and Etiologic Factors

Ulnar styloid impaction (USI) syndrome is characterized by the impaction of the triquetrum against the ulnar styloid, causing chondromalacia, synovitis, and ulnar-sided wrist pain. Anatomically, the tip of the ulnar styloid is covered by the meniscus homologue. When an excessively long ulnar styloid abuts the triquetrum, in the presence of an intact anatomy, the meniscus homologue will be interposed between the tip of the ulnar styloid and the triquetrum. Therefore, in the early stages when the TFCC is intact, a soft tissue impingement rather than bone-to-bone impaction is in effect.[22,23] USI occurs when the TFCC has eroded and exposes the tip of the ulnar styloid, which is in direct contact with the triquetrum. In full pronation, the volar aspect of the triquetrum faces the tip of the ulnar styloid. In the presence of an excessively long ulnar styloid, flexion and ulnar deviation of the wrist can cause impingement of the meniscus homologue between the 2 bones. Such a mechanism of impingement occurs with prolonged typing. In full supination, the dorsal aspect of the triquetrum faces the tip of the ulnar styloid. Flexion and ulnar deviation of the wrist only increases the distance between the triquetrum and the ulnar styloid. Therefore, in the supinated wrist, the impingement can only occur with wrist extension and ulnar deviation.

Biyani and colleagues[24] studied the radiographs of 400 subjects without wrist symptoms and described 5 morphologic variants, the commonest being an elongated process. They defined a standard ulnar styloid process to be 3 to 6 mm in length with a medial angulation not exceeding 15°. Giachino and colleagues[25] reviewed the radiographs of 1000 subjects without bony trauma and found that the ulnar styloid length, measured from the base of the ulnar styloid to the tip, in a line parallel with the long axis of the ulna, ranged from 0.0 to 14.8 mm with a mean of 6.31 mm (SD 1.82 mm). They identified 56 subjects with USI and classified the etiologic factors as follows:

1. Impaction of the triquetrum by a long ulnar styloid occurs with a congenitally long ulnar styloid process, or distal radial growth arrest and Madelung deformity, or styloid overgrowth from a nonunion (**Fig. 6**).
2. Impaction of the triquetrum on a normal ulnar styloid occurs when the carpus moves proximally, as in collapse of the proximal carpal row following a wrist fusion; in Kienböck disease; when the radius moves proximally, as in distal radius malunion with a loss of radial length; the carpus ulnarly translocates; or the hand-wrist-radius complex moves ulnarly as an intact unit, which occurs after full or partial ulnar head excision.
3. Dynamic styloid impaction occurs based on ligamentous laxity, instability, or loading activities such as racquet sports and golf.
4. There is a combination of the above.

Diagnosis

The syndrome occurs in supination because the carpus and radius rotate around the ulnar head, which moves the ulnar styloid radially and, therefore, closer to the triquetrum. The patient with symptomatic USI will typically complain of ulnar-sided wrist pain, aggravated by wrist extension and certain positions, such as having their hands on their hips or in their back pockets, repetitively turning pages, or forcing the lower hand position as in the slap-shot in ice hockey. There may be a history of trauma to the distal radius or ulna, prior wrist surgery to the carpus, or generalized ligamentous laxity.

On examination, there is point tenderness to palpation of the ulnar styloid tip. Typically, pain is increased by direct palpation precisely over the tip of the ulnar styloid. The pain is deep and volar to the ECU tendon. USI may be confused with UCI, which also presents as ulnar-sided pain. UCI is a consequence of ulnar head and lunate impaction. In this latter instance, the pain is ulnar and dorsal, and increased by local palpation over the proximal ulnar aspect of the lunate. The tenderness is not over the ulnar styloid. UCI and USI may both be present. When seen on a lateral radiograph, the carpus is volar to the styloid. Wrist dorsiflexion brings the triquetrum closer to the styloid and can cause impingement. Topper and colleagues[22] described a provocative test that consists of wrist dorsiflexion and pronation, followed by rotation of the forearm into full supination while maintaining dorsiflexion. Radiographic signs suggestive of USI include ulnar styloid sclerosis, growth, flattening, small kissing cysts, and (occasionally) loose bodies. A bone scan may show increased uptake about the styloid process. An MRI can show focal subchondral sclerosis and chondromalacia of the styloid tip and proximal triquetrum.[25]

Treatment

Nonoperative treatment includes NSAIDs, therapy, splinting, and corticosteroid injections. Operative management varies. In the presence of a long styloid, an excision of the ulnar styloid suffices. When USI is the result of a combination of factors and when multiple diagnoses are present, the surgical treatment varies and a simple excision of the ulnar styloid is no longer the only procedure necessary.

Arthroscopic-Assisted Ulnar Styloid Excision Technique

Bain and Bidwell[26] have described an arthroscopic-assisted technique for an ulnar styloid excision in stylocarpal impaction, in which the long ulnar styloid affects the triquetrum. This can also be combined with an arthroscopic wafer resection. With the arthroscope in the 3 to 4 portal, a 22-gauge needle is introduced into the 6U portal. This is then substituted by a 3.5-mm burr. The burr is placed onto the tip of the ulnar styloid, which is confirmed fluoroscopically. The resection is then done percutaneously until sufficient ulnar styloid has been removed to prevent impingement (see **Fig. 6**).

Outcomes

There are no reported series of an arthroscopic-assisted resection of the ulnar styloid. Topper

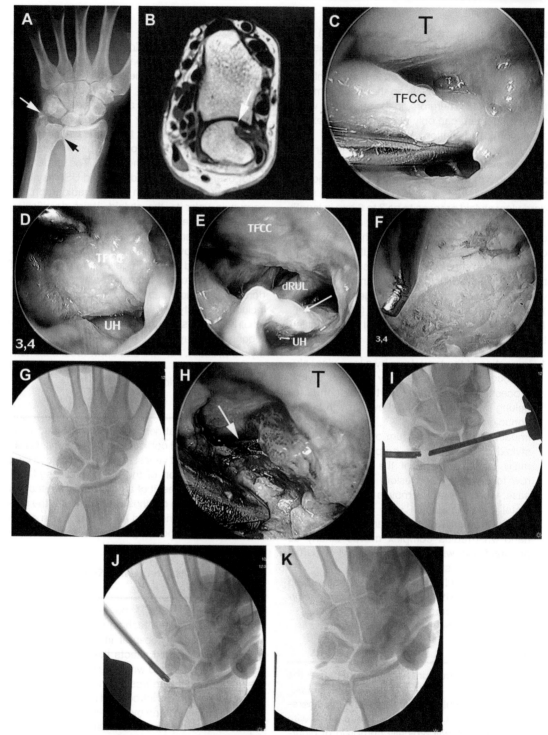

Fig. 6. A 53-year-old man with ulnar styloid impingement. (*A*) Ulnar styloid impingement (*white arrow*) and pre-existing early DRUJ osteoarthritis (*black arrow*) plus a nonunion of the ulnar styloid tip. (*B*) Coronal CT scan shows preservation of the ulnocarpal joint space but a small osteophyte (*arrow*). (*C*) View from the 3 to 4 portal of a long flap tear of the TFCC. T, triquetrum. (*D*) Elevation of the TFCC tear reveals the ulnar head (UH). (*E*) The scope is advanced into the DRUJ to demonstrate an unstable flap of articular cartilage (*arrow*), which is separated off from the ulnar head (UH). The deep radioulnar ligament (dRUL) is still firmly attached. (*F*) A wafer resection of the ulnar head is performed. (*G*) The ulnar styloid is localized with a 22-gauge needle fluoroscopically. (*H*) The needle (*arrow*) is visualized from the 3 to 4 portal as it pierces the ulnar capsule overlying the tip of the ulnar styloid. (*I*) Position of the burr is checked fluoroscopically and arthroscopically. (*J*) Ulnar styloid is resected percutaneously. (*K*) After completion of wafer resection and ulnar styloidectomy. (© 2017 David J. Slutsky)

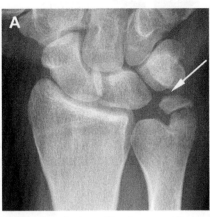
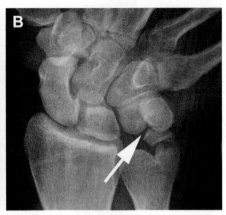

Fig. 7. (*A*) AP Radiograph view of impingement between the triquetrum and a nonunited ulnar styloid fragment (*arrow*). (*B*) Note the impingement with the triquetrum during ulnar deviation (*arrow*). (© 2017 David J. Slutsky)

and colleagues[22] reported good results in 7 out of 8 subjects following an open ulnar styloid excision; the VAS pain score improved from 3.5 to 1.3. Zahiri and colleagues[27] treated 5 subjects with USI due to a long ulnar styloid with an ulnar styloidectomy. All 5 subjects had complete relief of wrist pain by 10 to 16 weeks after surgery. The subjects remained symptom free at a mean follow-up of 36 months.

Ulnar Styloid Nonunions

An ulnar styloid nonunion occasionally results in symptomatic USI (**Fig. 7**).[28] A recent meta-analysis of 6 studies involving 365 subjects that compared the outcomes after distal radius fractures with a united versus a nonunited ulnar styloid process found no relation between the nonunion of the ulnar styloid process and function.[29] Although ulnar styloid fractures are a common feature of the distal radius fracture pattern, symptomatic nonunions of the ulnar styloid are found in a minority of these injuries. They may occur in isolation or be associated with a TFCC tear. In this case, it is uncertain whether the nonunion or the TFCC is the cause of pain. Similarly, it is unknown whether resecting the nonunion or repairing the TFCC or both are responsible for any pain relief. In these cases, it is the author's preference to scope the DRUJ and evaluate the attachment of the deep radioulnar ligament (**Fig. 8**). If the deep foveal ligaments are intact, a simple excision will suffice.

Reeves[30] reviewed 197 subjects with a prior distal radius fracture. He found that 7 of 12 subjects with persistent wrist pain had radiographic evidence of an ulnar styloid nonunion (**Fig. 9**). Four of the 7 subjects had relief of their pain with excision of the ulnar styloid nonunion. Burgess and Watson[31] reported on 9 subjects with chronic

ulnar-sided wrist pain and radiographic evidence of a hypertrophic ulnar styloid nonunion. All of the subjects were treated with a subperiosteal excision of the nonunion fragment. This procedure relieved the localized pain without changing either radiocarpal or DRUJ stability. Hauck and colleagues[28] classified type 1 as a nonunion associated with a stable DRUJ and type 2 as a nonunion with DRUJ subluxation. Protopsaltis and Ruch[32] reported on 8 subjects (6 with a prior history of a distal radius fracture) with symptomatic ulnar styloid nonunions and TFCC tears who improved following an arthroscopic TFCC repair and open excision of the ulnar styloid fragment (**Fig. 10**). The time from injury to surgery ranged from 8 to 120 months. Diagnostic arthroscopy demonstrated 2 consistent findings in all 8 subjects: all had avulsion of the ulnar margin of the

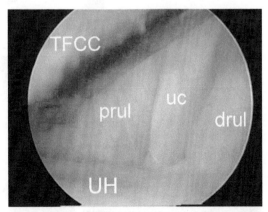

Fig. 8. Arthroscopic view from the volar DRUJ portal of an intact deep radioulnar ligament in a patient with an ulnar styloid nonunion. The conjoined palmar (prul) and dorsal (drul) radioulnar ligaments, and the ulnar collateral (uc) ligaments, are well attached to the ulnar head (UH). (© 2017 David J. Slutsky)

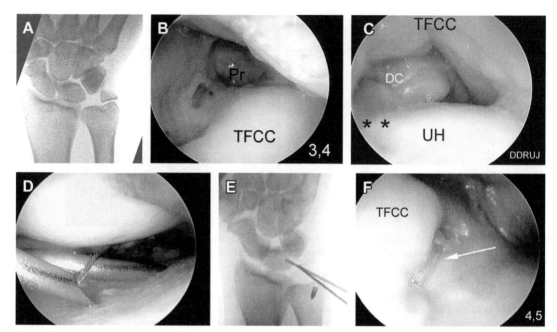

Fig. 9. Ulnar styloid nonunion with DRUJ instability. (*A*) 39-year-old woman with a symptomatic ulnar styloid nonunion and volar DRUJ instability. (*B*) Radiocarpal view demonstrating a normal appearing TFCC, but the hook test was positive. PR, pisiform recess. (*C*) DRUJ arthroscopy through the volar DRUJ portal demonstrates an empty fovea sign with an absence of the deep radioulnar ligament attachment (*asterisks*). DC, dorsal capsule; UH, ulnar head. (*D*) Arthroscopic-assisted foveal reattachment. (*E*) Fluoroscopic view of the bone anchor and suture placement using 18-gauge needles after an open excision of the nonunited ulnar styloid. (*F*) View of the TFCC reattachment with a horizontal mattress suture (*arrow*). (© 2017 David J. Slutsky)

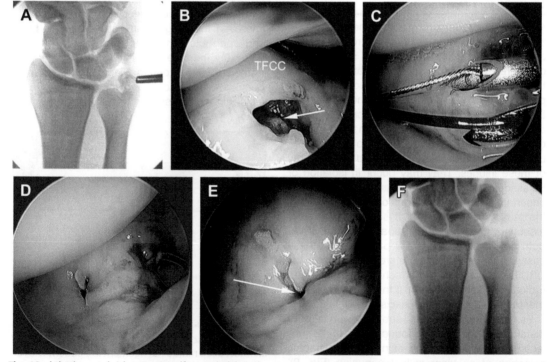

Fig. 10. (*A*) Ulnar styloid nonunion (forceps). (*B*) Arthroscopic view demonstrating a TFCC tear with exposure of the ulnar head (*arrow*). (*C*) Insertion of an absorbable suture. (*D*) Following suture repair of the TFCC tear. (*E*) Traction on the suture closes the TFCC tear (*arrow*). (*F*) AP view after an open resection of the nonunited styloid. (© 2017 David J. Slutsky)

TFCC from the ECU subsheath and a full-thickness chondral injury on the dorsum of the triquetrum. Three 2 to 0 absorbable sutures were used for arthroscopic outside-in technique to repair the peripheral margin of the avulsed articular disc to the capsule and the ECU subsheath. After placement of the sutures, the ulnar styloid fragment was dissected subperiosteally through a 1 cm incision, and excised. The TFCC repair sutures were then tied down to the capsule and retinaculum. The wrist was immobilized in 60° of supination with a custom-molded orthosis for 4 weeks followed by motion. Seven of 8 subjects were available for final follow-up evaluation at an average of 23 months (range, 11–28 months). The mean postoperative DASH score was 3.69 (SD 9.68; $P<.05$) over the mean preoperative DASH score of 32.3 (SD 11.5). The VAS improved from a preoperative mean of 6.14 (SD 1.49) to a postoperative mean of 1.0 (SD 0.83; $P<.05$). No subject had DRUJ instability at the time of the last office visit.

REFERENCES

1. Palmer AK, Glisson RR, Werner FW. Relationship between ulnar variance and triangular fibrocartilage complex thickness. J Hand Surg Am 1984;9(5): 681–2.
2. Hara T, Horii E, An KN, et al. Force distribution across wrist joint: application of pressure-sensitive conductive rubber. J Hand Surg Am 1992;17(2): 339–47.
3. Werner FW, Glisson RR, Murphy DJ, et al. Force transmission through the distal radioulnar carpal joint: effect of ulnar lengthening and shortening. Handchir Mikrochir Plast Chir 1986;18(5):304–8.
4. Mikic ZD. Age changes in the triangular fibrocartilage of the wrist joint. J Anat 1978;126(Pt 2):367–84.
5. Viegas SF, Ballantyne G. Attritional lesions of the wrist joint. J Hand Surg Am 1987;12(6):1025–9.
6. Tomaino MM. Ulnar impaction syndrome in the ulnar negative and neutral wrist. Diagnosis and pathoanatomy. J Hand Surg Br 1998;23(6):754–7.
7. Friedman SL, Palmer AK, Short WH, et al. The change in ulnar variance with grip. J Hand Surg Am 1993;18(4):713–6.
8. Steinborn M, Schurmann M, Staebler A, et al. MR imaging of ulnocarpal impaction after fracture of the distal radius. AJR Am J Roentgenol 2003;181(1): 195–8.
9. Cerezal L, del Pinal F, Abascal F. MR imaging findings in ulnar-sided wrist impaction syndromes. Magn Reson Imaging Clin N Am 2004;12(2):281–99, vi.
10. Meftah M, Keefer EP, Panagopoulos G, et al. Arthroscopic wafer resection for ulnar impaction syndrome: prediction of outcomes. Hand Surg 2010;15(2):89–93.
11. Wnorowski DC, Palmer AK, Werner FW, et al. Anatomic and biomechanical analysis of the arthroscopic wafer procedure. Arthroscopy 1992;8(2):204–12.
12. Osterman AL, Seidman GD. The role of arthroscopy in the treatment of lunatotriquetral ligament injuries. Hand Clin 1995;11(1):41–50.
13. Tomaino MM, Elfar J. Ulnar impaction syndrome. Hand Clin 2005;21(4):567–75.
14. Gupta R, Bingenheimer E, Fornalski S, et al. The effect of ulnar shortening on lunate and triquetrum motion–a cadaveric study. Clin Biomech (Bristol, Avon) 2005;20(8):839–45.
15. Iwatsuki K, Tatebe M, Yamamoto M, et al. Ulnar impaction syndrome: incidence of lunotriquetral ligament degeneration and outcome of ulnar-shortening osteotomy. J Hand Surg Am 2014;39(6): 1108–13.
16. Markolf KL, Tejwani SG, Benhaim P. Effects of wafer resection and hemiresection from the distal ulna on load-sharing at the wrist: a cadaveric study. J Hand Surg Am 2005;30(2):351–8.
17. Slutsky DJ. Distal radioulnar joint arthroscopy and the volar ulnar portal. Tech Hand Up Extrem Surg 2007;11(1):38–44.
18. Yin HW, Qiu YQ, Shen YD, et al. Arthroscopic distal metaphyseal ulnar shortening osteotomy for ulnar impaction syndrome: a different technique. J Hand Surg Am 2013;38(11):2257–62.
19. Slade JF 3rd, Gillon TJ. Osteochondral shortening osteotomy for the treatment of ulnar impaction syndrome: a new technique. Tech Hand Up Extrem Surg 2007;11(1):74–82.
20. Bornotoin MA, Nagle DJ, Martinez A, et al. A comparison of combined arthroscopic triangular fibrocartilage complex debridement and arthroscopic wafer distal ulna resection versus arthroscopic triangular fibrocartilage complex debridement and ulnar shortening osteotomy for ulnocarpal abutment syndrome. Arthroscopy 2004;20(4):392–401.
21. Vandenberghe L, Degreef I, Didden K, et al. Ulnar shortening or arthroscopic wafer resection for ulnar impaction syndrome. Acta Orthop Belg 2012;78(3): 323–6.
22. Topper SM, Wood MB, Ruby LK. Ulnar styloid impaction syndrome. J Hand Surg Am 1997;22(4): 699–704.
23. Ruland RT, Hogan CJ. The ECU synergy test: an aid to diagnose ECU tendonitis. J Hand Surg Am 2008; 33(10):1777–82.
24. Biyani A, Mehara A, Bhan S. Morphological variations of the ulnar styloid process. J Hand Surg Br 1990;15(3):352–4.
25. Giachino AA, McIntyre AI, Guy KJ, et al. Ulnar styloid triquetral impaction. Hand Surg 2007;12(2): 123–34.

26. Bain GI, Bidwell TA. Arthroscopic excision of ulnar styloid in stylocarpal impaction. Arthroscopy 2006; 22(6):677.e1-3.

27. Zahiri H, Zahiri CA, Ravari RK. Ulnar styloid impingement syndrome. Int Orthop 2010;34(8):1233–7.

28. Hauck RM, Skahen J 3rd, Palmer AK. Classification and treatment of ulnar styloid nonunion. J Hand Surg Am 1996;21(3):418–22.

29. Wijffels MM, Keizer J, Buijze GA, et al. Ulnar styloid process nonunion and outcome in patients with a distal radius fracture: a meta-analysis of comparative clinical trials. Injury 2014;45(12):1889–95.

30. Reeves B. Excision of the ulnar styloid fragment after Colles' fracture. Int Surg 1966;45(1):46–52.

31. Burgess RC, Watson HK. Hypertrophic ulnar styloid nonunions. Clin Orthop Relat Res 1988;(228):215–7.

32. Protopsaltis TS, Ruch DS. Triangular fibrocartilage complex tears associated with symptomatic ulnar styloid nonunions. J Hand Surg Am 2010;35(8): 1251–5.

Arthroscopic Evaluation of Associated Soft Tissue Injuries in Distal Radius Fractures

Tommy Lindau, MD, PhD (Hand Surgery)

KEYWORDS

- Arthroscopy • Chondral • DRU joint • Lunotriquetral ligament • Scapholunate ligament • TFCC

KEY POINTS

- A fall onto an outstretched hand may cause a wide spectrum of injuries, such as a simple sprain, radial styloid fracture in isolation, or a radial styloid fracture as part of a greater arch injury, thereby forming part of a complete or incomplete perilunate dislocation mechanism.
- Displaced radius fractures in nonosteoporotic patients have a high incidence of associated soft tissue injuries. Associated injuries affect the long-term outcome, and arthroscopic evaluation is paramount to establish a correct and complete diagnosis and facilitate early treatment.
- After falls, arthroscopy can diagnose triangular fibrocartilage complex injuries, inter-carpal scapholunate and lunotriquetral ligament tears and chondral lesions. Once evaluated and graded, the appropriate surgical treatment of these lesions can be added to the fracture fixation.
- Undetected associated injuries may explain the absence of improved outcome in studies comparing volar locking plate fixation and early mobilization versus external fixation. Possibly, further improved outcome may follow if arthroscopy is used in conjunction with volar locking plate fixation.
- Arthroscopy as an adjunct in the management of distal radius fractures has been available for more than 20 years, but still requires experience and management in expert centers. Successful management of this simple but complex fracture requires:
  - Thorough understanding of the anatomy.
  - Understanding the relevance of individual fracture fragments.
  - Awareness of associated soft tissue injuries.

INTRODUCTION

The outcome of distal radius fracture treatment can still not be fully predicted. There is no scientific evidence for anything that is done in the management of distal radius fractures.[1]

Arthroscopic evaluation is superior in assessing the intra-articular step-off as well as the rotation of articular fracture fragments. It is also possible to identify and evaluate chondral and ligament injuries (**Table 1**).[2–4] There is a high incidence of soft tissue injuries associated with distal radius fractures, which are frequently missed when the fracture is managed by conventional methods of treatment (see **Table 1**).[2,3] These injuries are to be expected because the radius is involved in the greater arch mechanism described by Mayfield and colleagues[5] in perilunate dislocations (**Fig. 1**). This

Conflict of Interest: The author has no conflict of interest.
Pulvertaft Hand Centre, University of Derby, Uttoxeter Road, Derby DE22 3SN, UK
E-mail address: tommylindau@hotmail.com

hand.theclinics.com

Table 1
Soft tissue injuries associated with distal radius fractures

Study, Year	Number and Type of Injury	TFCC Injury (%)	SL Injury (%)	LT Injury (%)
Geissler et al,[2] 1996	60, intra-articular	49	32	15
Lindau et al,[3] 1997	50, intra-articular and extraarticular	78	54	16
Richards,[17] 1997	118, intra-articular and extraarticular	35 (intra-articular) 53 (extraarticular)	21 (intra-articular) 7 (extraarticular)	7 (intra-articular) 13 (extraarticular)
Mehta,[18] 2000	3, intra-articular	58	85	61
Hanker,[19] 2001	173, intra-articular	61	8	12

Abbreviations: LT, lunotriquetral; SL, scapholunate; TFCC, triangular fibrocartilage complex.

condition is particularly noted in nonosteoporotic patients who more often present with intra-articular fractures caused by a severe, high-energy trauma, whereas such associated injuries are uncommon in osteoporotic patients, in whom most fractures are extraarticular and caused by low-energy trauma. Hence, arthroscopy should be considered in younger patients with high-energy trauma, in particular radial styloid fractures, in order to detect these injuries in addition to improving intra-articular congruency by arthroscopically fine-tuned reduction and fixation of these fragments (see **Fig. 1**).

INDICATIONS FOR ARTHROSCOPY IN DISTAL RADIUS FRACTURES

- The main indication for arthroscopy in the management of distal radius fractures is an intra-articular step-off of more than 1 mm after an attempted closed reduction.
- Second, radius fractures with associated scaphoid fractures and/or obvious ligament injuries benefit from arthroscopic evaluation. Radiological signs may suggest associated soft tissue injuries, such as widening of intercarpal joint spaces and/or radiographic disruption of the carpal arches of the Gilula lines; the 3 arches that can be drawn along the proximal and distal carpal rows (see **Fig. 1**).
- Third, a radiological widening of the distal radioulnar (DRU) joint may be another sign of a ligament injury to the triangular fibrocartilage complex (TFCC) that may need arthroscopic evaluation.
- Simple radial styloid fractures are most often 2-part fractures and may be part of an incomplete greater arch injury according to the

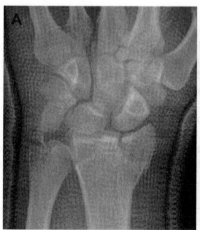 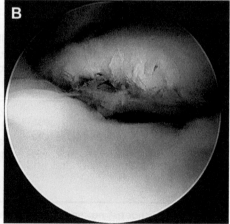

Fig. 1. (*A*) Radius fracture with associated scapholunate (SL) ligament injury diagnosed with the ring sign of the scaphoid. (*B*) Arthroscopic view of the fracture affecting the ridge between the lunate (*left* in image) and scaphoid facets of the radius.

Mayfield mechanism, but without a dislocation of the lunate[5] (see **Fig. 1**).

- Complex, impacted fractures such as die-punch fractures warrant arthroscopic evaluation, reduction, and fixation.
- Three-part or 4-part intra-articular fractures or even more complex injuries with high-grade intra-articular comminution (so-called explosion fractures) are challenging but benefit from expert arthroscopic management.

THE ARTHROSCOPIC PROCEDURE: DRY OR WET?

The dry arthroscopic technique minimizes the risk of further soft tissue swelling and secondary compartment syndrome, compared with the wet technique with continuous saline irrigation, but it may make the procedure slightly more cumbersome.[6] Dry should not be taken literally, because there might be intra-articular debris and hemarthrosis, which must be cleared by irrigating the joint before continuing with a dry arthroscopy technique.[6] If a dry arthroscopy technique is preferred, the air valve should be kept open to permit free circulation of air through the joint and the suction should be turned off unless needed.

THE ARTHROSCOPIC PROCEDURE: ARTHROSCOPIC EVALUATION

- Safe portals have to be established, occasionally with fluoroscopic assistance bearing in mind not to further displace any fracture fragments.
- The examination starts by evaluating the radiocarpal joint surface regarding intra-articular congruency and possible need for optimizing the provisional reduction.
- In this respect, a 2-mm probe is helpful, inserted through the 4-5 or the 6-R portal, to accurately evaluate the gap, separation, and step-off of fragments.
- Once articular congruity is achieved, associated ligament or cartilage injuries are evaluated: integrity of the scapholunate (SL) ligament, the lunotriquetral (LT) ligament, and the TFCC or any other intra-articular disorder is visualized and the sequence of surgery can be planned.
- TFCC injuries seem to be the most common associated ligament injury. They are found in around three-quarters of these fractures (see **Table 1**).[2,3]

- SL ligament injuries are the second most frequent injuries. They are found in between one-third and one-half of cases (see **Table 1**).[2,3]
- LT ligament tears are less common and are seen in about one-sixth of the fractures (see **Table 1**).[2,3]
- Chondral lesions have been found[3] with a possible long-term development of secondary osteoarthritis (OA).[7]

TRIANGULAR FIBROCARTILAGE COMPLEX INJURIES

TFCC injuries are the most common associated intra-articular injuries in distal radius fractures in nonosteoporotic patients (see **Fig. 2**, **Table 1**; **Table 2**).[2,3] Cadaveric studies suggest that a displacement of the distal radius has to be more than 4 mm of radial shortening, down to 0° of radial inclination and a dorsal tilt of a minimum of 10° in order for an ulnar attachment of TFCC to be compromised.[10] In a 1-year outcome study, peripheral tears to the TFCC caused instability and subsequent worse outcome[11] (see **Fig. 2B**). However, in a recent 15-year prospective longitudinal outcome study of untreated TFCC tears, this seemed to be less of a clinical problem than was anticipated, because only 1 patient needed a stabilizing procedure because of painful instability.[12]

In the absence of scientific evidence, clinical experience supports advice regarding TFCC treatment in association with distal radius fractures (see **Table 2**; the principles regarding management and technical aspects are discussed elsewhere in this issue).

INTERCARPAL LIGAMENT INJURIES

Intercarpal ligament injuries to the SL and LT ligaments associated with distal radius fractures can be considered to be incomplete greater arch injuries, as described by Mayfield and colleagues[5] (see **Fig. 1**). It is important to evaluate and diagnose these ligament injuries. In the absence of arthroscopy, fluoroscopic assessment in ulnar and radial deviation of the wrist can diagnose severe intercarpal ligament injuries as disrupted Gilula lines. Arthroscopic evaluation not only diagnoses them but also allows grading based on a combined radiocarpal and midcarpal assessment[2,3] (**Fig. 4**, **Tables 3** and **4**). Depending on the grading, severity is better defined and further management is decided.

The ligament injuries are directly visualized at radiocarpal arthroscopy and are classified as partial or complete (see **Fig. 4**A, **Tables 3** and **4**). The

Table 2
Classification of triangular fibrocartilage complex tears with explanation of biomechanical problems with the tear and suggested treatment

Type of Tear	Understanding the Tear	Treatment
Central perforation tears (**Fig. 2**A) (Palmer,[8] 1989)	• Stable • This treatment does not change the overall rehabilitation plan	• Debridement (suction punch, shaver, radiofrequency probe) • Care should be taken to avoid jeopardizing the stability provided by the important palmar and dorsal ulnoradial ligaments
Peripheral tears (see **Fig. 2**B) (Palmer,[8] 1989)	• May cause DRU joint instability • Distal tears are avulsed from the capsule and subsheath to ECU • Proximal tears are avulsed from the fovea of the ulnar head • Proximal tears cannot be seen at radiocarpal arthroscopy • Combined distal and proximal tears cause instability of the DRU joint	• Distal tears: debride and possibly suture back to the capsule and ECU subsheath[9] • Proximal tears: reattachment to the fovea of the ulna[9] • Combined tears should also be reattached[9] • Reattachment can be done with arthroscopy assistance or with an open technique with similar good outcome (**Fig. 3**) Arthroscopically assisted reattachment: • Two or three 2/0 absorbable (polydioxanone) sutures are passed through the periphery of the TFCC and fixed to the distal ulna, either through drill holes or with one of the many suture anchors • The repair is protected from supination and pronation for 4 wk, followed by 2–4 wk in a short-arm cast
Ulnocarpal ligament tears (Palmer,[8] 1989)	• Very rare[3]	Reinsertion technique: • Simplest option: directly through the palmar approach in line with the exposure of the critical corner in the intermediate column • This repair should be protected for 4 wk in relation to the rehabilitation for the fracture
Radial avulsion tears (Palmer,[8] 1989)	• Uncommon • Often associated with a dorsoulnar fracture fragment • May cause instability of the DRU joint	Reattachment technique: • A dorsal fracture should be fixed • Because of the distal radius fracture, the technique based on drill holes through the radius is not suitable • A miniopen dorsoradial approach is done and ligament is reattached with suture anchors

Abbreviation: ECU, extensor carpal ulnaris.

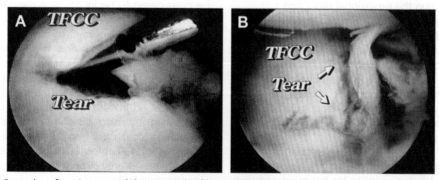

Fig. 2. (*A*) Central perforation tear of the triangular fibrocartilage (TFCC) ligament. This condition may be painful and debridement should be considered, but it never leads to instability of the DRU joint. (*B*) Peripheral TFCC tear that showed increased instability and a worse outcome 1 year after injury. Fifteen years after these injuries, only 1 patient needed secondary reattachment, suggesting that it may not always need repair.

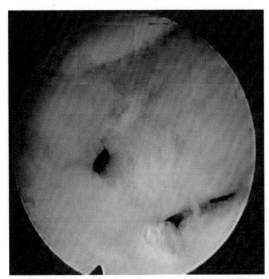

Fig. 3. Repair of the peripheral tear has to be through the fovea of the ulnar head to regain stability. Suture anchors, drill holes, and other techniques are available.

ligaments are examined along their dorsal, membranous, and palmar portions.

From the midcarpal joint, the joint space, not the ligament, is evaluated for widening/gap and step-off (see **Fig. 4**B). A probe with known size (eg, 1-mm thickness and 2-mm tip length) is useful to gauge the widenings/gaps and steps more accurately (see **Tables 3** and **4**). The widening/gap and the step-off reflect the degree of mobility of the affected intercarpal joint, as a consequence of the ligamentous injury previously seen at radiocarpal arthroscopy. This mobility is not necessarily a pathologic mobility but may be an inherent constitutional

hypermobility or laxity. Once the traction is released, the evaluated joint can be tested by checking signs of pathologic excessive mobility with the arthroscope in the midcarpal joint. Thus, the intercarpal ligament injury can be fully classified and graded for improved management (see **Tables 3** and **4**).

SCAPHOLUNATE LIGAMENT INJURIES

SL ligament injuries occur in half of displaced distal radius fractures, at least in the nonosteoporotic population[3] (see **Table 1**). If left untreated, complete high-grade SL tears are likely to progress first to SL dissociation and symptomatic carpal instability.[13] This condition in the long term leads to posttraumatic scapholunate advanced collapse (SLAC) osteoarthritis. Because of the long-term consequences of untreated SL tears, it is important to detect SL tears early and to consider treatment. If found and treated early, arthroscopic reduction and percutaneous pinning is the simplest option and has a good outcome in 85% of patients. It is noteworthy that there is no strong evidence (level 1 or 2) for management of these injuries and published recommendations are mainly experience based.[14]

Grade I to III Scapholunate Injuries

Low-grade incomplete injuries are best managed with immobilization, because most patients are asymptomatic at 1 year[13] and there are no long-term findings for SLAC wrist and so forth.[14] Therefore, the rehabilitation protocol for mobilization of the distal radius fracture after volar locking plate fixation may have to be adjusted depending on the severity of the SL injury.[15]

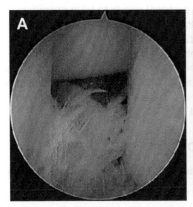
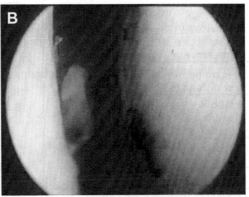

Fig. 4. (*A*) Arthroscopic view from the radiocarpal portal with a so-called drive-through sign; that is, the scope can be passed through the SL ligament that is completely torn (a grade IV SL tear). (*B*) Midcarpal arthroscopy shows a step and a gap that can be measured for grading, in this case a grade 3 tear.

Table 3
Arthroscopic classification of scapholunate ligament tears according to Geissler and colleagues[2]

Grade	Radiocarpal Joint	Midcarpal Instability	Step-off
1	Hemorrhage of inter-carpal ligament, no attenuation	None	None
2	Incomplete partial or full tear, no attenuation	Slight gap (<3 mm)	Midcarpal only
3	Ligament attenuation; incomplete partial or small full tear	Probe can be passed between carpal bones	Midcarpal and radiocarpal
4	Complete tear	Gross instability; 2.7-mm scope can be passed through (drive-through sign)	Midcarpal and radiocarpal

From Geissler WB, Freeland AE, Savoie FH, et al. Intracarpal soft-tissue lesions associated with an intra-articular fracture of the distal end of the radius. J Bone Joint Surg Am 1996;78(3):357–65; with permission.

Grade IV Scapholunate Injuries

Radiographic SL dissociation and long-term SLAC wrist is more likely with these injuries if untreated, and consequently early treatment is important.[16]

Grade IV complete intercarpal injuries can be treated with arthroscopic reduction and percutaneous Kirschner wire (K-wire) pinning provided there are no radiological signs of dissociation because this implies that the secondary stabilizers have been injured as well (**Fig. 5**). While protecting the sensory branches of the radial nerve, a skin incision is made slightly palmar to the anatomic snuffbox. K-wires into the scaphoid are used as a joystick to achieve arthroscopic reduction, which can be assessed from the midcarpal joint. Once reduction is achieved, the K-wire is advanced into the lunate. An additional K-wire should be inserted into the scaphocapitate joint (see **Fig. 5**). Pins can be removed at 6 weeks.[16]

More importantly, if grade IV complete SL injuries are found with radiologically visible dissociation already on the trauma film, then the treatment rationale should most likely be with an open repair.[16] Open direct repair is followed by protective K-wires as described earlier. During closure, a dorsal intercarpal capsulodesis can be added to augment the repair.

LUNOTRIQUETRAL LIGAMENT INJURIES

The incidence of LT ligament injuries is about 1 in 6 (see **Table 1**). So far, there is no evidence that LT tears lead to long-term problems when associated with distal radius fractures.[13,14]

Stable LT incomplete injuries (grades I–III) may benefit from immobilization if the fracture mobilization protocol needs to be reconsidered.

Grade IV complete injuries may need arthroscopic debridement of the tear and percutaneous pinning of the joint. K-wires are introduced from a dorsoulnar approach. The LT dissociation is reduced with a joystick maneuver and 2 or 3 K-wires are advanced across the joint. Wires are kept for 6 weeks.

Table 4
The Lindau classification system for intercarpal scapholunate and lunotriquetral ligament injuries and mobility of the joints

	Radiocarpal Arthroscopy Ligament Appearance	Midcarpal Arthroscopy Appearance	
Grade		Diastasis (mm)	Step-off (mm)
1	Hematoma or distension	0	0
2	As above and/or partial tear	0–1	<2
3	Partial or total tear	1–2	<2
4	Total tear	>2	>2

From Lindau T, Arner M, Hagberg L. Intra-articular lesions in distal fractures of the radius in young adults. A descriptive arthroscopic study in 50 patients. J Hand Surg Br 1997;22(5):639; with permission.

CHONDRAL LESIONS

Acute chondral lesions[3] can be seen as:

- Subchondral hematomas (with or without cartilage cracks)
- Avulsed cartilage flakes
- Complete avulsions of the cartilage

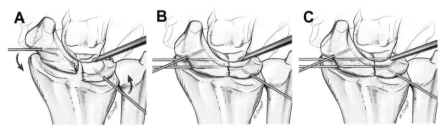

Fig. 5. Repair of a grade III to IV SL tear can be done with an arthroscopy-assisted technique. (*A*) One K-wire in the scaphoid and lunate respectively is used and (*B*) a joystick maneuver (*arrows*) is used with the scope in the midcarpal joint to secure adequate reduction of the joint. (*B, C*) K-wires are inserted into the scaphoid and, once reduction has been achieved, the wires are advanced over the SL joint and a final wire is inserted into the capitate to protect the torn ligament and allow healing. (*From* Lindau T. Arthroscopic management of scapholunate dissociation. In: del Piñal F, Luchetti R, Mathoulin C, editors. Arthroscopic management of distal radius fractures. 1st edition. Berlin: Springer; 2010; with permission.)

There is some evidence that subchondral hematoma can lead to the development of early onset of mild radiographic OA.[7] There is currently no other treatment option than debridement for these injuries. A tempting, but unproven, option is the microfracture treatment, as used in the knee joint. Chondral lesions may lead to treatment changes; a comminuted intra-articular fracture might be treated with a primary partial wrist fusion instead of a lengthy attempt at reducing a multifragmentary joint surface with loss of cartilage, because there is increased awareness of an expected bad outcome with these associated lesions. Together with the associated ligament injuries, chondral lesions reflect the complexity of distal radial fractures, especially in the nonosteoporotic population.[6]

OUTCOMES

At present, there is no scientific evidence that arthroscopy is necessary in the management of distal radius fractures. However, there seems to be increasing support regarding the benefit of arthroscopy in the management of distal radius fractures.[9,11–15] Furthermore, there is limited experience in arthroscopically assisted treatment of associated injuries. However, TFCC repairs in conjunction with distal radius fixation resulted in a high degree of patient satisfaction and good to excellent clinical outcomes.[9]

SUMMARY

There is an increasing awareness of the complexity of distal radius fracture; it should not only be seen as a bony injury but as a bony consequence of the energy passing the wrist while breaking the radius. The main advantage of arthroscopically assisted management of distal radius fractures is to improve intra-articular accuracy to less than 1 mm of incongruence. The second advantage is that this can be combined with complete evaluation, management, and treatment of TFCC, intercarpal ligament, and cartilage injuries. The third advantage is that the surgeon has complete control of all fracture-related and treatment-related factors in distal radius fractures by arthroscopic assistance. It is my hope that this concept will continue to evolve for the benefit of patients.

REFERENCES

1. Cochrane Library; Handoll H, Elstub L, Elliott J, et al. Cochrane Bone, Joint and Muscle Trauma Group. About The Cochrane Collaboration (Cochrane Review Groups (CRGs)) 2008, Issue 4.
2. Geissler WB, Freeland AE, Savoie FH, et al. Intracarpal soft-tissue lesions associated with an intra-articular fracture of the distal end of the radius. J Bone Joint Surg Am 1996;78:357–65.
3. Lindau T, Arner M, Hagberg L. Intraarticular lesions in distal fractures of the radius in young adults. A descriptive arthroscopic study in 50 patients. J Hand Surg Br 1997;22:638–43.
4. Cognet JM, Martinache X, Mathoulin C. Arthroscopic management of intra-articular fractures of the distal radius. Chir Main 2008;27:171–9 [in French].
5. Mayfield JK, Johnson RP, Kilcoyne RF. The ligaments of the human wrist and their functional significance. Anat Rec 1976;86:417–28.
6. del Piñal F. Technical tips for (dry) arthroscopic reduction and internal fixation of distal radius fractures. J Hand Surg Am 2011;36:1694–705.
7. Lindau T, Adlercreutz C, Aspenberg P. Cartilage injuries in distal radial fractures. Acta Orthop Scand 2003;74:327–31.
8. Palmer AK. Triangular fibrocartilage complex lesions: a classification. J Hand Surg 1989;14A:594–606.

9. Ruch DS, Yang CC, Smith BP. Results of acute arthroscopically repaired triangular fibrocartilage complex injuries associated with intra-articular distal radius fractures. Arthroscopy 2003;19:511–6.

10. Scheer JH, Adolfsson LE. Patterns of triangular fibrocartilage complex (TFCC) injury associated with severely dorsally displaced extra-articular distal radius fractures. Injury 2012;43:926–32.

11. Lindau T, Adlercreutz C, Aspenberg P. Peripheral tears of the triangular fibrocartilage complex cause distal radioulnar instability after distal radial fractures. J Hand Surg Am 2000;25:464–8.

12. Mrkonjic A, Geijer M, Lindau T, et al. The natural course of traumatic triangular fibrocartilage complex tears in distal radial fractures: a 13-15 year follow-up of arthroscopically diagnosed but untreated injuries. J Hand Surg Am 2012;37:1555–60.

13. Forward D, Lindau T, Melsom D. Intercarpal ligament injuries associated with fractures of the distal radius. Arthroscopic assessment and 12 month follow-up. J Bone Joint Surg Am 2007;89:2334–40.

14. Mrkonjic A, Lindau T, Geijer M, et al. Arthroscopically diagnosed scapholunate ligament injuries associated with distal radial fractures. A 13- to 15-year follow-up. J Hand Surg Am 2015;40:1077–82.

15. Ono H, Katayama T, Furuta K, et al. Distal radial fracture arthroscopic intraarticular gap and step-off measurement after open reduction and internal fixation with a volar locked plate. J Orthop Sci 2012;17(4):443–9.

16. Chennagiri RJR, Lindau T. Assessment of scapholunate instability and review of evidence for management in the absence of arthritis. J Hand Surg Eur 2013;38:727–38.

17. Richards RS, Bennett JD, Roth JH, et al. Arthroscopic diagnosis of intra-articular soft tissue injuries associated with distal radial fractures. J Hand Surg [Am] 1997;22:772–6.

18. Mehta JA, Bain GI, Heptinstall RJ. Anatomical reduction of intra-articular fractures of the distal radius. An arthroscopically assisted approach. J Bone Joint Surg (Br) 2000;82-B:79–86.

19. Hanker GJ. Radius fractures in the athlete. Clin Sports Med 2001;20:189–201.

Arthroscopic-Assisted Reduction of Intra-articular Distal Radius Fracture

Yukio Abe, MD, PhD*, Kenzo Fujii, MD

KEYWORDS

• Wrist • Distal radius fracture • Intra-articular fracture • Arthroscopy • Articular step-off

KEY POINTS

- Wrist arthroscopy is an efficient adjunct for intra-articular distal radius fracture fixation. However, performing wrist arthroscopy during the plate fixation is troublesome with the vertical traction applied and released.
- To facilitate the procedure, the authors developed a surgical technique, plate presetting arthroscopic reduction technique (PART), using a palmar locking plate. Since July 2005, they have performed PART for 248 intra-articular distal radius fractures with good and excellent results.
- Arthroscopic-assisted reduction of intra-articular fragments is superior to fluoroscopic assisted. PART also allows detection of intra-articular migration of fracture fragments, screw protrusion, and associated soft tissue injuries.

INTRODUCTION

Distal radius fracture (DRF) is one of the most common injuries not only for hand surgeons but also for general orthopedic or trauma surgeons. Although manual reduction and cast immobilization had been the main treatment traditionally, surgical intervention is often needed for irreducible fractures or uncontrolled fracture reduction. Numerous surgical procedures have been described for these fractures; however, the latest development of a palmar locking plate (PLP) fixation markedly changed the treatment of DRF.[1–3] PLP fixation creates a more rigid mechanical construct and allows early mobilization with the goal of an improved functional outcome. The functional outcome of DRF is considered to be affected by the extra-articular alignment, anatomic reduction of the articular surface, intra-articular soft tissue injuries, and postoperative complications.[4–12] Wrist arthroscopy is currently recognized as an important adjunctive procedure in the management of DRF, because arthroscopically assisted reduction provides excellent visualization of the articular condition not only with regard to anatomic restoration of articular fragments but also to evaluate and treat intra-articular soft tissue injuries.[13–15] It would be easier if used in conjunction with percutaneous pinning and external fixation. However, wrist arthroscopy becomes troublesome when PLP fixation is performed because vertical traction has to be both applied and released during the surgery. Therefore, the authors have developed a plate presetting arthroscopic reduction technique (PART) using a PLP that can simplify the combination of plating and arthroscopy.[16–18] This article describes the procedure of PART and its effectiveness for the treatment of DRF.

Department of Orthopaedic Surgery, Saiseikai Shimonoseki General Hospital, 8-5-1, Yasuoka-cho, Shimonoseki 759-6603, Japan
* Corresponding author.
E-mail address: handsurgeonabe@jcom.home.ne.jp

Hand Clin 33 (2017) 659–668
http://dx.doi.org/10.1016/j.hcl.2017.07.011

hand.theclinics.com

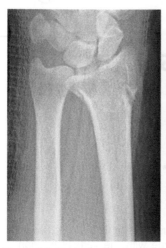
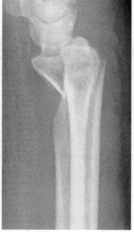
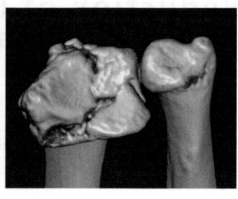

Fig. 1. 3D CT is valuable for making a plan of how to reduce the fragments.

INDICATIONS/CONTRAINDICATIONS

Although various factors affect the prognosis of treatment of DRF, accurate restoration of the alignment of the radius with its carpal and ulnar articulations, anatomic reduction of articular surface, and treatment of associated intra-articular soft tissue injury are the most important factors. Wrist arthroscopy has the advantage not only of a direct visualization of the reduction of intra-articular fragments but also of the possibility to manage intra-articular soft tissue injuries. Intra-articular soft tissue injuries were found to have almost the same incidence in both extra-articular and intra-articular DRF in the authors' institute, and they consider wrist arthroscopy for any type of DRF. However, they consider that low-activity patients, extra-articular fractures in the elderly, open fractures, and DRF associated with other multiple fractures are contraindications for PART.

SURGICAL TECHNIQUE
Preoperative Planning

Besides the standard posteroanterior and lateral radiographs, oblique radiographs at 45° of supination and pronation of the forearm, and computed tomography (CT), including 3-dimensional (3D) reconstruction, are valuable in deciding a surgical strategy for the treatment of DRF (**Fig. 1**).

Preparation and Patient Positioning

The arthroscopy monitor, the fluoroscopy and the arthroscopic equipment, including a small-diameter arthroscope with a 30° field of vision, a shaver, and a radiofrequency device must be positioned conveniently (**Fig. 2**). Even though dry arthroscopy was recently recommended to

prevent extravasation and for its convenience,[19] the authors prefer wet technique. A palmar approach is used to apply the plate before the arthroscopic procedure. Saline can flow away readily through the palmar incision, especially in an intra-articular fracture. Therefore, the authors are less concerned about swelling during the arthroscopy. Blood clots and debris can be easily removed. The wet technique can also prevent the heat problem in using a radiofrequency device. The patient, who has been placed under general or regional anesthesia, is placed in the supine position with the arm draped freely over a hand table. A tourniquet is wrapped around the upper arm and is inflated.

Surgical Approach

Exposure
A longitudinal skin incision is made between the flexor carpi radialis (FCR) tendon and the radial artery (so-called Henry approach; **Fig. 3**). The length

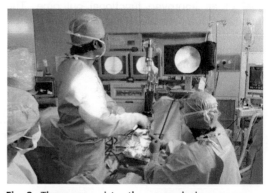

Fig. 2. The scene wrist arthroscopy during surgery.

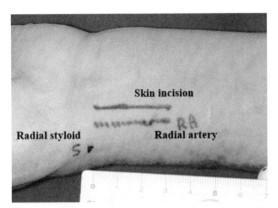

Fig. 3. The skin incision is set just ulnar side to the radial artery; its length is usually approximately 3 cm.

of the skin incision can vary according to the severity of comminution at the palmar cortex. The shortest skin incision is about 2.5 cm for a simple metaphyseal fracture. The radial artery is retracted radially, and the FCR tendon is retracted ulnarly together with the median nerve. Retracting

the flexor pollicis longus muscle ulnarly exposes the pronator quadratus muscle, which is split in its distal one-third for fracture site exposure and reduction.

Fracture reduction

The fracture of the palmar site is reduced by manipulating the fragments using a periosteal elevator. As the palmar cortex of the radius is generally less comminuted, reduction of the palmar cortex is an indicator of anatomic reduction. If severe comminution of palmar cortex is recognized, the use of an external fixator with ligamentotaxis temporarily would be beneficial to maintain the reduction. Several intrafocal pins are inserted to reduce the alignment radially and dorsally (**Fig. 4**A, a, b, c). After anatomic reduction is achieved possibly including the articular surface, the fragments are subsequently fixed under fluoroscopy with several interfragmental pins percutaneously (see **Fig. 4**A, d, e). Typically, for an intra-articular fracture, at least 4 to 5 Kirschner wires (K-wires), 1.5 mm in

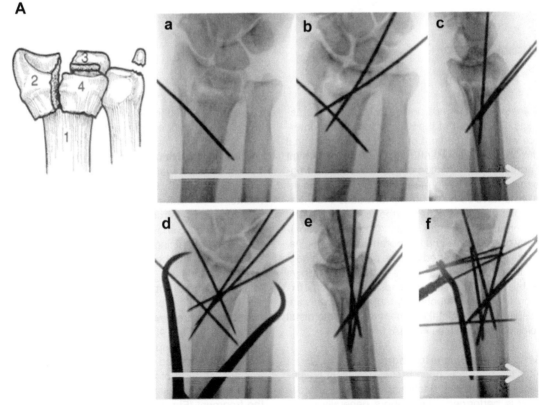

Fig. 4. (*A*) The sequence of fracture reduction and fixation for typical C3 fracture. Fracture reduction is acquired with manipulation and some intrafocal pinnings (*a*: intra-focal pinning from radial side, *b, c*: from dorsal side). Reduction is fixed with some interfragmental pinnings (*d, e*: interfragmental pinnings with tenaculum clump), and a PLP is provisionally fixed (*f*). (*B*) Arthroscopic reduction of step-off (*g*: before reduction, *h*: after reduction). A PLP is finally fixed (*i, j*). *Yellow arrows* indicate the order of reduction and temporary fixation. *Red arrow* indicates the arthroscopic reduction of the intra-articular fragment.

B

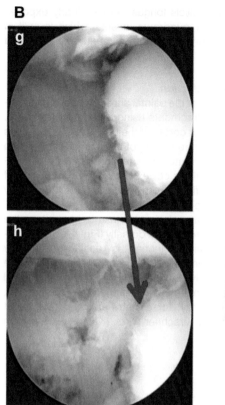

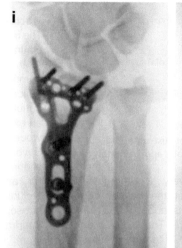

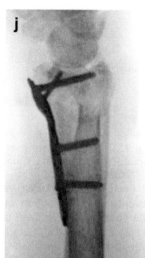

Fig. 4. *(continued)*

diameter, are inserted from the radial and dorsal aspects. Placement of the K-wires should not interfere with the placement of the PLP. The intrafocal pins are quite important to maintain the alignment if arthroscopic reduction of the intra-articular fragments has to be performed, because interfragmental pins have to be removed to reduce the intra-articular fragments. After temporary fixation of the fracture by K-wires, the locking plate is preset palmarly on the radius and temporarily fixed with pins. A screw is then inserted into the proximal fragment through the oval hole of the plate, which allows slight adjustment of the plate position at the final fixation. In addition, subchondral supporting wires are inserted into the distal fragment through the distal holes of the plate (see **Fig. 4**A, f).

Wrist arthroscopic inspection

After the plate has been preset, the wrist is suspended in a vertical traction tower. Wrist arthroscopy is performed. The authors generally use 2 dorsal portals to evaluate and treat the intra-articular fragments and soft tissue injuries, the 3-4 portal (between the extensor pollicis longus tendon and the extensor digitorum communis tendons) and the 4-5 portal (between the extensor

digitorum communis tendons and the extensor digiti minimi tendon). In addition, the authors sometimes use the palmar portal through the gliding floor of the FCR tendon to inspect the palmar segment tear of the scapholunate interosseous ligament (SLIL) and dorsal fracture fragments.[20,21] A 2.3-mm arthroscope with a 30° field of vision is introduced through the 3-4 portal, and a probe or a shaver is inserted through the 4-5 portal. The remaining hematoma in the joint should be removed for better visualization. The intra-articular condition, such as fracture fragments and soft tissue structures, is thoroughly inspected.

Fragments that are not reduced by the initial manipulation are now reduced under arthroscopic control (see **Fig. 4**B, g, h). K-wires preventing reduction of the displaced intra-articular fragment have to be removed or can be used as a joystick. Residual step-off of the fragment can be reduced by joystick maneuver using a K-wire inserted to the fragment (**Fig. 5**A). Fragments just separated from each other are reduced by percutaneous tenaculum clamping (**Fig. 5**B). Central depression is reduced by pushing up from the intramedullary canal using a probe inserted at the dorsal or palmar fracture site (**Fig. 5**C). Free fragments,

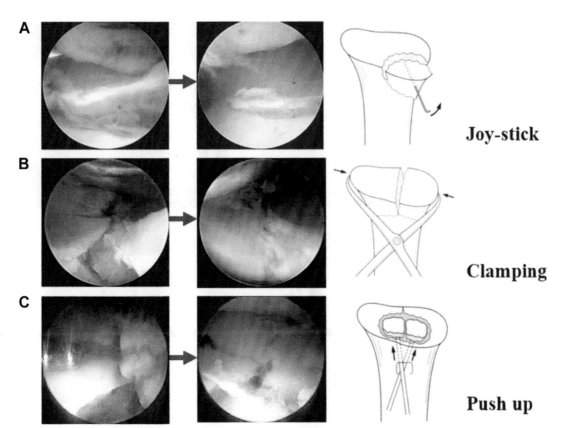

Fig. 5. (*A*) The step-off of the fragments is reduced by joystick maneuver. (*B*) Fragments, which are separated from each other, are reduced by tenaculum clamping technique. (*C*) The central depression is reduced by pushing up from the intramedullary. (*Adapted from* Abe Y. How to perform wrist arthroscopy with volar locking plate fixation for distal radius fracture. MB Orthop 2014;27(1):81; with permission.)

which are too small to fix, are removed. After reduction of the fragments is achieved, temporary K-wire fixation is performed again. These K-wires are removed after inserting locking screws through the distal plate holes.

After reduction of the intra-articular fragments arthroscopically, associated soft tissue injuries should be evaluated and treated. The necessity of initial treatment of soft tissue injury is still controversial. The authors' principles are, if an SLIL injury is recognized, midcarpal arthroscopy is performed to evaluate scapholunate stability with a probe (**Fig. 6**). Similarly, if distal radioulnar joint (DRUJ) instability is suspected, DRUJ arthroscopy should be performed to confirm a foveal tear of the triangular fibrocartilage complex (TFCC). Their strategy for the treatment of an SLIL injury is percutaneous pinning for grade III instability, repair of the dorsal part of SLIL, and augmentation using a dorsal intercarpal ligament for grade IV instability according to Geissler classification.[7] For foveal tear of TFCC,[22] the authors

perform the primary repair arthroscopically (**Fig. 7**). These procedures are basically indicated for younger and active patients. As soon as intra-articular fragments and soft tissue injuries are treated, vertical traction is removed, and the PLP is subsequently and securely fixed to the distal radius (see **Fig. 4**B, i, j). Since the introduction of the PLP, the authors rarely perform bone grafting for dorsal bone defects. However, artificial bone graft would facilitate bone union in the severely comminuted fracture at the metaphysis, or severely osteoporotic bone. The wound is irrigated; a drain is inserted, and the overlying skin is closed.

Postoperative Care

Early rehabilitation can be allowed because PLP provides rigid fixation. A dorsal splint is applied just after surgery; the splint is removed, and active wrist motion is started on the first day after surgery. Passive motion and grasping exercises are

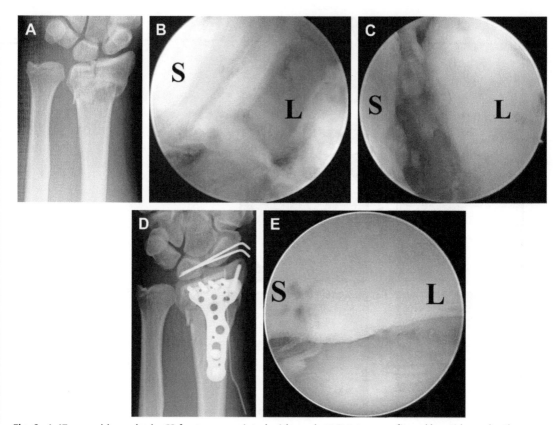

Fig. 6. A 47-year-old man had a C2 fracture associated with grade III SLIL tear confirmed by midcarpal arthroscopy (*A*: preoperative radiograph; *B*: SLIL was torn from the lunate attachment through viewing from the radiocarpal arthroscopy; *C*: scapholunate gap was recognized through the midcarpal arthroscopy). The fracture was reduced and fixed with a PLP. (*D*) Simultaneously, the scapholunate joint was transfixed with 2 K-wires. The K-wires were removed 12 weeks after surgery. (*E*) Six months after surgery, at the time of plate removal, SLIL was confirmed to be completely healed. S, scaphoid; L, lunate.

started from the second day with the therapist. Forearm rotation exercises are prohibited in patients who have ulnar side injuries, such as unfixed distal ulna fracture, ulnar styloid fracture, and TFCC repairs, until 3 weeks after surgery.

Complications

The authors have never experienced severe complications from arthroscopic reduction procedures, such as tendon rupture, major neurovascular injury, or compartment syndrome, in more than 450 cases. There were several complaints of numbness at the dorsal wrist after the surgery. However, the symptoms improved in 3 to 6 months.

The Advantages of Wrist Arthroscopy

From July 2005 to August 2016, PART was performed in 248 wrists of 242 consecutive intra-articular DRF patients. The 61 men and 181 women ranged in age from 17 to 86 year old (average age, 62.7 years old). The authors classified all the fractures using the AO/ASIF (Association for Osteosynthesis/Association for the Study of Internal Fixation) classification system. The fractures consisted of 8 B3, 113 C1, 18 C2, and 109 C3 fractures. From these experiences, the authors recognized several advantages of arthroscopic surgery for DRF (**Box 1**). First, during PART, anatomic reduction of the articular surface is initially achieved under fluoroscopy, and reduction is reconfirmed by arthroscopy. In this process, the authors could recognize the difference between fluoroscopic and arthroscopic reduction (**Fig. 8**). They hypothesized that after fluoroscopic reduction there will be no remaining gap and step-off of 2 mm or more in 231 intra-articular fractures. However, under arthroscopy, the authors recognized more than 2-mm residual displacement in 49 wrists (21.2%). The residual displacement in the coronal plane was frequently observed.

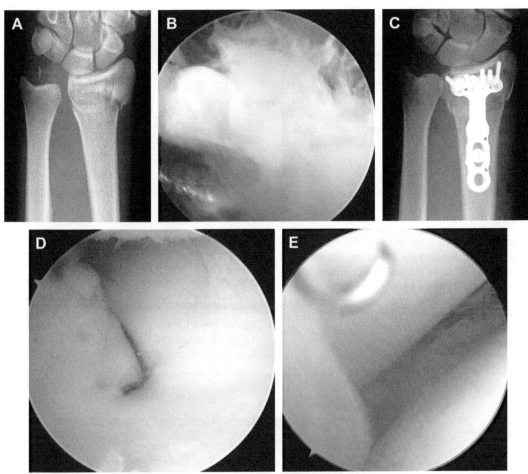

Fig. 7. (*A*) An 18-year-old man suffered a C3 fracture of the right radius and a C1 fracture on the left radius. (*B*) There was associated complete TFCC foveal tear as shown in DRUJ arthroscopy. (*C*) The fracture was reduced and fixed with PART. (*D*) In addition, the TFCC foveal tear was arthroscopically repaired. Function of the wrist was returned to almost normal 3 months after the surgery. (*E*) TFCC healing was confirmed with DRUJ arthroscopy at the time of plate removal 6 months after the initial surgery.

Box 1
The advantage of wrist arthroscopy in the surgical treatment of distal radius fracture

1. Accurate reduction of intra-articular fragments is possible compared with fluoroscopic reduction.

2. Intra-articular fragments (free body) undetected with radiograph and CT can be recognized.

3. Screw protrusion into joint surface can be monitored.

4. Intra-articular soft tissue injury associated with fracture can be evaluated and treated.

Second, during arthroscopy, the authors identified fracture fragments that could not be seen on preoperative radiographs and CT scan (**Fig. 9**). In 248 intra-articular fractures, they arthroscopically could visualize free fracture fragments, including small cancellous bone chips in 23 wrists (9.3%). If these fragments were not removed, they might produce wrist pain because of impingement.

Third, a PLP produces maximal mechanical support when the distal screws are inserted into the subchondral zone of the distal radius. If the plate placement is too distal, screws may protrude into the joint surface. Wrist arthroscopy is able to monitor any screw protrusion into the joint (**Fig. 10**).

Finally, investigating the intra-articular soft tissue situation, using wrist arthroscopy is one great

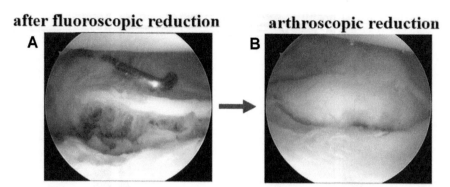

Fig. 8. (*A*) Remaining step-off after fluoroscopic reduction can (*B*) be easily reduced by arthroscopic reduction.

advantage. In 248 intra-articular fractures, SLIL injury was recognized in 81 wrists (32.7%). Of these, grade III or IV instability according to the Geissler classification was recognized in 19 wrists, and pinning or primarily repair was performed in 5 wrists. Traumatic TFCC tear was recognized in 102 wrists (41.1%). The TFCC foveal tear was repaired primarily in 3 wrists.

Outcomes

Two hundred four wrists of 199 patients with intra-articular DRF treated with PART were followed up for more than 1 year. The follow-up period ranged from 12 to 70 months (average 15 months). The age of the 51 men and 148 women ranged from 17 to 85 years old (average age, 62 years old). The fractures consisted of 7 B3, 92 C1, 15 C2,

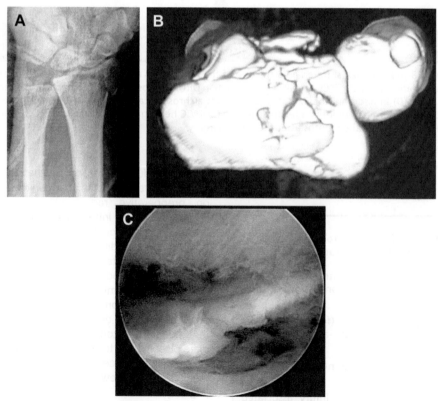

Fig. 9. A huge chondral fragment was not recognized in the (*A*) radiograph and (*B*) CT preoperatively, but was identified (*C*) arthroscopically.

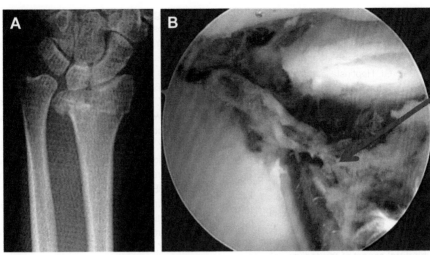

Fig. 10. (*A*) A C3 DRF was provisionally fixed with K-wires and a PLP. (*B*) A K-wire inserted to fix a PLP was protruded into the joint. *Arrow* indicates K-wire for temporary fixation was protruded into the joint.

and 90 C3 fractures. The mean palmar tilt was 7.5° (range: −5° to 25°), radial inclination 26.0° (range: 18°–33°), and ulnar variance 1.4 mm (range: −3° to 8.5 mm). The mean extension range of the wrist was 69° (range: 50°–85°), and the mean flexion range was 64° (range: 35°–85°). The mean pronation range of the forearm was 83° (range: 70°–90°), and the mean supination range was 89° (range: 75°–95°). The mean grip strength was 91.5% (range: 38%–133%) of the opposite side. The final results according to the Mayo Modified Wrist Score were 155 excellent (76.0%), 45 good (22.0%), 3 fair (1.5%), and 1 poor (0.5%). The mean Disabilities of the Arm, Shoulder and Hand

score at final follow-up was 3.4 points (range: 0–33.0) (**Table 1**). There were few complications: 5 gross displacements of the distal fragment, 2 extensor pollicis longus tendon ruptures, and 1 complex regional pain syndrome. The final results of these 8 cases were 4 good, 3 fair, and 1 poor.

REFERENCES

1. Chen NC, Jupiter JB. Current concepts review. Management of distal radius fractures. J Bone Joint Surg 2007;89A:2051–62.
2. Chung KC, Watt AJ, Kotsis SV, et al. Treatment of unstable distal radius fractures with the volar locking plate systems. J Bone Joint Surg 2006; 88A:2687–94.
3. Willis AA, Kutsumi K, Zobitz ME, et al. Internal fixation of dorsally displaced fractures of the distal part of the radius. J Bone Joint Surg 2006;88A: 2411–7.
4. Catalano LW, Barron OA, Glickel SZ. Assessment of articular displacement of distal radius fractures. Clin Orthop 2004;423:79–84.
5. Cheng HS, Hung LK, Ho PC, et al. An analysis of cause and treatment outcome of chronic wrist pain after distal radius fractures. Hand Surg 2008; 13:1–10.
6. Fernandez DL, Geissler WB. Treatment of displaced articular fractures of the radius. J Hand Surg 1991; 16A:375–84.
7. Geissler WB, Freeland AE, Savoie FH, et al. Intracarpal soft-tissue lesions associated with an intra-articular fracture of the distal end of the radius. J Bone Joint Surg 1996;78A:357–65.
8. Knirk JL, Jupiter JB. Intra-articular fractures of the distal end of the radius in young adults. J Bone Joint Surg 1986;68A:647–59.

Table 1		
Final results of 204 intra-articular fractures treated with plate presetting arthroscopic reduction technique		
Radiologic evaluation	Palmar tilt	7.5° (−5°–25°)
	Radial inclination	26.0° (18°–33°)
	Ulnar variance	1.4 mm (−3–8.5 mm)
Functional evaluation	Extension	69° (50°–85°)
	Flexion	64° (35°–85°)
	Pronation	83° (70°–90°)
	Supination	89° (75°–95°)
	Grip strength	91.5% (38%–133%)
MMWS		E: 76.0%, G: 22.0% F: 1.5%, P: 0.5%
DASH		3.4 (0–33.0)

Abbreviations: DASH, disabilities of the arm, shoulder and hand; E, excellent; G, good; F, fair; MMWS, Mayo Modified Wrist Score; P, poor.

9. Lindau T, Arner M, Hagberg L. Intra articular lesions in distal fractures of the radius in young adults. A descriptive arthroscopic study in 50 patients. J Hand Surg 1997;22B:638–43.

10. Mehta JA, Bain GI. Heptinstall. Anatomic reduction of intra-articular fractures of the distal radius. J Bone Joint Surg 2000;82B:79–86.

11. Richards RS, Bennett JD, Roth JH, et al. Arthroscopic diagnosis of intra-articular soft tissue injuries associated with distal radius fractures. J Hand Surg 1997;22A:772–6.

12. Trumble TE, Schmitt SR, Vedder NB. Factors affecting functional outcome of displaced intra-articular distal radius fractures. J Hand Surg 1994; 19A:325–40.

13. Doi K, Hattori Y, Otsuka K, et al. Intra-articular fractures of the distal aspect of the radius: arthroscopically assisted reduction compared with open reduction and internal fixation. J Bone Joint Surg 1999;81A:1093–110.

14. Lindau T. Principles and practice of wrist surgery, the role of wrist arthroscopy in distal radius fractures. Philadelphia: Saunders; 2010.

15. Ruch DS, Vallee J, Poehling GG, et al. Arthroscopic reduction versus fluoroscopic reduction in the management of intra-articular distal radius fractures. Arthroscopy 2004;20:225–30.

16. Abe Y, Tsubone T, Tominaga Y. Plate presetting arthroscopic reduction technique for the distal radius fractures. Tech Hand Up Extrem Surg 2008; 12:136–43.

17. Abe Y, Yoshida K, Tominaga Y. Less invasive surgery with wrist arthroscopy for distal radius fracture. J Orthop Sci 2013;18:398–404.

18. Abe Y. Plate presetting and arthroscopic reduction technique (PART) for treatment of distal radius fractures. Handchir Mikrochir Plast Chir 2014;46: 278–85.

19. del Pinal F. Technical tips for (dry) arthroscopic reduction and internal fixation of distal radius fractures. J Hand Surg 2011;36A:1694–705.

20. Abe Y, Doi K, Hattori Y, et al. A benefit of the volar approach for wrist arthroscopy. Arthroscopy 2003; 19:440–5.

21. Abe Y, Doi K, Hattori Y, et al. Arthroscopic assessment of the volar region of the scapholunate interosseous ligament through a volar portal. J Hand Surg 2003;28A:69–73.

22. Abe Y, Tominaga Y, Yoshida K. Various patterns of traumatic triangular fibrocartilage complex tear. Hand Surg 2012;17:191–8.

Arthroscopic Management of Intra-articular Malunion in Fractures of the Distal Radius

Francisco del Piñal, MD, PhD[a],*, James Clune, MD[b]

KEYWORDS

- Arthroscopic-assisted osteotomy • Inside-out osteotomy • Distal radius malunion
- Arthroscopic arthrolysis • Intra-articular malunion radius

KEY POINTS

- Intra-articular malunions of the distal radius are time sensitive. Delaying treatment for more than 3 months can result in irreversible cartilage damage.
- Arthroscopic treatment of intra-articular malunions allows for better visualization, precision, and preservation of capsular blood supply than open techniques.
- Dry arthroscopy allows for adequate visualization of the wrist joint without excessive edema caused by wet arthroscopy.
- Resection arthroplasty is an acceptable alternative to wrist arthrodesis in certain cases.

INTRODUCTION

Intra-articular malunion after a distal radius fracture can be debilitating. The diagnosis is often elusive and patients may arrive in your office in a delayed fashion. Unfortunately, during the delay, irreversible damage to the cartilaginous surfaces may occur.[1–3] Patients are often diagnosed with complex regional pain syndrome, as there is chronic pain after the distal radius fracture that is in fact a malunion and being missed. This is unfortunate because the malunion, when diagnosed early, can be successfully treated and panarthrodesis can be avoided.

Traditional treatment for the malunion of the articular surfaces after a distal radius fracture was pioneered in the 1990s.[4–9] Intervention involved re-cutting the displaced fragments and reducing them anatomically under fluoroscopic guidance. Osteotomies were made volarly or dorsally based on the location of the malunion. These are considered "outside-in" techniques.

There are reports of excellent results with the outside-in approach.[7–9] However, the capsular window must be made very large to allow for adequate visualization during osteotomy, and even then, it is somewhat blind, especially when treating a volar shear malunion, as the volar ligaments must be maintained. Additionally, once the malunion is reduced, the joint space becomes extremely narrow. Maintenance of reduction can be relied on only with "feeling" and fluoroscopy.[10]

Arthroscopic treatment of intra-articular malunions was developed in an effort to better maintain the blood supply to the surrounding tissue and to attain better visualization of the osteotomy sites. At first, "wet" arthroscopy was implemented; however, visualization remained difficult. Dry arthroscopy resulted in a much better visualization and has become our gold standard for the treatment of distal radius malunions.[11,12]

Disclosure Statement: Nothing to disclose.
[a] Private Practice, Madrid, Spain; [b] Section of Plastic Surgery, Yale School of Medicine, 330 Cedar Street Boardman Building, New Haven, CT 06509, USA
* Corresponding author. Calle Serrano 58-1B, Madrid E-28001, Spain
E-mail addresses: drpinal@drpinal.com; pacopinal@gmail.com

Hand Clin 33 (2017) 669–675
http://dx.doi.org/10.1016/j.hcl.2017.07.004

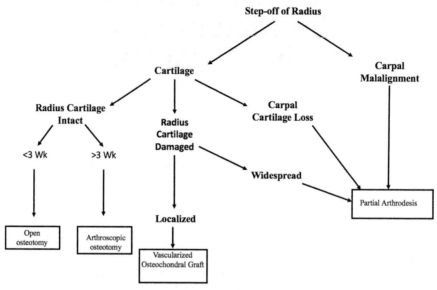

Fig. 1. Decision tree for treatment of intra-articular distal radius malunions.

We describe our arthroscopic method for the treatment of intra-articular malunions of the distal radius.

INDICATIONS AND CONTRAINDICATIONS

Candidates for traditional "outside-in" osteotomies are also eligible for arthroscopic-guided "inside-

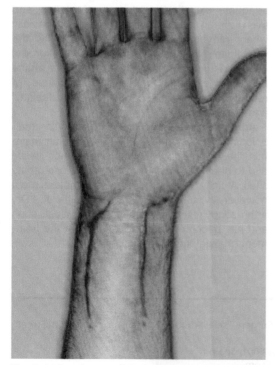

Fig. 2. Volar-ulnar and limited Henry approach for a complex multipiece malunion. (© Dr Piñal, 2010.)

out" osteotomy.[13] A preoperative computed tomography (CT) scan is essential for decision making and operative planning.

Traditionally, a patient with a malunion and an intra-articular step-off of 2 mm or more would be a candidate for an osteotomy, whether there was pain or not.[1] A more controversial approach would include patients with a step-off of 1 mm.[14,15] In fact, if a patient is young and active, a step-off at the lunate or scaphoid fossa will produce symptoms even if it is only a 1-mm step-off. On the other hand, in a low-demand patient or if the step-off is not at the lunate and scaphoid fossa, but in the sagittal crest, it may be possible to avoid a procedure to correct an area that may not undergo much cartilage wearing. These situations should be considered on a case-by-case basis.

Timing is also important. Beyond 6 to 8 weeks after the fracture, the fracture sites are filled up with mature bone rather than scar and granulation tissue, which makes osteotomies more difficult. Some would suggest waiting and would intervene when the patient finally has symptoms of cartilage wear. However, in our opinion, this treatment approach burns the bridge, as the major contraindication to intra-articular osteotomy is the loss of the radius or carpal articular cartilage. Waiting has no benefit, and solutions have to be sought to prevent further cartilage wear. When the radius cartilage is worn but the carpals are fine, our preferred approach is to reconstruct the radius by means of a vascularized osteochondral graft.[16,17] If both the radius and carpal bones have loss of cartilage, resection arthroplasty is our best option and we experienced very pleasing postoperative outcomes.[18] If the damage is widespread, then the only alternative is arthrodesis. In most cases, it is radio-scapho-lunate fusion, which also can be performed arthroscopically.[19–23] Thus, there is no doubt in our opinion that early intervention is superior. However, one should not give up on any patient who presents in a delayed fashion, as surprisingly, some patients still benefit from osteotomy, or other forms of reconstruction (**Fig. 1**).[18]

TECHNIQUE

1. Exsanguinate the arm and stabilize with the table strap.
2. A volar-ulnar incision is used if dealing with a volar-ulnar shear malunion. A Henry approach is used for the typical intra-articular malunion, but both approaches (volar-ulnar and volar-radial) may be needed to have full access of the volar radius in multipiece malunions (**Fig. 2**). With the arm flat on the table, the extra-articular callus is removed. Do not attempt to go directly to the joint at this point. This may result in splitting the cartilage in the wrong location.
3. If a plate is the method of fixation, it can be provisionally placed with a single screw.
4. The hand is placed in traction with the fingers upward. We use the system as shown in **Fig. 3**; 12 to 15 kg of traction is applied. It is important that the hands can be readily placed on the table and quickly put back to the traction system and vice versa. The system we previously described and demonstrated in **Fig. 3**C allows for sterile transfer of the hand between the table and the traction system any time.[11]

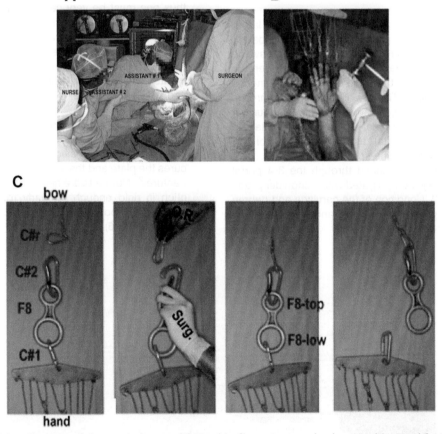

Fig. 3. (*A*) Arrangement of the surgical team. (*B*) Hand in finger traps and volar portal in use. (*C*) Method for maintaining sterility while allowing for rapid transfer of the hand from the vertical traction system to flat on the table, and vice versa. The hand is placed in finger traps. All the components of the vertical traction system are sterile except C#r. The operating room staff connects the hook C#r with the carabiner 2 (C#2) held by the surgeon. After this initial connection, the surgeon can release and reattach carabiner #1 (C#1) from the lower part of the figure of 8 (F8-low) without contamination of the sterile field. C, carabiner; F, figure of 8; OR, operation room staff; Surg, surgeon. (© Dr Piñal, 2006.)

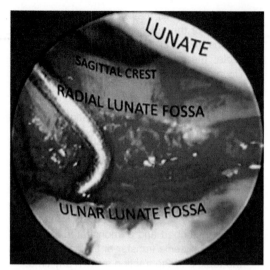

Fig. 4. Shoulder probe evaluation of the step-off and condition of the cartilage. (© Dr Piñal, 2010.)

5. The dorsal 3-4 and 6R portals are made larger than usual to permit passage of the osteotomes. We use a 15′ blade to make transverse incisions in the skin only, and then widen the portal sites with scissors to avoid cutaneous nerve injury. The dry arthroscopic technique must be used, otherwise saline will pour out through the portals. We also always place a volar-radial portal, as described by Doi and colleagues,[14] when necessary (**Fig. 3**B).
6. The scope is placed through the 3-4 portal and the joint is palpated with a shoulder probe (**Fig. 4**). Condition of the cartilage and degree of step-off are evaluated and correlated with the preoperative CT scan.

7. Once the joint has been deemed salvageable, the camera is moved through the 6R portal and the 3-4 and volar-radial portals are used for instrumentation. Debridement is achieved with shavers (2.9-mm gator microblade TM, ref C9961; ConMed Linvatec, Largo, FL). A clear view will be obtained only if all the scar and debris in and around the joint capsule are removed. The joint will need to be flushed with saline to obtain a better view.
8. Bone is cut with a 15° or 30° shoulder periosteal elevator and straight and curved osteotomes (**Fig. 5**) Curved osteotomes are necessary, as straight instruments cannot be manipulated in the tight space of the joint.
9. Osteotomes for osteotomy of volar fragments are typically introduced dorsally and dorsal fragments are treated with a volar approach. The osteotome is used to gently but fully mobilize the displaced fragments. The tendons are all under tension due to the traction, thus one must be very careful not to cut the tendon with the sharp osteotomes. Small curettes, shaver, or burr can be used to trim the newly formed bone, callus, and scar tissue that are prohibiting perfect reduction. Fragments can be hooked with a shoulder probe and pulled upward to restore articular alignment.
10. Once a proper reduction is achieved, the plate is applied on the distal radius. One surgeon holds the bones in position while the other secures the plate and the screws as for an acute fracture.[24] No grafts are necessary, as the fixation is rigid enough for early mobilization. Various methods of fracture stabilization can be used (**Fig. 6**).

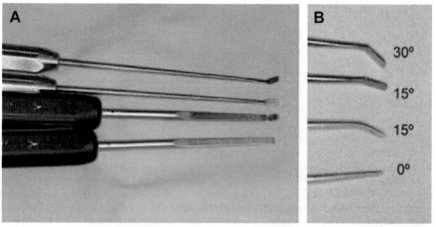

Fig. 5. (*A*) Two shoulder periosteal elevators and 2 osteotomes. (*B*) Different degrees of angulation help for making cuts in a narrow space. (© Dr Piñal, 2009.)

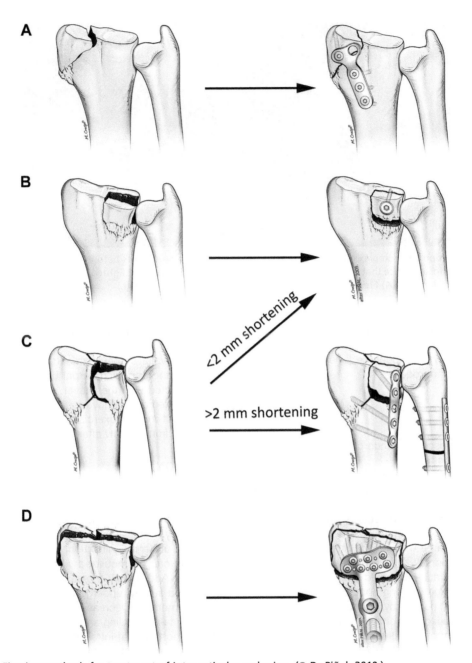

Fig. 6. Fixation methods for treatment of intra-articular malunion. (© Dr Piñal, 2010.)

11. Portals are closed with Steri-Strips. The wrist and hand are immobilized for 48 hours and then gentle range of motion is begun (**Fig. 7**).

ARTHROSCOPIC RESECTION ARTHROPLASTY

In step 6, the surgeon inspects the cartilage to determine if it is severely damaged. Traditionally, if a load-bearing section of the cartilage is destroyed, partial or total wrist arthrodesis may be the procedure of choice. However, we advocate a resection arthroplasty.[18]

An arthroscopic resection arthroplasty relies on removal of the articular portion of the radius at the location of the step-off, and thus the site of arthritis. The remaining radiocarpal joint and non-traumatized cartilage is preserved. The procedure is similar to other motion-preserving procedures, such as 4-corner fusion and proximal row

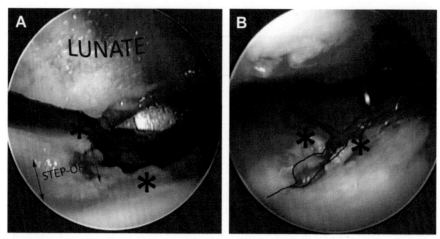

Fig. 7. Correction of a complex old malunion. The asterisks mark the same spots before and after the osteotomy in the lunate fossa. Notice that although step-offs have been leveled, gaps (highlighted by the lines) are unavoidable in old malunions. (*A*) Pre-reduction. (*B*) After reduction. (© Dr. Piñal, 2010.)

carpectomy in that the healthy areas remain to serve as the load-bearing surface.

Our experience with this procedure has been favorable and the procedure is less drastic than a total wrist arthrodesis.

PROCEDURE

1. Dry arthroscopy is undertaken through the 3-4 and 6R portals.
2. The radiocarpal joint is debrided with a 2.9-mm shaver until enough space is created to visualize the joint surface.
3. Thick adhesions and scar is encountered and the purpose of aggressive debridement is to create a large working space. Additionally, the natural dorsal sulcus between the capsule and proximal row should be recreated.
4. With a large working space, the articular surface can be clearly assessed. The step-off and denuded area should be clearly visualized.
5. A 2.9-mm burr is used to resect the section of the intra-articular step-off (**Fig. 8**).

6. The depth of resection should be approximately 0.5 mm below the normal joint surface. Care is taken to avoid the volar rim of the radius and the volar carpal ligaments. The mirror image on the opposing carpal bone also should be resected with the shaver. All debris should be irrigated and removed.
7. Range-of-motion exercises should be implemented immediately after the surgery.

DISCUSSION

Distal radius intra-articular malunions must be precisely evaluated. Our opinion is that the most accurate method of evaluation is with dry wrist arthroscopy. The articular deformity is clearly delineated under magnification, and small irregular fragments can be mobilized with delicate instrumentation. Additionally, the capsule and thus fragment blood supply, undergoes minimal disruption with this method. Decreased capsular disruption allows for faster healing and earlier mobilization.

It is important that intra-articular malunions be treated expeditiously. After 3 months, there may

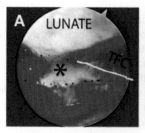
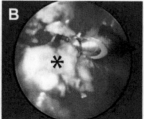
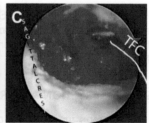

Fig. 8. (*A*) Damage to lunate caused by the protruding volar-ulnar fragment (*asterisk*). (*B*) Debridement with 2.9-mm burr. (*C*) Fifty percent of the anterior lunate fossa has been removed. (© Dr Piñal, 2012.)

be severe cartilaginous damage and thus the realignment of fragments may be of little use. If a patient presents after 3 months, it would be worth evaluating arthroscopically before intervention to gain a better understanding of the damage caused by the prolonged altered joint mechanics. If the cartilage in areas of significant carpal contact is preserved, osteotomies may be undertaken. Otherwise, a reconstructive osteochondral graft or partial arthrodesis should be considered.

REFERENCES

1. Knirk JL, Jupiter JB. Intra-articular fractures of the distal end of the radius in young adults. J Bone Joint Surg Am 1986;68:647–59.
2. Bradway JK, Amadio PC, Cooney WP. Open reduction and internal fixation of displaced, comminuted intra-articular fractures of the distal end of the radius. J Bone Joint Surg Am 1989;71A:839–47.
3. Catalano LW III, Cole RJ, Gelberman RH, et al. Displaced intra-articular fractures of the distal aspect of the radius: long term results in young adults after open reduction and internal fixation. J Bone Joint Surg Am 1997;79A:1290–302.
4. Fernandez DL. Reconstructive procedures for malunion and traumatic arthritis. Orthop Clin North Am 1993;24:341–63.
5. Gonzalez del Pino J, Nagy L, Gonzalez Hernandez E, et al. Intraarticular osteotomies for complex malunited fractures: indications and surgical technique. Rev Ortop Traumatol 2000;44: 406–17. [in Spanish].
6. Marx RG, Axelrod TS. Intraarticular osteotomy of distal radial malunions. Clin Orthop 1996;327:152–7.
7. Prommersberger KJ, Ring D, del Pino J, et al. Corrective osteotomy for intra-articular malunion of the distal part of the radius: surgical technique. J Bone Joint Surg Am 2006;88A(Suppl 1):202–11.
8. Ring D, Prommersberger KJ, González del Pino J, et al. Corrective osteotomy for intra-articular malunion of the distal part of the radius. J Bone Joint Surg Am 2005;87:1503–9.
9. Saffar P. Treatment of distal radius radial intraarticular malunions. In: Saffar PH, Cooney WP III, editors. Fractures of the distal radius. London: Martin Dunitz; 1995. p. 249–58.
10. Lutsky K, Boyer MI, Steffen JA, et al. Arthroscopic assessment of intra-articular distal radius fractures after open reduction and internal fixation from a volar approach. J Hand Surg 2008;33A:476–84.
11. del Piñal F, Garcia-Bernal FJ, Delgado J, et al. Correction of malunited intra-articular distal radius fractures with an inside-out osteotomy technique. J Hand Surg 2006;31A:1029.
12. del Piñal F, Garcia-Bernal FJ, Pisani D, et al. Dry arthroscopy of the wrist: surgical technique. J Hand Surg 2007;32A:119–23.
13. del Piñal F, Cagigal L, Garcia-Bernal FJ, et al. Arthroscopically guided osteotomy for management of intra-articular distal radius malunions. J Hand Surg Am 2010;35(3):392–7.
14. Doi K, Hattori Y, Otsuka K, et al. Intra-articular fractures of the distal aspect of the radius: arthroscopically assisted reduction compared with open reduction and internal fixation. J Bone Joint Surg Am 1999;81A:1093–110.
15. Trumble TE, Schmitt SR, Vedder NB. Factors affecting functional outcome of displaced intra-articular distal radius fractures. J Hand Surg 1994; 19A:325–40.
16. del Piñal F, Garcia-Bernal JF, Delgado J, et al. Reconstruction of the distal radius facet by a free vascularized osteochondral autograft: anatomic study and report of a case. J Hand Surg 2005; 30A:1200–10.
17. del Piñal F, Klausmeyer M, Moraleda E, et al. Vascularized graft from the metatarsal base for reconstructing major osteochondral distal radius defects. J Hand Surg Am 2013;38(10):1883–95.
18. del Piñal F, Klausmeyer M, Thams C, et al. Arthroscopic resection arthroplasty for malunited intra-articular distal radius fractures. J Hand Surg Am 2012;37(12):2447–55.
19. Ho PC. Arthroscopic partial wrist fusion. Tech Hand Up Extrem Surg 2008;12(4):242–65.
20. del Piñal F, Tandioy-Delgado F. (Dry) arthroscopic partial wrist arthrodesis: tips and tricks. Handchir Mikrochir Plast Chir 2014;46(5):300–6.
21. del Piñal F. Reconstruction of the distal radius facet by a free vascularized osteochondral autograft. In: Slutsky DJ, Osterman AL, editors. Fractures and injuries of the distal radius and carpus. Philadelphia: Saunders; 2009. Available at: www.expertconsultbook.com/W9.
22. Saffar P. Radio-lunate arthrodesis for distal radial intraarticular malunion. J Hand Surg 1996;21B:14–20.
23. Garcia-Elias M, Lluch A, Ferreres A, et al. Treatment of radiocarpal degenerative osteoarthritis by radioscapholunate arthrodesis and distal scaphoidectomy. J Hand Surg 2005;30A:8–15.
24. Del Piñal F. Technical tips for (dry) arthroscopic reduction and internal fixation of distal radius fractures. J Hand Surg Am 2011;36:1694–705.

Scaphoid Union
The Role of Wrist Arthroscopy

Jeff Ecker, BMedSc (Hons), MBBS, FRACS[a,b,c,*]

KEYWORDS

- Scaphoid • Arthroscopy • Union • Nonunion

KEY POINTS

- Radiographs and computed tomography scans do not always provide sufficient information to know whether a scaphoid fracture or bone graft has united.
- Arthroscopic surgery provides additional information that assists in determining whether a fracture or bone graft has united, partially united or has united.
- When to use wrist arthroscopy and how to perform wrist arthroscopy to evaluate scaphoid fracture and scaphoid nonunion is described.

RATIONALE

It can be difficult to know whether a scaphoid fracture or bone graft has united. In some cases, the information obtained from radiographs, computed tomography (CT) scans, and MRI scans may not be enough to make a confident diagnosis of scaphoid union. This problem affects both scaphoid fractures and scaphoid nonunions that have been bone grafted. When this occurs, arthroscopic examination of the fracture or bone graft provides additional information to diagnose whether the scaphoid has united, partially united, or has not united.

Radiographs often do not show enough detail to confidently know whether union has occurred. A double-line sign on MRI represents the fracture line coupled with a revascularization front and is nearly always associated with union.[1] MRI imaging does not clearly show whether bone union has occurred. Internal fixation devices (screws, K-wires, or both) create interference and make it difficult to see the fracture or bone graft site clearly.

Trabecular bone bridging on CT studies is currently the best way to evaluate scaphoid union. It is usually possible to define scaphoid union and nonunion, but there is an intermediate state of partial union for which it is still uncertain how much trabecular bridging is required and if the trabecular bridging is mechanically strong enough to allow return to full activity.[2,3] It has been postulated that if 50% of the fracture has been bridged by trabeculae then the fracture or bone graft can be considered to have united.[2,3] Very rarely, bone may appear to be bridging the fracture site, but it is the cancellous bone of the proximal pole impacting into the cancellous bone of the distal scaphoid, which can give the impression of union (see case 3).

When it is uncertain whether a scaphoid fracture or a bone grafted internally fixed scaphoid has united, the options are limited and comprise of the following:

1. Continue wrist immobilization in a splint until there is interval change in the appearance of the CT scan demonstrating increased trabeculae crossing the scaphoid fracture or bone graft.
2. Remove the splint, mobilize the wrist, and perform follow-up CT scans to ensure the scaphoid has united. In other words, perform a trial of motion.
3. Conduct an arthroscopic examination of the midcarpal surface of the scaphoid to probe

[a] Western Orthopaedic Clinic, Perth, Western Australia, Australia; [b] Hand and Upper Limb Centre, Perth, Western Australia, Australia; [c] Curtin University of Technology, Perth, Western Australia, Australia
* 25 Queenslea Drive, Claremont, Western Australia 6010, Australia.
E-mail address: rooms@ecker.com.au

Hand Clin 33 (2017) 677–686
http://dx.doi.org/10.1016/j.hcl.2017.07.001
0749-0712/17/© 2017 Elsevier Inc. All rights reserved.

hand.theclinics.com

and manipulate the fracture or bone graft to determine if it is stable or mobile.

If at arthroscopy the scaphoid is stable and trabeculae can be seen crossing the fracture or bone graft on CT scan, then the options are:

1. Remove the splint and mobilize the wrist.
2. Immobilize the wrist in a thermoplastic splint or cast for a longer period of time and perform a further CT scan to assess if there is an interval increase in the amount of bone trabeculae bridging the scaphoid fracture or bone graft.
3. If there is no internal fixation then consider internal fixation of the scaphoid with a headless compression screw.
4. If the scaphoid has been internally fixed and there is a solid fibrous nonunion that is stable, the nonunion can be arthroscopically excised leaving around the internal fixation and performing an arthroscopic top-up graft (see case 4).

Alternatively, if the scaphoid fracture is unstable there is a nonunion of the scaphoid, and if it has been internally fixed, the fixation devices are loose. Although this can pose a difficult surgical problem, arthroscopy simplifies management because the diagnosis is clear.

SURGICAL TECHNIQUE

There is often extensive arthrofibrosis obscuring the scaphoid fracture or bone graft. This fibrotic tissue has to be removed with a shaver to get a good view of the fracture or bone graft site. To complicate matters, the bone is often soft and incorrect introduction of arthroscopic instruments can damage the cartilage and carpal bones. The technique involves the use of a wrist tower to apply traction across the wrist. A 1.9 mm arthroscope is inserted into the midcarpal joint using an ulnar midcarpal joint portal. A radial midcarpal joint portal is made to insert the shaver, probe, and a burr if required. The position of the radial midcarpal joint portal is important. To place the radial midcarpal joint portal in the optimal position, an 18-gauge needle is inserted while viewing through the ulnar midcarpal portal. Once the needle can be inserted along the line of the fracture, the radial midcarpal joint portal can be made confidently knowing that the instruments can easily access the entire fracture.

Case Studies

Case 1
A 36-year-old man presented acutely with a trans-scaphoid perilunate fracture dislocation that was arthroscopically reduced and internally fixed with 3.0 mm headless compression screw and an anti-rotation K-wire. Three months after surgery it was uncertain whether the scaphoid fracture had united (**Fig. 1**).

The antirotation K-wire was removed and the scaphoid examined arthroscopically (**Fig. 2**). The fracture was viewed from the midcarpal surface of the scaphoid and was stable on probing under direct vision.

The patient was advised to remove his splint, start a wrist proprioceptive exercise program, and use his wrist normally.

Eighteen months after surgery a CT scan showed increased bone crossing the fracture site and a united scaphoid (**Fig. 3**).

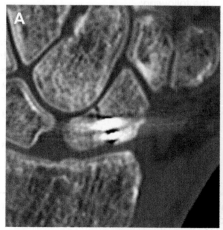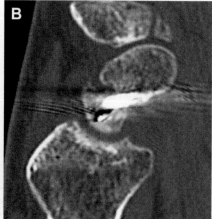

Fig. 1. (*A*, *B*) Three months after arthroscopic reduction and internal fixation of a trans-scaphoid perilunate fracture dislocation with compression screw and antirotation K-wire. A small amount of bone can be seen bridging the scaphoid fracture and it is uncertain whether the fracture has united.

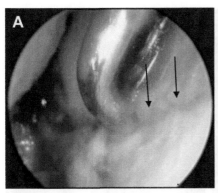
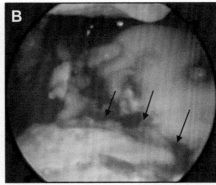

Fig. 2. (A, B) The fracture (*arrows*) was solid on probing and it felt like there was bone bridging the fracture site.

Summary In this case, on CT scans it was uncertain if there was a partial scaphoid union or nonunion. Arthroscopic surgery revealed that the scaphoid fracture and screw were stable. Based on this information, the patient was instructed to remove his splint, start therapy and exercises, and use his wrist. Follow-up imaging demonstrated solid scaphoid union.

Case 2

A 24-year-old man presented with a nonunion of the proximal one-third of the scaphoid and a dorsal intercalated segment instability deformity (**Fig. 4**). It was thought that this was the result of an injury that occurred 15 months before his initial presentation.

The nonunion was arthroscopically excised, reduced, bone grafted, and internally fixed with 4 by 1.2 mm K-wires inserted from distal to proximal into the scaphoid. Fourteen weeks after the internal fixation and bone grafting it was uncertain whether the scaphoid had united (**Fig. 5**).

Arthroscopic examination of the fracture revealed that the midcarpal joint surface of the fracture was filled with vascular tissue (**Fig. 6**). K-wires were removed.

The scaphoid moved as an integral unit after removal of the K-wires and the bone graft fracture site felt like it was filled with bone on probing. An exchange screw was inserted percutaneously from distal to proximal through the same incision that was used to remove the K-wires. This was done under image intensification and arthroscopic visualization. Postoperatively, the patient removed his splint, started a proprioceptive wrist exercise program, and used his wrist normally. Radiographs at 15 months demonstrated solid scaphoid union (**Fig. 7**).

Summary Although the CT scan was suggestive of partial union of the bone graft site, this was uncertain. Wrist arthroscopy revealed that the bone graft scaphoid complex was stable after removal of the K-wires. An exchange headless compression

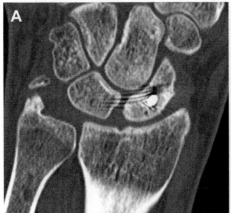
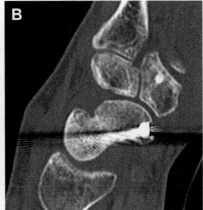

Fig. 3. (A, B) CT scan 18 months after arthroscopic reduction and internal fixation showing interval increase in bone crossing the scaphoid fracture demonstrating a solidly united scaphoid.

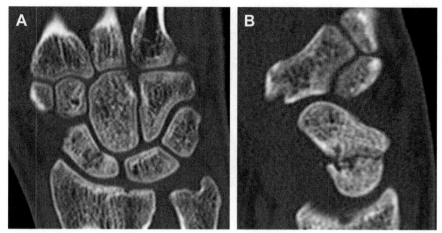

Fig. 4. (*A, B*) A CT scan showing a 15-month old nonunion of the proximal one-third of the scaphoid with a flexion deformity at the nonunion site.

screw was inserted, the patient removed his thermoplastic splint, started an exercise program, and used his wrist normally. Follow-up imaging demonstrated solid union of the bone graft.

Case 3

A 26-year-old presented with a 6-month old transscaphoid dorsal perilunate fracture dislocation (**Fig. 8**). The carpal dislocation and the scaphoid

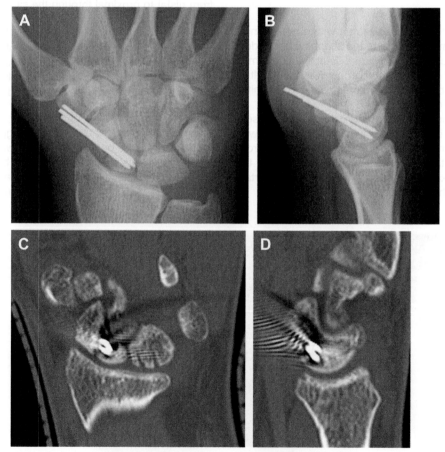

Fig. 5. (*A, B*) Radiographs and (*C, D*) CT scans show the fracture site 14-weeks after internal fixation of the scaphoid with 4 × 1.2 mm K-wires. It is uncertain whether the fracture has united.

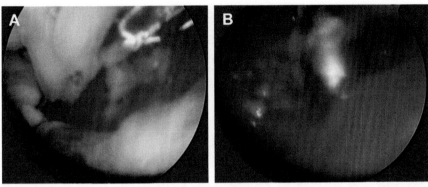

Fig. 6. (*A*) Vascular tissue in the fracture site. (*B*) After removal of K-wires, debridement of the fracture site and probing, the scaphoid moved as an integral unit.

were reduced using a bone distractor inserted into the distal shaft of the radius and the index finger metacarpal, and the scaphoid was internally fixed with a headless compression screw and an antirotation K-wire. In addition, the midcarpal joint was neutralized with K-wires inserted from the scaphoid into the distal carpal row, from the triquetrum into the proximal carpal row, and from the lunate into the distal carpal row. The operation was performed using an open dorsal approach (**Fig. 9**).

Seven months after the operation, the scaphoid had shortened at the fracture site as evidenced by the proximal end of the headless compression screw protruding through the proximal pole of the scaphoid and the distal end of the screw protruding through the distal scaphoid. There appeared to be bone crossing the fracture but it was uncertain whether the scaphoid had united (**Fig. 10**).

Wrist arthroscopy was performed and the scaphoid fracture identified with a probe from the midcarpal surface of the scaphoid. Once the fibrous tissue was excised using a shaver, it was clear that the scaphoid had not united and the headless compression screw and antirotation wire were loose (**Fig. 11**).

The headless compression screw and K-wire were removed using an open dorsal approach and a 1 cm dorsal wrist arthrotomy over the proximal pole of the scaphoid. The nonunion was arthroscopically excised, bone grafted, and internally fixed with 3 percutaneous K-wires inserted from a distal to proximal direction (**Fig. 12**).

The scaphoid fracture united 10 weeks after the arthroscopic bone graft and internal fixation (**Fig. 13**).

Summary In this case, it was uncertain whether the scaphoid fracture had partially united or

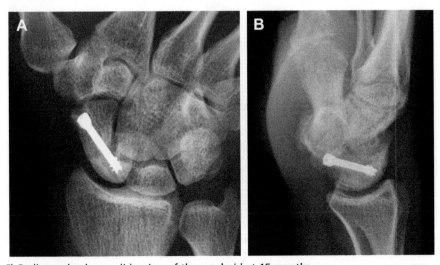

Fig. 7. (*A, B*) Radiographs show solid union of the scaphoid at 15 months.

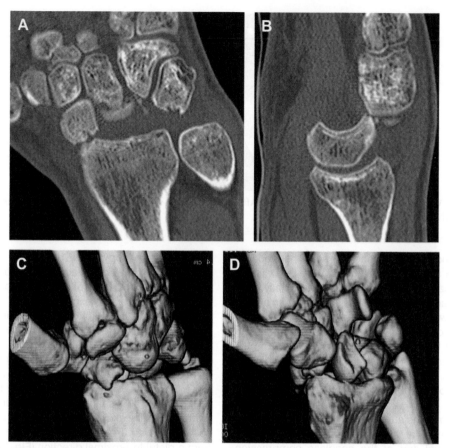

Fig. 8. (*A*, *B*) CT scan of 6-month-old dorsal trans-scaphoid perilunate fracture dislocation. (*C*, *D*) Three-dimensional rendering CT of 6-month-old dorsal trans-scaphoid perilunate fracture dislocation.

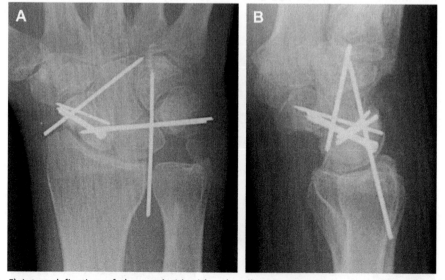

Fig. 9. (*A*, *B*) Internal fixation of the scaphoid with a headless compression screw, antirotation K-wire. The scaphoid fixation was neutralized with K-wires inserted from the scaphoid into the distal carpal row, the triquetrum, lunate and scaphoid, and from the lunate into the hamate.

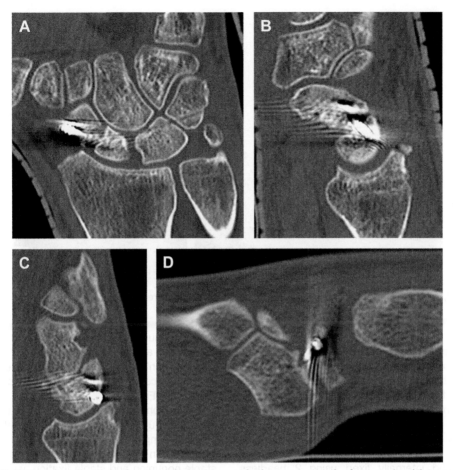

Fig. 10. (*A, B*) CT scan at 7 months showing what appears to be bone crossing the fracture site. (*C*) Screw protruding through the proximal pole of the scaphoid. (*D*) Screw protruding through the distal scaphoid.

whether there was a nonunion. Arthroscopic wrist surgery resolved the uncertainty by identifying an impacted nonunion with loose fixation. Rarely, a nonunion can shorten and impact such that the proximal and distal surfaces of the fracture compress and simulate union on CT scan. Arthroscopic bone graft and internal fixation resulted in scaphoid union.

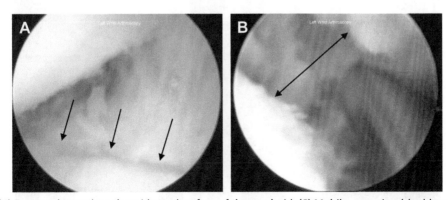

Fig. 11. (*A*) Fracture (*arrows*) on the midcarpal surface of the scaphoid. (*B*) Mobile nonunion (*double arrow*) after debridement of the fibrous tissue.

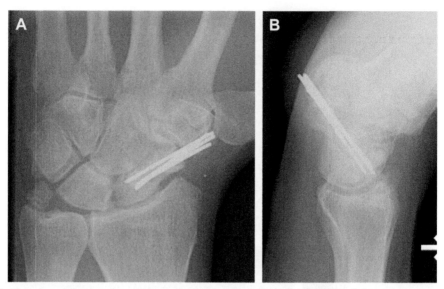

Fig. 12. (*A*, *B*) Radiographs showing arthroscopic bone graft and K-wire fixation of the nonunion.

Case 4

A 17-year-old elite footballer fractured his scaphoid at the junction of the middle and proximal one-third and the fracture was treated in a cast. The fracture did not unite.

An open reduction and internal fixation and bone graft was performed that did not unite. A second operation was performed, the fixation was removed, the scaphoid nonunion was bone grafted and internally fixed using 2 headless compression screws inserted from a proximal to distal direction. The fracture did not unite and he was referred for a free vascularized medial femoral bone graft (**Fig. 14**).

Arthroscopic examination revealed a stable fibrous union. The fixation was not removed, the

fibrous nonunion was excised using a 3.5 mm burr to cut around the shafts of the 2 headless compression screws and the bone defect was arthroscopically packed with iliac crest cancellous bone graft (**Fig. 15**).

The scaphoid united 10 weeks after arthroscopic top-up graft (**Fig. 16**) and he returned to playing competitive football 3 months after the operation. In this case, arthroscopy confirmed a stable nonunion and stable fixation, which meant that the fibrous scaphoid nonunion could be excised and iliac crest cancellous bone graft compressed around the screws.

Summary Wrist arthroscopy confirmed that there was a stable fibrous union, bone was not bridging

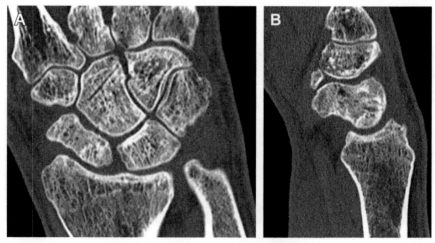

Fig. 13. (*A*, *B*) CT scan of the united scaphoid after removal of the K-wires.

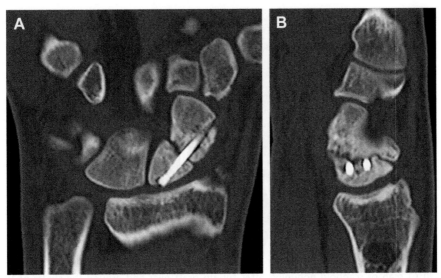

Fig. 14. (*A, B*) Nonunited scaphoid with 2 headless compression screws. There was no lucency around the screws indicating that screws were not loose.

the fracture, and the internal fixation was stable. The patient had missed 2 years of competitive football and wanted to return to playing football as soon as possible. Based on the arthroscopic findings, the nonunion was excised and a bone graft performed, leaving the screws in situ. The scaphoid united soundly 10 weeks after the top-up bone graft.

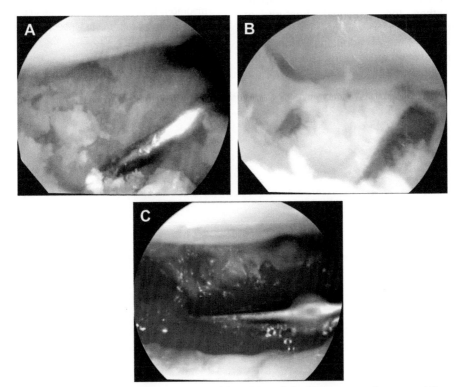

Fig. 15. (*A*) The probe identifying the nonunion site. (*B*) Excision of the fibrous nonunion around the screws. The bone was excised with a 3.5 mm burr cutting around the shafts of the headless compression screws. (*C*) Cancellous iliac crest bone graft was inserted and compressed into the nonunion.

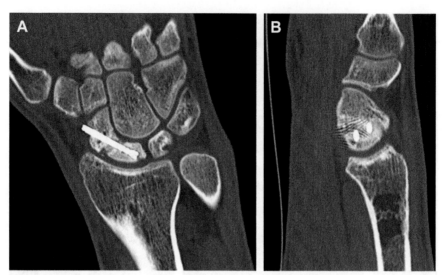

Fig. 16. (*A, B*) CT scan of scaphoid nonunion after top-up graft over and around the shafts of the headless compression screws.

SUMMARY

In most cases, scaphoid fracture or bone graft union can be identified on CT scan and the use of wrist arthroscopy to confirm scaphoid fracture or bone graft union is unnecessary.

When CT imaging does not clearly demonstrate whether the scaphoid fracture or bone graft has united, arthroscopic wrist surgery can be used to obtain additional information to determine whether the fracture or bone graft has united, partially united, or has not united.

REFERENCES

1. Hackney LA, Dodds SD. Assessment of scaphoid fracture healing. Curr Rev Musculoskelet Med 2011; 4(1):16–22.

2. Grewal R, Suh N, MacDermid J. Use of computed tomography to predict union and time to union in acute scaphoid fractures treated nonoperatively. J Hand Surg Am 2013;38(5):872–7.

3. Singh HP, Forward D, Davis TR, et al. Partial union of acute scaphoid fractures. J Hand Surg Br 2005;30(5): 440–5.

Arthroscopic Scapholunate Ligament Reconstruction, Volar and Dorsal Reconstruction

Fernando Corella, PhD[a,b,c,]*, Miguel Del Cerro, MD[b],
Montserrat Ocampos, PhD[a,b], Clara Simon de Blas, PhD[d],
Ricardo Larrainzar-Garijo, PhD[a,c]

KEYWORDS

- Scapholunate instability • Wrist arthroscopy • Scapholunate ligament • Carpal instability

KEY POINTS

- Patients suitable for this surgery should fulfill 3 criteria: complete tear of the scapholunate (SL) ligament, easily reducible instability, and presence of clinical symptoms.
- Contraindications for this technique are the presence of degenerative lesions or other associated ligament injuries.
- The technique reconstructs both the dorsal and volar portion of the SL ligament with a 3-mm graft from the flexor carpi radialis tendon.
- The graft is fixed to the scaphoid and lunate tunnels with interference screws.
- Early mobilization rehabilitation protocols include midcarpal motion exercise at 2 weeks, full range of motion exercise at 4 weeks, and proprioception exercises at 6 weeks after the surgery.

 Video content accompanies this article at http://www.hand.theclinics.com/.

INTRODUCTION: NATURE OF THE PROBLEM

Scapholunate (SL) ligament instability is the most common form of carpal instability. Patients usually have dorsal wrist pain, decreased grip strength, and impaired wrist function. Untreated SL instability can result in a predictable sequence of degenerative changes in the wrist.[1]

SL instability can be treated by an arthroscopic or an open technique. Arthroscopic SL ligament debridement, thermal shrinkage, and SL pinning were reported with the benefit of limited damage to healthy soft tissues.[2–5] For SL ligament reconstruction, a wide variety of open procedures have been described.[6–8] All of the open procedures required a wide dorsal dissection, which resulted in considerable damage to the soft tissues and a reduction in joint mobility.

Conflict of Interest: F. Corella, M. Ocampos and M. Del Cerro are consultant in Arthrex Company.
Disclosures: None of the authors of the article receive funding, grants, or in-kind support in support of the research or the preparation of the article.
[a] Orthopedic and Trauma Department, Infanta Leonor University Hospital, C/ Gran Vía del Este N° 80, Madrid 28031, Spain; [b] Hand Surgery Unit, Beata María Ana Hospital, C/Doctor Esquerdo, 83, Madrid 28007, Spain; [c] Surgery Department, School of Medicine, Complutense University of Madrid, Plaza de Ramón y Cajal S/N, Madrid 28040, Spain; [d] Computer Sciences and Statistics Department, Rey Juan Carlos University of Madrid, Calle Tulipán, s/n, Madrid 28933, Spain
* Corresponding author. C/Gran Vía Del Este N° 80, Madrid 28031, Spain.
E-mail address: fernando.corella@gmail.com

hand.theclinics.com

Arthroscopic SL ligament reconstruction was described in 2011[9,10] and combined the advantages of arthroscopic (minimally invasive surgery) and open techniques (reconstruction of the ligament). It serves the 3-fold purpose of anatomic reconstruction, avoidance of open surgery and detachment of the joint capsule, and a reliable and sturdy reconstruction for early mobilization.

ANATOMIC RECONSTRUCTION

The SL interosseous ligament consists of 3 subregions: the dorsal, palmar, and proximal (listed in order of decreasing strength).[11–13] The dorsal part was thought to be the strongest and different techniques of dorsal SL ligament reconstruction were commonly described. However, these reconstruction with only 1 dorsal fixation point between the 2 bones cannot preclude SL volar widening or sagittal rotation (**Fig. 1**). With an additional reconstruction on the volar side, the second strongest SL portion is also restored and 2 fixation points between the 2 bones can be created. Reconstructing both the dorsal and the volar SL portions becomes logical biomechanically and is gaining attention in recent years.[10,14–17]

In addition to restoring the portions of the SL ligament, restoring the scaphoid alignment is also important. Short and colleagues[18,19] demonstrated that the scaphoid bone was not only flexed, but also pronated in SL instability. Scaphoid pronation creates a static stress at the dorsum of the wrist. It also produces a dynamic stress as the scaphoid is dorsally translated over the dorsal rim of the radius at wrist extension and radial deviation. This explains why patients with SL instability would have dorsal wrist pain, especially with wrist hyperextension or Watson's stress test, and it explains why degenerative changes begin not in a radial styloid but in the dorsum of the scaphoid fossa. This dorsal displacement over the dorsal rim of the radius can be checked arthroscopically with the arthroscopic scaphoid 3-dimensional test.[20] An anatomic reconstruction should not only reconstruct the SL ligament (both dorsal and volar), but also supinate the scaphoid, and prevent dorsal translation of the scaphoid over the scaphoid fossa.

AVOIDANCE OF OPEN SURGERY AND DETACHMENT OF THE JOINT CAPSULE

Arthroscopic SL reconstruction is a minimally invasive technique that obviates the need for extensive open dissection and capsulotomy (**Fig. 2**). Postoperative fibrosis, scarring, and stiffness are

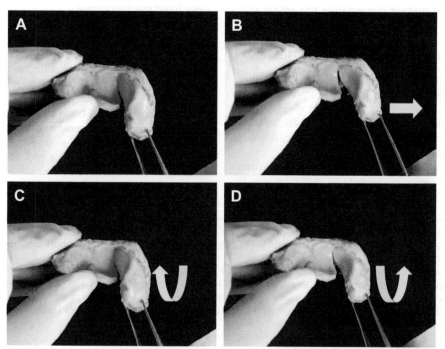

Fig. 1. (*A*) Right wrist specimen in which the dorsal portion of the scapholunate ligament was maintained. (*B–D*) With only a single connection between the 2 bones, neither volar opening nor sagittal rotation could be avoided.

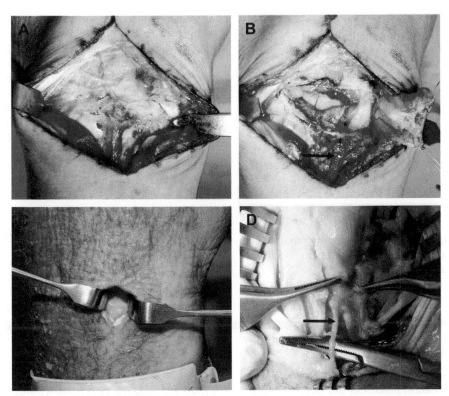

Fig. 2. (*A, C*) Comparison of the size of the surgical wounds between a classical dorsal approach and the approach in arthroscopic scapholunate ligament reconstruction. (*B, D*) Surgical extensiveness in an open capsulotomy. The *black arrow* points to the posterior interosseous nerve (PIN). The PIN is sectioned during the dorsal approach and is preserved during arthroscopic SL ligament reconstruction (dissection performed in a cadaver specimen).

minimized in this way. The dorsal intercarpal ligament is not detached from the bones, which is one of the most important SL secondary stabilizers. Its injury has been shown to result in an evolution of a dynamic instability into a static one.[21,22]

In addition, with this technique, the posterior interosseous nerve (PIN) is preserved. The abductor pollicis longus, extensor carpi radialis, flexor carpi radialis (FCR), and flexor carpi ulnaris are important dynamic stabilizers of the SL joint.[23–28] The PIN is the main nerve of these dynamic stabilizers.[26,29,30] Preservation of the PIN is important to maintain function in these muscles. Cadaveric studies of this arthroscopic technique demonstrated that the damage to the soft tissues was minimal and no PIN was injured in any of the specimens[9] (see **Fig. 2**). Ho and associates[16] and Carratalá and coworkers[31] have also performed SL ligament reconstruction without violation of the joint capsule.

RELIABLE AND STURDY RECONSTRUCTION FOR EARLY MOBILIZATION

As in knee or ankle ligament reconstruction surgeries, with arthroscopic SL reconstruction the

graft is fixed directly onto the bone with interferential screws. A K-wire is not used. This allows midcarpal motion in 15 days and a full range of motion in 4 weeks.

In 2011, three of our authors described an anatomic study and the technique of arthroscopic reconstruction of the dorsal portion of the SL ligament and the secondary stabilizers.[9] In 2013, a modification of this procedure with an additional volar portion of SL reconstruction was published.[10] We now elaborate on the "surgical tips" and technical modifications to make arthroscopic SL ligament reconstruction easier. Clinical and radiologic results of the first 27 patients are demonstrated.

INDICATIONS AND CONTRAINDICATIONS

Patients who have the following 3 criteria are suitable candidates for arthroscopic SL reconstruction (**Box 1**):

1. Arthroscopically complete SL ligament tear, that is, European Wrist Arthroscopy Society classification grade IIIC, IV, or V SL lesions.[32]

Box 1
Indications and contraindications of arthroscopic ligamentoplasty

Indications

Complete lesion of the scapholunate ligament

Very easily reducible instability

With clinical impact

Contraindications

Presence of degenerative lesions

Presence of associated ligament injuries

2. Very easily reducible instability, that is, the scaphoid can be easily reduced and positioned by an arthroscopic probe.
3. The presence of clinical symptoms, that is, pain, a decrease in the grip strength, and/or impairment of wrist function.

Patients who have the following conditions are contraindicated for the surgery:

1. The presence of degenerative lesions, especially chondral lesions in the dorsal scaphoid fossa, that is, scaphoid lunate advanced collapse stage 1 changes. These lesions are difficult to be diagnosed with MRI or radiographs. Their presence should always be verified with arthroscopy.
2. The presence of associated ligament injuries, especially lunotriquetral injury. Combined SL and lunotriquetral lesions make the lunate bone floating,[33] which can be identified by the rocking chair sign.[34]

SURGICAL TECHNIQUE AND PROCEDURE
Preoperative Planning

Careful preoperative history taking and physical examination are essential. Patients have dorsal wrist pain at the SL interval and dorsal scaphoid fossa that worsen with wrist hyperextension. Grip strength is weak. The scaphoid shift test, resisted finger extension test, and SL ballottement test are positive.[35] Imaging studies include radiographs—posteroanterior (PA) and lateral views—and a dynamic radiograph with clenched fist. MRI is also useful. Diagnostic arthroscopic assessment is essential to confirm that arthroscopic SL reconstruction is indicated (Video 1).

Preparation and Patient Positioning

The operation is performed under regional anesthesia (axillary block) or general anesthesia with a pneumatic tourniquet placed at the upper arm close to the armpit. The patient is placed supine with the affected arm on a hand table. The wrist is maintained in vertical traction during the whole procedure. The traction tower commonly used is an Arc Wrist Tower (Acumed, Hillsboro, OR), which maintains a vertical traction and leaves the volar side of the wrist free. Positioning and set-up is shown in **Fig. 3**. The C-arm is entered parallel to the floor from the volar side of the wrist. With the suspended hand in pronation or supination, a PA or lateral view is easily obtained.

Surgical Approach

Arthroscopic dorsal radiocarpal portals (3/4 and 6R) and dorsal midcarpal portals (radial and ulnar) are used. Two 1.5-cm longitudinal incisions are made. One is dorsal central overlying the fourth extensor tendon compartment, another is volar central, which is the same incision and approach used for the volar central portal.[36] Two more incisions are used to retrieve a tendon graft. One is overlying FCR and scaphoid (radial distal), another one is 10 cm proximally over the FCR tendon (radial proximal; **Fig. 4**).

Surgical Procedure

The surgical technique can be divided into 5 steps (Video 2).

Step 1: Bone tunnels

The tunnels are created with a 1 mm K-wire through the 3/4 portal. This step consumes time and it is difficult to insert such a small K-wire through the portal. A 14-G abbocath needle is helpful to guide the K-wire insertion. The exact position of the K-wire should be from the origin of the SL ligament on the proximal scaphoid to the scaphoid tubercle (**Fig. 5**). Because the insertion point is not exactly under the portal site, the abbocath needle is inserted through the portal into the joint and is slid distally over the scaphoid. Once the position is confirmed, the tip of the needle is fixed into the bone and the direction is adjusted under fluoroscopic guidance. When the direction is satisfactory in both the PA and lateral view, a 1-mm K-wire is introduced through the abbocath needle by another surgeon (**Fig. 6**).

A 1.5-cm longitudinal incision (dorsal central) is made over the fourth extensor compartment between the 3/4 and 6R portals. This incision is directly over the lunate bone. The extensor retinaculum is opened longitudinally. Extensor

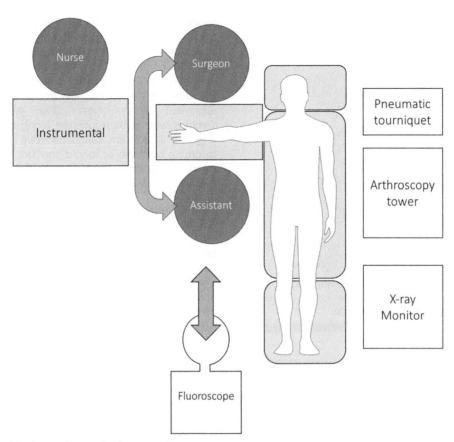

Fig. 3. Positioning and setup in the operation room.

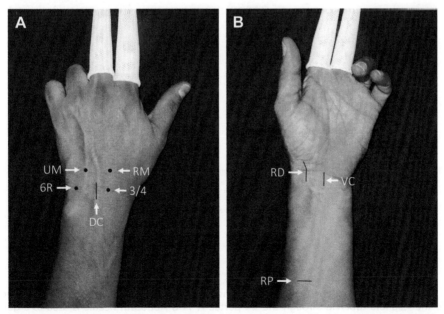

Fig. 4. (*A, B*) Portals and incisions used for the technique. DC, dorsal central incision; RD, radial distal incision; RM, radial midcarpal portal; RP, radial proximal incision; UM, ulnar midcarpal portal; VC, volar central incision.

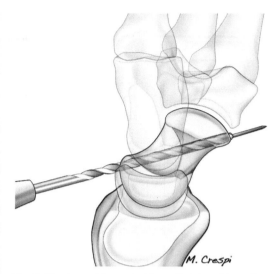

Fig. 5. The tunnel is created from the dorsal insertion of the scapholunate ligament on the proximal scaphoid to the scaphoid tubercle.

tendons are retracted to the radial side. The dorsal joint capsule is exposed (Figs. 7 and 8). An abbocath needle is then used as a guide. The tunnel is centered on the lunate in the PA view and is parallel to the distal articular surface of the lunate in the lateral view irrespective to the alignment of the lunate (Fig. 9). Another 1-mm K-wire is then inserted along the needle (Fig. 10). A 2.5-mm cannulated drill bit is used to create both the scaphoid and lunate tunnels. A drill guide should be used to avoid injury to the extensor tendons.

Step 2: Preparation to retrieve the graft

As the FCR tendon graft passed through the scaphoid tunnel, it would be intra-articular. A loop should be placed inside the joint to prepare later retrieval of the graft. An arthroscope is placed through the 6R portal to visualize the dorsal and radial side of the wrist. At the dorsal central wound with the extensor tendon

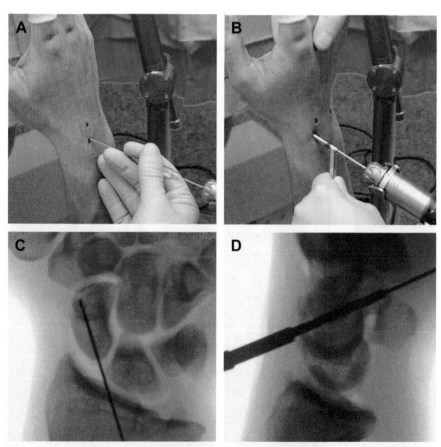

Fig. 6. (A, B) The tunnel is created from the dorsal insertion of the scapholunate ligament on the proximal scaphoid to the scaphoid tubercle through the 3/4 portal. A 14-G Abbocath needle is used as a guide for the K-wire. A cannulated 2.5-mm drill bit is inserted with the protection of a drill guide. (C, D) Posteroanterior and lateral fluoroscopic views.

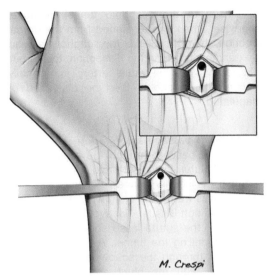

M. Crespi

Fig. 7. A 1.5-cm longitudinal incision (dorsal central) is made over the fourth extensor compartment. This incision is directly over the lunate bone. The extensor retinaculum is opened longitudinally and the extensor tendons are retracted to the radial side. Through this incision, the lunate tunnel is performed. Lately, the entrance of the lunate tunnel is united with the radiocarpal joint, which ensures that the graft will pass smoothly through the capsule and the joint into the bone tunnel.

retracted, the capsular vent made for the lunate bone tunnel is extended proximally to the radiocarpal joint under arthroscopic guidance. The entrance of the lunate tunnel is then united

with the radiocarpal joint, which ensures that the graft will pass smoothly through the capsule and the joint into the bone tunnel (see **Fig. 7**). A Curved SutureLasso (Arthrex, Naples, FL) is introduced through this incision, and its loop is retrieved from the 3/4 portal (**Figs. 11** and **12**).

Step 3: Harvesting the flexor carpi radialis tendon graft

The graft is an FCR hemitendon that is 3 mm wide and 8 to 10 cm long. The scaphoid tunnel exits radial to the FCR. To ensure that the radial side of the FCR is obtained, the graft should be harvested from the distal to the proximal as the FCR fibers have a constant torsion by an average of 180° in the wrist and forearm level.

The distal incision (radial distal) is a 2-cm longitudinal incision from the proximal wrist crease to the scaphoid tunnel. The proximal incision (radial proximal) is a 2 cm transverse incision over the FCR, 10 cm proximal to the distal one. At the radial distal wound, a 2O′ monofilament suture is passed through the FCR, capturing 3 mm of the radial side of the tendon. In the radial proximal wound, the tendon sheath is opened and a Suture Passing Wire (Arthrex) is passed distally under the tendon sheath and retrieved in the radial distal wound. The threads of the 2O′ monofilament sutures are loaded to the passing wire and brought to the radial proximal wound. By pulling

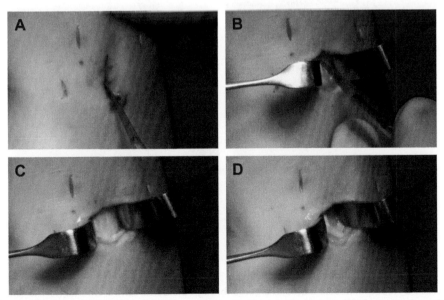

Fig. 8. (*A*) 1.5 cm longitudinal incision (dorsal central) is made over the lunate. (*B*) The extensor retinaculum is opened longitudinally. (*C*) The extensor tendons of the fourth compartment are identified. (*D*) The tendons are retracted to the radial side, exposing the articular capsule.

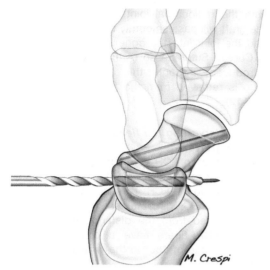

Fig. 9. The lunate tunnel is created parallel to its distal articular surface and centered on the lunate.

the threads from the radial proximal wound, the FCR is cut and the graft is obtained. The graft is cut at the proximal end and retrieved in the radial distal wound (**Fig. 13**). The graft is further

split distal to the scaphoid tunnel because, otherwise, when it is tensioned from the dorsal direction, the graft will flex the scaphoid instead of extending it. During the dissection, the superficial branch of the radial artery is normally encountered. It should then be dissected or coagulated.

Step 4: Graft passage and fixation
The graft is passed through the tunnels using a Straight SutureLasso (Arthrex). Graft passage through the bone tunnels consumes time because it is frequently caught by the adjacent capsule or soft tissue. To avoid trapping the soft tissue, the suture lasso should be passed right after drilling the tunnel. A 1-mm K-wire is introduced through the scaphoid tunnel at the 3/4 portal, with the blunt end forward. The tunnel is drilled again with a 3-mm cannulated drill. The K-wire is left inside the tunnel. The sharp end of the K-wire, at the dorsal side of the wrist, is inserted to the hole of the lasso tip and guides the lasso through the bone tunnel to the volar side. The graft is then captured by the loop and brought to the 3/4 portal (**Fig. 14**).

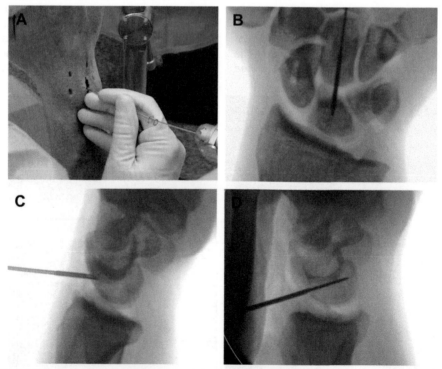

Fig. 10. (A) A 14-G Abbocath needle is used as a guide through the dorsal central wound. (B) The tunnel is at the center of lunate in the posteroanterior view, and (C, D) parallel to the distal lunate articular surface. The position of the K-wire and drill should be inclined in a proximal to distal direction if there is a dorsal intercalated segment instability deformity.

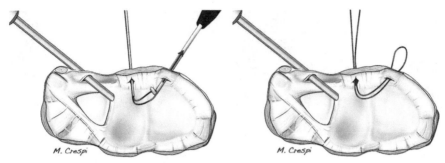

Fig. 11. Through the dorsal central wound, a Curved SutureLasso is introduced into the joint and the loop is retrieved from the 3/4 portal. (*Courtesy of* Arthrex, Naples, FL.)

The graft is then fixed to the tunnel with a 3 × 8 mm Bio-Tenodesis screw (Arthrex) inserted from the volar side while traction is applied to the graft from the dorsal side (**Fig. 15**). The interference screw is too small to be cannulated. Screw insertion can be difficult because the bone tunnel can be occluded by the graft and the soft tissues. It should follow the graft entrance site and fluoroscopic guidance of its direction is important (**Fig. 16**). The graft located in the 3/4 portal is passed through the loop of the Curved Suture-Lasso (Arthrex) to the dorsal central wound (**Fig. 17**A, B).

A volar central incision is then made.[36] Extensor tendons of the fourth compartment and flexor tendons are retracted. A K-wire is inserted from the volar to the dorsal direction, with the sharp tip forward. The tunnel is redrilled with a 3-mm cannulated drill bit. The graft must not be trapped when the drill exits at the dorsal side. The SutureLasso is introduced to the tunnel following the K-wire and captures the graft, bringing it to the volar central wound (see **Fig. 17**C–H).

The arthroscope is inserted and the ulnar midcarpal portal is viewed. Wrist traction is released. With the tendon graft pulled from the volar side, if the scaphoid is supinated, the step-off and gapping between the scaphoid and lunate disappear, extension deformity of the lunate is corrected, and the arthroscopic 3-dimensional test[20] becomes negative (**Figs. 18** and **19**). A Bio-Tenodesis screw is then inserted into the lunate tunnel, either under fluoroscopic control or arthroscopic control with the scope entering through the 6R portal (**Fig. 20**).

Step 5: Volar reconstruction
There are 2 major differences between the current technique and the previous technique[10] we described. Previously, the graft was fixed volarly with a capsuloligamentous suture as described by Del Piñal,[14] which is time consuming. Now the graft is directly fixed to the scaphoid at the SL ligament footprint using a Micro-corkscrew 2/0 (Arthrex), which is a small anchor of 1 mm predrilling.

Previously, the graft was passed intra-articularly in the same way as the dorsal side. Because there is a close proximity of the bone, volar joint capsule, and the Testut ligament, the volar joint space is limited (**Fig. 21**). Passing the tendon graft intra-articularly is not only time consuming, but also difficult. Currently, the graft is passed

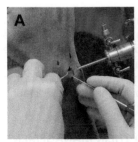
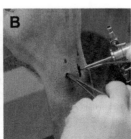
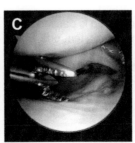
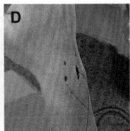

Fig. 12. (*A*) The arthroscope is placed in the 6R portal. A curved SutureLasso is introduced into the joint through the dorsal central wound. (*B, C*) The loop is retrieved from the 3/4 portal. (*D*) The loop is positioned now inside the joint, between the bones and capsule. (*Courtesy of* Arthrex, Naples, FL.)

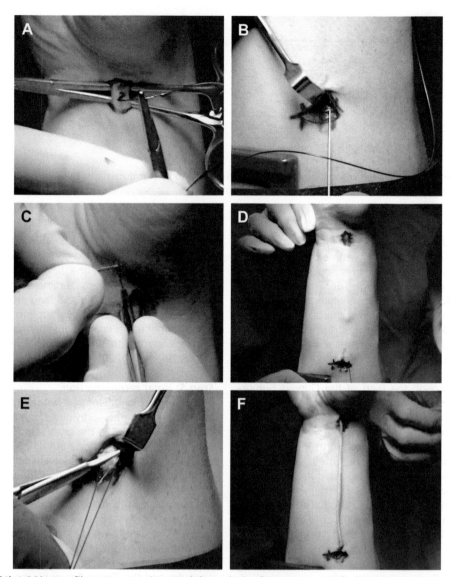

Fig. 13. (*A*) A 2O′ monofilament suture is passed through the flexor carpi radialis (FCR), capturing 3 mm of the radial side of the tendon. (*B*) Proximally, the tendon sheath is opened and a suture passing wire is advanced distally and retrieved in the distal wound. (*C*) The loop of the passing wire is loaded with the 2O′ monofilament threads. (*D*) The threads are taken to the proximal wound, cutting the FCR. (*E, F*) The graft is cut in the proximal wound and retrieved in the distal wound. (*Courtesy of* Arthrex, Naples, FL.)

in an extraarticular manner. A loop is passed over the capsule underlying the flexor tendons from the radial distal wound to the volar central wound. The graft is captured by the loop and brought to the radial distal wound and fixed with the 2O' threads of the anchor (**Figs. 22** and **23**, Video 2).

Graft reinforcement
Graft resistance and strength can be increased with the use of a 1.3-mm SutureTape (Arthrex). The procedure is the same as the SutureTape

passed and fixed along with the tendon graft. The only difference is that, after the graft is fixed to the scaphoid bone with the anchor, the volar portion of the SutureTape that exits from the lunate tunnel is sutured to the portion that exits from the scaphoid tunnel (**Figs. 24** and **25**, Video 3).

COMPLICATIONS AND THEIR MANAGEMENT

There are 3 major theoretic risks: tunnel breakage and fracture, damage of delicate structures

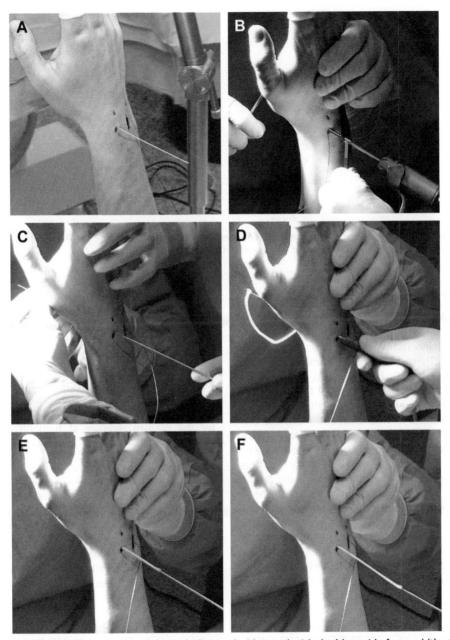

Fig. 14. (*A*) A 1-mm K-wire is introduced through the scaphoid tunnel with the blunt side forward (the tip should be at the 3/4 portal). (*B*) The tunnel is drilled again with a 3-mm drill bit. (*C*) The SutureLasso is introduced following the K-wire. (*D*) The graft is captured with the loop. (*E, F*) The graft is brought easily to the 3/4 portal. (*Courtesy of* Arthrex, Naples, FL.)

around the portals or tunnels, and avascular necrosis of scaphoid or lunate.

Tunnel Breakage and Fracture

It is essential to check frequently that the K-wire is at the correct position before drilling.

Damage of Delicate Structures Around the Portals or Tunnels

In a preliminary cadaver study, the distance between the portals, tunnels, and the structures at risk was demonstrated and can be used as a reference.[9]

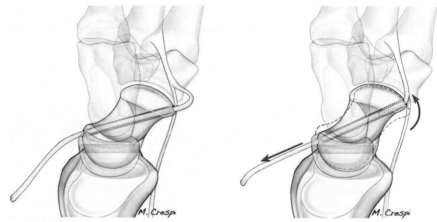

Fig. 15. The graft is pulled from the dorsal side. The scaphoid is therefore extended. A 3 × 8 mm Bio-Tenodesis screw is introduced from the volar side. (*Courtesy of* Arthrex, Naples, FL.)

Avascular Necrosis of Scaphoid or Lunate

The scaphoid tunnel entry site, which is at the insertion of the dorsal SL ligament, is far from the vessel insertion point at the waist of the scaphoid. There have been numerous operations reported with bone tunnels made at the scaphoids. Avascular necrosis of the scaphoids was reported rarely. With the arthroscopic procedure, and the limited dissection and the surrounding vascularity being well-preserved, the risk of avascular necrosis should be even lower. Avascular necrosis of the lunate may be more worrisome. However, the lunate vascular supply originates along various ligamentous insertions.[37] Because the tunnel is located in the middle of the lunate where its capsuloligamentous structure is not detached, vascular damage should be unlikely.

None of our patients had experienced any of these complications.

A complication that occurs more frequently is pain at the volar tunnel at the scaphoid over the FCR tendon, which is generally treated with a corticosteroid injection.

Two patients who had screw migration in the scaphoid tunnel also presented with similar pain at the same region. The screws were noticed to have migrated because they were palpable at the wrist dorsum. The symptoms disappeared after the screws removal at 6 months after the surgery.

Postoperative Care

The use of interference screw makes the reconstruction stronger. A K-wire was not used. The mobilization protocol can be started early. Dart-throwing exercise avoids overloading the graft. This motion mainly involves the midcarpal joint with limited movement in the proximal carpal row[38,39] and induces minimal elongation and

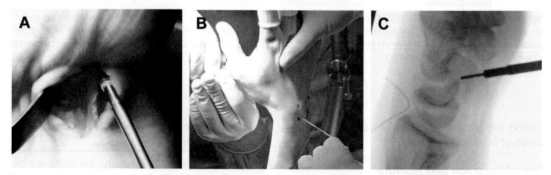

Fig. 16. (*A*) The Bio-Tenodesis screw is introduced from the volar side into the scaphoid tunnel following the graft. (*B*) While traction is applied from dorsal, the screw is introduced from volar. (*C*) Fluoroscopy is used to check the correct direction and position of the screw. (*Courtesy of* Arthrex, Naples, FL.)

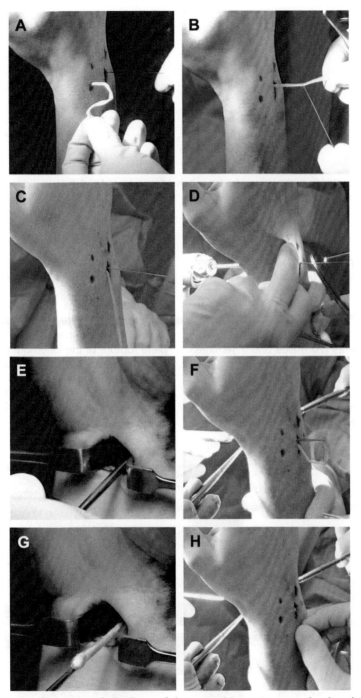

Fig. 17. (*A*, *B*) The graft is brought with the loop of the Curved SutureLasso to the dorsal central wound. (*C*) The K-wire is inserted from the volar to the dorsal in the lunate tunnel. (*D*) The tunnel is drilled with a 3-mm cannulated drill bit from volar. (*E*) The SutureLasso is introduced to the lunate tunnel following the K-wire. (*F*) The graft is captured and (*G*, *H*) taken easily to the volar central wound. (*Courtesy of* Arthrex, Naples, FL.)

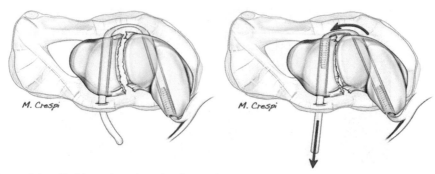

Fig. 18. The graft is pulled from the volar side. The scaphoid is supinated and the gap is closed. The screw is introduced from the dorsal side.

tension on the scapholunate ligament.[40] The postoperative mobilization protocol is shown in (**Fig. 26**).

OUTCOMES

A total of 27 patients (20 males and 7 females) were treated between 2011 and 2016. The average age was years 33.5 years (range, 18–51; SD, 9.25). All patients had a chronic lesion (>3 months from injury). The dominant hand was affected in 66.7%. Before surgery,

all patients reported having pain, a decrease in grip strength, and a decline in the wrist function.

Arthroscopy was performed in all cases to confirm a complete rupture of the SL ligament without degenerative changes or without a complete rupture of the lunotriquetral ligament. There were 14 grade IIIC and 13 grade IV lesions with instability assessed by the European Wrist Arthroscopy Society classification.[32] The preoperative and postoperative clinical data are detailed in **Table 1**.

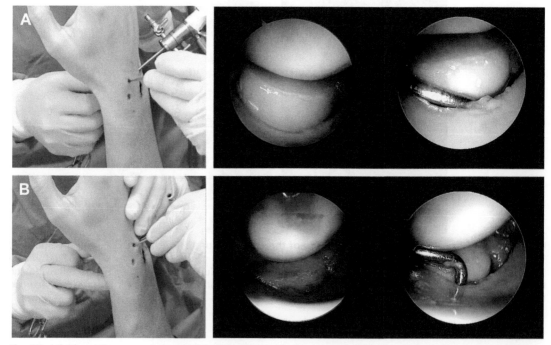

Fig. 19. (A) The arthroscope is located in the ulnar midcarpal portal. Wrist traction is released. (A) Without pulling the graft, there is a step-off and gapping. (B) With the graft being pulled, step-off and gapping disappear.

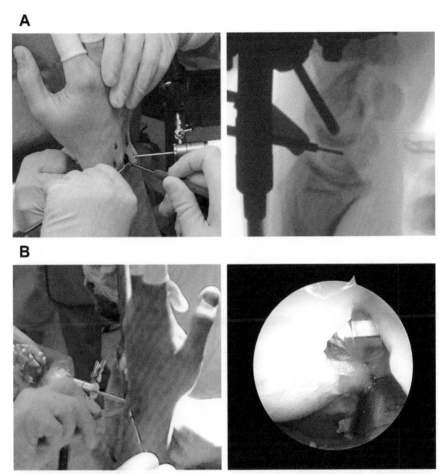

Fig. 20. Insertion of the Bio-Tenodesis screw can be performed (*A*) under fluoroscopic control, or (*B*) under arthroscopic control with the scope at the 6R portal viewing the lunate tunnel. (*Courtesy of* Arthrex, Naples, FL.)

Clinical results showed no difference between the preoperative and 6-month postoperative range of motion. There was a significant increase in the average grip strength 6 months after surgery, which increased as time elapses from surgery. A significant decrease in the average visual analog scale and Disability of the Arm, Shoulder and Hand scores after surgery was observed, and they decreased as time progresses after surgery.

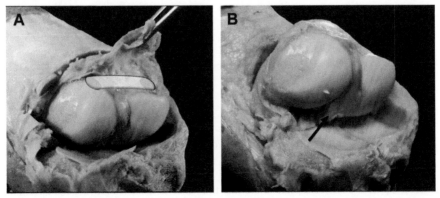

Fig. 21. (*A*) There is enough space between the bones and the dorsal joint capsule. A graft (*drawn on white*) can easily be placed in the correct position. (*B*) There is limited space because there is a close proximity of the bones, Testut ligament, and volar joint capsule (*black arrow*).

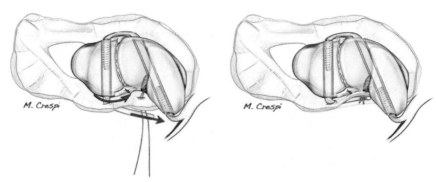

Fig. 22. The graft is passed over the capsule and is directly fixed to the scaphoid at the SL ligament footprint using a Micro-corkscrew 2/0. (*Courtesy of* Arthrex, Naples, FL.)

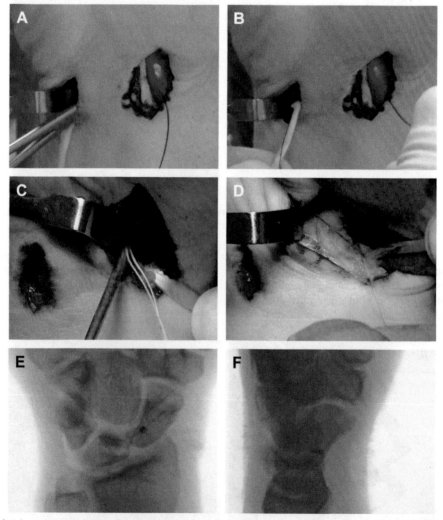

Fig. 23. (*A*) A loop is passed over the capsule and under the flexor tendons from the radial distal (RD) wound to the volar central (VC) wound. (*B*) The graft is captured with the loop and brought from the VC wound to the radial distal wound. (*C*) A Micro-corkscrew 2/0 is inserted at the SL ligament footprint. (*D*) The graft is sutured with the 2O′ threads. (*E, F*) Fluoroscopic control. (*Courtesy of* Arthrex, Naples, FL.)

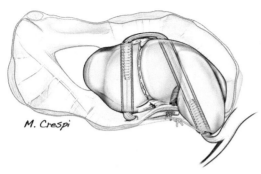

M. Crespi

Fig. 24. Graft resistance and strength can be increased with the use of a 1.3 mm SutureTape. The SutureTape is passed and fixed with the screws along with the tendon graft. After the graft is fixed to the scaphoid bone with the anchor, the volar portion of the SutureTape that exits from the lunate tunnel is sutured to the portion that exits from the scaphoid tunnel. (*Courtesy of* Arthrex, Naples, FL.)

A static instability was detected in 11 patients (41%), whereas a dynamic instability was presented in 16 patients (59%). In patients with static instability, the mean preoperative SL angle was 72.3° (range, 60–86; SD, 9.44) and the mean preoperative gap was 4.19 mm (range, 3.1–5.5; SD, 0.99). In patients with dynamic instability, the mean preoperative gap was 2.87 mm (range, 2.1–5.2; SD, 0.84). The preoperative and postoperative radiographic parameters are detailed in **Table 2**.

A significant decrease in the average overall gap after surgery and in the average overall SL angle after surgery for static patients were found. Also there was a significant decrease in the average overall gap for dynamic patients. Despite a significant improvement in the SL angle and the gap, the gap remained open in many patients with static instability. However, the clinical result in patients with an open gap was satisfactory. Some clinical results and the explanation of why the gap was not related to the clinical result are demonstrated in Video 4.

SUMMARY

Arthroscopic SL volar and dorsal ligament reconstruction achieves an anatomic reconstruction, avoids an open procedure and capsular detachment, and provides a strong construct for early mobilization. Proper patient selection for this operation is important. It reconstructs both the dorsal and volar portion of the SL ligament with a 3-mm graft of the FCR tendon, which is fixed to the scaphoid and lunate tunnels with interference screws. Early postoperative mobilization can be started. Clinical results show improvement in grip strength, visual analog scale, Disability of the Arm, Shoulder and Hand scores and the range of motion can be preserved.

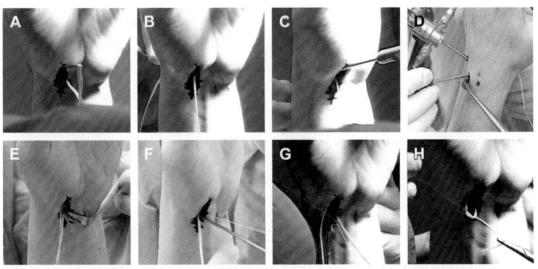

Fig. 25. (*A, B*) A-1.3 mm SutureTape is passed through the 3-mm scaphoid tunnel together with the graft. A portion of the SutureTape remains in the radial distal (RD) wound. (*C, D*) The fixation in the scaphoid and lunate are performed with a 3 × 8 Bio-Tenodesis screw. (*E*) Both the graft and the SutureTape are taken to the RD wound. (*F*) The anchor is introduced in the scaphoid. (*G*) The graft is sutured with the 20′ threads. (*H*) The portion of the SutureTape that exits from the lunate tunnel is sutured to itself, and exits from the scaphoid tunnel. (*Courtesy of* Arthrex, Naples, FL.)

TIME	INMOBILIZATION	MOVEMENTS
<2 Wk	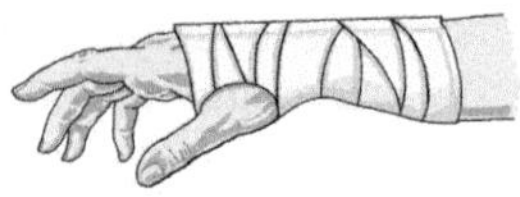	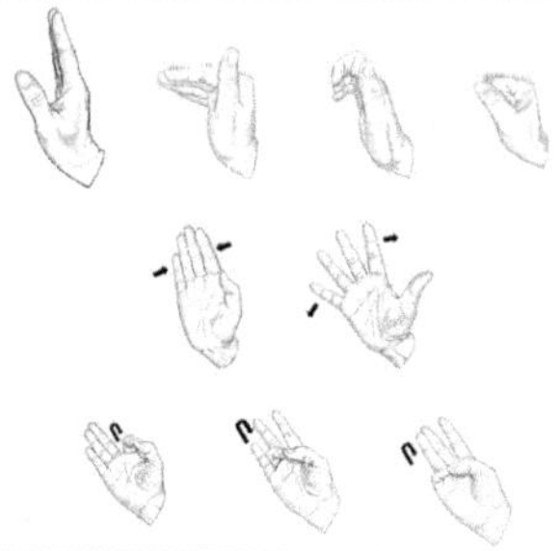
2 – 4 Wk	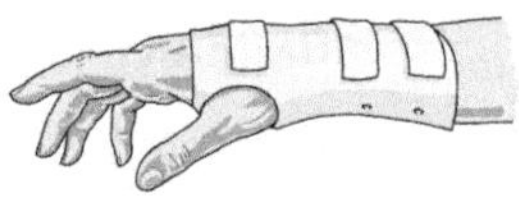	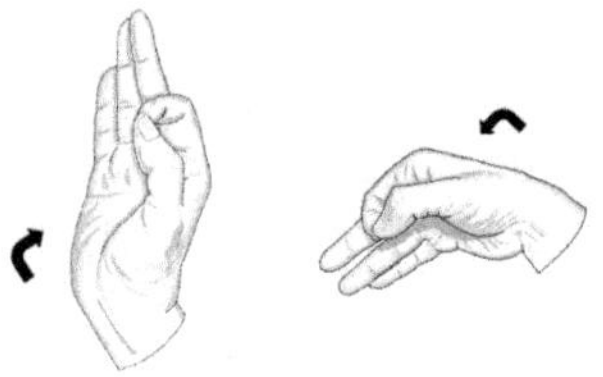
4– 6 Wk	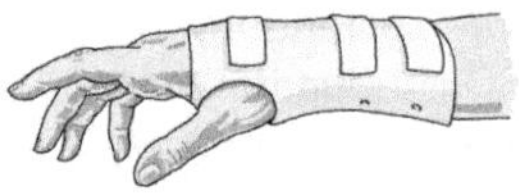	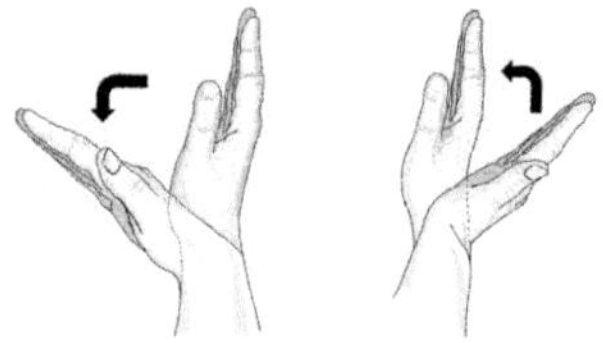
6 – 10 Wk	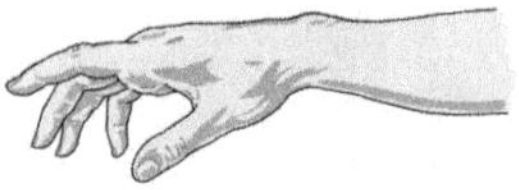	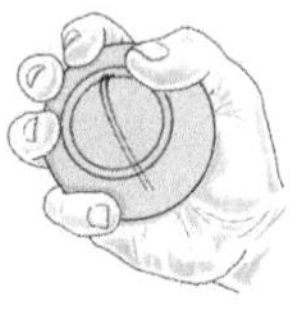
>10 Wk	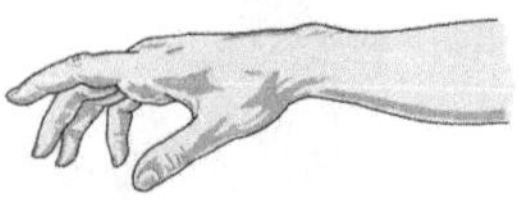	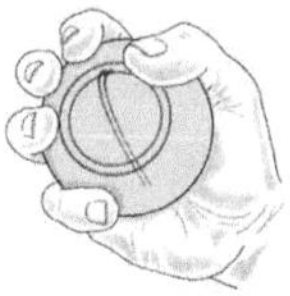

Fig. 26. Postoperative rehabilitation protocol. Less than 2 weeks: Dorsal slab. Six packs fingers exercises. "No" strength in gripping. At 2 to 4 weeks: Thermoplastic splint. Remove splint 30 for minutes 4 times a day for exercises. Exclusively midcarpal motion (dart throwing motion). At 4 to 6 weeks: Nocturnal thermoplastic splint. Progressively full range of motion exercises. At 6 to 10 weeks: Off splint. Exercises with "progressive" strength in gripping. Proprioception exercises: "power ball." Strengthening exercises with a 1-kg weight (supinator muscles). Greater than 10 weeks: Increase weight up to 3 kg (supinator muscles). After 12 weeks, normal activity without restriction. Avoid contact sports until month 4 or 5.

Table 1
Descriptive statistics for wrist extension, wrist flexion, grip strength, VAS, and DASH on each time period

Variable	Preoperative	3 mo AS	6 mo AS	1 y AS	≥2 y AS
			Time		
Wrist extension					
Average	83	73↓[b]	84	87	89
SD	6.7	11.8	5.7	4.4	3.1
n	27	26	23	19	10
Wrist flexion					
Average	80	67↓[b]	79	81	84
SD	11.4	12.1	8.4	7.3	6.1
n	27	26	23	19	10
Grip strength					
Average	33	29	37↑[a]	39↑[a]	46↑[a]
SD	11.1	10.7	10.4	12.9	9.4
n	27	25	23	18	9
VAS					
Average	5	1.9↓[b]	1.2↓[b]	1.1↓[b]	0.4↓[b]
SD	19.4	15.0	11.7	12.4	0.4
n	27	25	22	18	10
DASH					
Average	35.3	24.8↓[b]	12.7↓[b]	10.5↓[b]	4.2↓[b]
SD	15.9	15.6	11.5	13.6	5.8
n	27	26	22	17	11

Abbreviations: AS, after surgery; DASH, Disability of the Arm, Shoulder and Hand; SD, standard deviation; VAS, visual analog scale.
[a] ↑ Significant increase.
[b] ↓ Significant decrease.

Table 2
Descriptive statistics for radiographic parameters

Type	Preoperative	Postoperative
		Time
Overall: Gap		
Average	3.47	2.94↓[a]
SD	1.11	1.21
n	22	22
Static		
Gap		
Average	4.19	3.66↓[a]
SD	0.99	1.33
n	10	10
Scapholunate ligament		
Average	72.3	68.6↓[a]
SD	9.44	9.39
n	10	10
Dynamic: gap		
Average	2.87	2.34↓[a]
SD	0.84	0.69
n	12	12

[a] ↓ Significant decrease.

SUPPLEMENTARY DATA

Supplementary data related to this article can be found online at http://dx.doi.org/10.1016/j.hcl. 2017.07.019.

REFERENCES

1. Watson HK, Ballet FL. The SLAC wrist- scapholunate advanced collapse pattern of degenerative arthritis. J Hand Surg Am 1984;9(3):358–65.

2. Lee JI, Nha KW, Lee GY, et al. Long-term outcomes of arthroscopic debridement and thermal shrinkage for isolated partial intercarpal ligament tears. Orthopedics 2012;35(8):1204–9.

3. Hirsh L, Sodha S, Bozentka D, et al. Arthroscopic electrothermal collagen shrinkage for symptomatic laxity of the scapholunate interosseous ligament. J Hand Surg Am 2005;30(6):643–7.

4. Darlis NA, Weiser RW, Sotereanos DG. Partial scapholunate ligament injuries treated with arthroscopic debridement and thermal shrinkage. J Hand Surg Am 2005;30(5):908–14.

5. Darlis NA, Kaufmann RA, Giannoulis F, et al. Arthroscopic debridement and closed pinning for chronic dynamic scapholunate instability. J Hand Surg Am 2006;31(3):418–24.

6. Michelotti BF, Adkinson JM, Chung KC. Chronic scapholunate ligament injury. Techniques in repair and reconstruction. Hand Clin 2015;31(3):437–49.

7. Manuel J, Moran SL. The diagnosis and treatment of scapholunate instability. Hand Clin 2010;26(1):129–44.

8. Kuo CE, Wolfe SW. Scapholunate instability: current concepts in diagnosis and management. J Hand Surg Am 2008;33(6):998–1013.

9. Corella F, Del Cerro M, Larrainzar-Garijo R, et al. Arthroscopic ligamentoplasty (bone-tendon-tenodesis). A new surgical technique for scapholunate instability: preliminary cadaver study. J Hand Surg Eur 2011;36(8):682–9.

10. Corella F, Del Cerro M, Ocampos M, et al. Arthroscopic ligamentoplasty of the dorsal and volar portions of the scapholunate ligament. J Hand Surg Am 2013;38(12):2466–77.

11. Sokolow C, Saffar P. Anatomy and histology of the scapholunate ligament. Hand Clin 2001;17(1):77–81.

12. Mataliotakis G, Doukas M, Kostas I, et al. Sensory innervation of the subregions of the scapholunate interosseous ligament in relation to their structural composition. J Hand Surg Am 2009;34(8):1413–21.

13. Logan SE, Nowak MD, Gould PL, et al. Biomechanical behavior of the scapholunate ligament. Biomed Sci Instrum 1986;22:81–5.

14. Del Piñal F. Arthroscopic volar capsuloligamentous repair. J Wrist Surg 2013;2(2):126–8.

15. Henry M. Reconstruction of both volar and dorsal limbs of the scapholunate interosseous ligament. J Hand Surg Am 2013;38(8):1625–34.

16. Ho P, Wing-yee Wong C, Tse W. Arthroscopic-assisted combined dorsal and volar scapholunate ligament reconstruction with tendon graft for chronic SL instability. J Wrist Surg 2015;4:252–63.

17. Eng K, Wagels M, Tham SK. Cadaveric scapholunate reconstruction using the ligament augmentation and reconstruction system. J Wrist Surg 2014;3(3):192–7.

18. Short WH, Werner FW, Sutton LG. Dynamic biomechanical evaluation of the dorsal intercarpal ligament repair for scapholunate instability. J Hand Surg Am 2009;34(4):652–9.

19. Short WH, Werner FW, Fortino MD, et al. A dynamic biomechanical study of scapholunate ligament sectioning. J Hand Surg Am 1995;20(6):986–99.

20. Corella F, Ocampos M, Del Cerro M. Arthroscopic scaphoid 3D test for scapholunate instability. J Wrist Surg 2017.

21. Elsaidi GA, Ruch DS, Kuzma GR, et al. Dorsal wrist ligament insertions stabilize the scapholunate interval: cadaver study. Clin Orthop Relat Res 2004;425:152–7.

22. Mitsuyasu H, Patterson RM, Shah MA, et al. The role the dorsal intercarpal ligament in dynamic and static scapholunate instability. J Hand Surg Am 2004;29(2):279–88.

23. Esplugas M, Garcia-Elias M, Lluch A, et al. Role of muscles in the stabilization of ligament-deficient wrists. J Hand Ther 2016;29(2):166–74.

24. Lluch A, Salvà G, Esplugas M, et al. Proprioception and neuromuscular control in carpal instabilities. Rev Iberoam Cir Mano 2015;43(1):70–8.

25. Salvà-Coll G, Garcia-Elias M, Llusá-Pérez M, et al. The role of the flexor carpi radialis muscle in scapholunate instability. J Hand Surg Am 2011;36(1):31–6.

26. Hagert E. Proprioception of the wrist joint: a review of current concepts and possible implications on the rehabilitation of the wrist. J Hand Ther 2010;23(1):2–17.

27. Salva-Coll G, Garcia-Elias M, Hagert E. Scapholunate instability: proprioception and neuromuscular control. J Wrist Surg 2013;2(2):136–40.

28. Salva-Coll G, Garcia-Elias M, Leon-Lopez MT, et al. Effects of forearm muscles on carpal stability. J Hand Surg Eur 2011;36(7):553–9.

29. Hagert E, Ljung BO, Forsgren S. General innervation pattern and sensory corpuscles in the scapholunate interosseous ligament. Cells Tissues Organs 2004;177(1):47–54.

30. Hagert E, Persson JKE, Werner M, et al. Evidence of wrist proprioceptive reflexes elicited after stimulation of the scapholunate interosseous ligament. J Hand Surg Am 2009;34(4):642–51.

31. Carratalá V, Lucas FJ, Alepuz ES, et al. Arthroscopically assisted ligamentoplasty for axial and dorsal reconstruction of the scapholunate ligament. Arthrosc Tech 2016;5(2):e353–9.

32. Messina JC, Van Overstraeten L, Luchetti R, et al. The EWAS classification of scapholunate tears: an anatomical arthroscopic study. J Wrist Surg 2013; 2(2):105–9.

33. Badia A, Khanchandani P. The floating lunate: arthroscopic treatment of simultaneous complete tears of the scapholunate and lunotriquetral ligaments. Hand (N Y) 2009;4(3):250–5.

34. Corella F, Del Cerro M, Ocampos M, et al. The "rocking chair sign" for floating lunate. J Hand Surg Am 2015;40(11):2318–9.

35. García-Elías M. Carpal instability.pdf. In: Wolfe SW, Hotchkiss RN, Pederson WC, et al, editors. Green's operative hand surgery. 6th edition. Philadelphia: Elsevier Churchill Livingstone; 2010. p. 465–522.

36. Corella F, Ocampos M, Cerro MD, et al. Volar central portal in wrist arthroscopy. J Wrist Surg 2016;5: 80–90.

37. Lamas C, Carrera A, Proubasta I, et al. The anatomy and vascularity of the lunate: considerations applied to Kienböck's disease. Chir Main 2007; 26(1):13–20.

38. Moritomo H, Apergis EP, Herzberg G, et al. 2007 IFSSH Committee Report of Wrist Biomechanics Committee: biomechanics of the so-called dart-throwing motion of the wrist. J Hand Surg Am 2007;32(9):1447–53.

39. Crisco JJ, Coburn JC, Moore DC, et al. In vivo radiocarpal kinematics and the dart thrower's motion. J Bone Joint Surg Am 2005;87(12):2729–40.

40. Upal MA, Crisco JJ, Moore DC, et al. In vivo elongation of the palmar and dorsal scapholunate interosseous ligament. J Hand Surg Am 2006;31(8): 1326–32.

Arthroscopic Management of Perilunate Injuries

Bo Liu, MD*, Shan-lin Chen, MD, Jin Zhu, MD,
Guang-lei Tian, MD

KEYWORDS

- Perilunate dislocation • Scaphoid fracture • Minimally invasive surgery • Wrist arthroscopy

KEY POINTS

- Perilunate injuries are rare but devastating injuries, often the result of high-energy trauma.
- The key to successful treatment of perilunate injuries is to achieve early anatomic reduction and maintain the carpal alignment.
- Arthroscopic management may encourage healing with less stiffness and is a favorable alternative in the treatment of perilunate injuries.

Perilunate injuries are severe wrist injuries, often the result of high-energy trauma. The pathway of injury may be strictly perilunar in so-called pure ligamentous perilunate dislocations (PLDs) through the lesser arc, or the injury may cause perilunate fracture dislocations (PLFDs) through the greater arc, which is commonly through the scaphoid (trans-scaphoid PLFDs).[1–3]

It is essential to identify these injuries acutely, because neglected injuries or late treatment usually leads to poor outcomes. The key to successful treatment of perilunate injuries is to achieve early anatomic reduction and maintain normal carpal alignment. Closed reduction and cast treatment have been shown to have unacceptable outcomes.[4] Surgical treatment with open reduction of the carpal bones, repair or reconstruction of the ligaments, and internal fixation of the fractures has been generally accepted for PLDs-PLFDs.[3–12] Open surgery, however, involves dissection of the important capsuloligamentous structures of the

wrist, which may lead to capsular scarring and joint stiffness. Open dissection could jeopardize the tenuous blood supply to scaphoid and the torn ligaments.

Recently, arthroscopic-assisted minimally invasive management of PLDs-PLFDs has been suggested by several investigators.[3,4,13–19] Combined with fluoroscopy, wrist arthroscopy allows anatomic reduction and precise percutaneous internal fixation of the carpal bones with minimal tissue dissection. This technique may encourage healing with less stiffness, and recent series have shown encouraging outcomes.[17–19] The purpose of this study is to review the technique and outcome of arthroscopic reduction and percutaneous fixation of a series of patients with acute PLD-PFLDs.[17]

PATIENTS

Of 40 consecutive patients with acute dorsal PLDs-PLFDs who were treated with arthroscopic-assisted

Disclosure Statement: The authors have nothing to disclose.
Department of Hand Surgery, Beijing Ji Shui Tan Hospital, 4th Clinical Hospital of Peking University, Beijing 100035, China
* Corresponding author.
E-mail address: bobliu7@hotmail.com

reduction and percutaneous fixation between 2012 and 2015, 31 patients have been followed-up for at least 1 year; 26 had trans-scaphoid dorsal PLFDs, and 5 had dorsal PLDs. The mean follow-up was 14.8 months (range 12–32 months). The mean age at the time of injury was 29 years (range 17–55 years). Dominant wrists were injured in 11 patients. The average time from injury to surgery was 8 days (range 2–20 days).

SURGICAL TECHNIQUE
Reduction of the Capitolunate Dislocation

Closed reduction of the dislocations of capitolunate joint had been attempted for all patients at the time of initial presentation. More than half (17 of 31) of the dislocations were reduced. For the remaining 14 dislocations, close reduction was tried again in the operation room under brachial plexus block before arthroscopy was performed; 8 dislocations were reduced under anesthesia but still failed in 6. Arthroscopic-assisted reduction of the capitolunate joint was then conducted when traction was applied by the arthroscopic traction tower. The 3-4 portal was used for initial inspection. Failure of close reduction was due to the volarly tilted lunate (along with proximal scaphoid fragment in trans-scaphoid PLFDs), which got stuck by the capitate or interposed torn palmar capsular ligaments. With finger-trap traction, a Freer elevator or a shoulder arthroscopic probe was used to reduce the dislocation arthroscopically by a shoehorn maneuver (**Fig. 1**). The authors found the 4-5 portal was convenient to apply this maneuver because the instrument was directly facing the subluxated lunate. All the 6 dislocations were arthroscopically reduced successfully by this technique.

Reduction and Fixation for Perilunate Dislocations

The 3-4 and 4-5 portals were used to examine and débride the radiocarpal joint. The initial view was usually obscured by the traumatic synovitis and capsuloligamentous edema. The authors used wet arthroscopy for articular distension, which facilitated synovectomy and débridement of intra-articular hematoma, torn ligament flaps, and bony or chondral debris and helped to establish a visual and working field. Fluid insufflation compressed the capillaries within the joint and synovitis and helped control the bleeding. Triangular fibrocartilage complex (TFCC) and volar intercarpal ligaments were examined by direct inspection and manual testing with an arthroscopic probe.

The midcarpal joint was examined through radial and ulnar midcarpal portals. Scapholunate (SL) and lunotriquetral (LT) ligaments were assessed with a probe. Any soft tissue or bony fragments interposed between SL and LT interval were débrided or removed to facilitate the reduction of the intercarpal joint.

Two Kirschner (K)-wires were placed toward lunate from scaphoid and triquetrum, respectively, under the guidance of fluoroscopy, without crossing the intercarpal interval (**Fig. 2A–D**). If the lunate was not in neutral position (ie, in volar or dorsal tilting), passively extended or flexed the wrist to restore the normal radiolunate angle and transfixed the radiolunate joint temporarily with a percutaneous K-wire inserted from dorsal distal radius (see **Fig. 2E**). Under direct visualization through midcarpal portal, reduction of the SL and LT intervals was conducted by manipulating the K-wires of the scaphoid and the triquetrum,

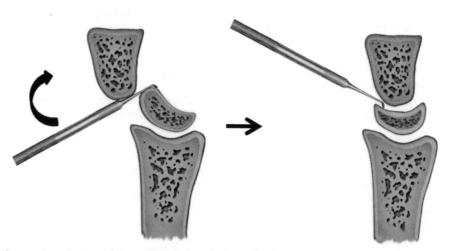

Fig. 1. Arthroscopic reduction of the capitolunate joint by a shoehorn maneuver.

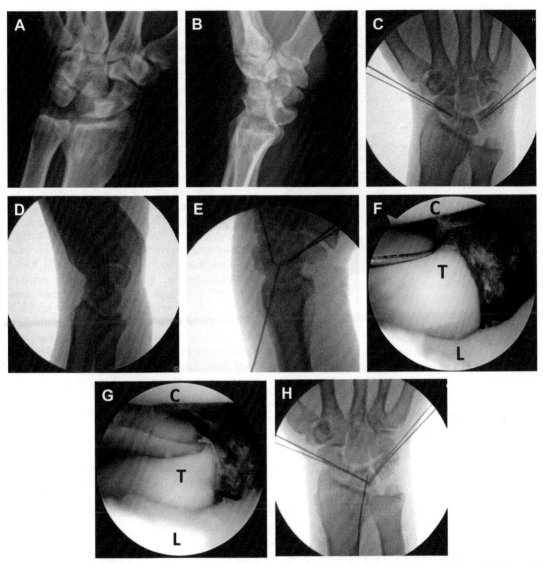

Fig. 2. (*A*) Posteroanterior (PA) radiographs and (*B*) lateral radiograph showing a PLD. (*C*) PA and (*D*) lateral radiograph showing the preparing of the K-wires. Note the dorsal tilting of the lunate. (*E*) The radiolunate joint was transfixed with a K-wire inserted from dorsal distal radius when the lunate was in neutral position. (*F*) Before correction of step and rotational deformity between the LT intervals. (*G*) The step and rotational deformity were corrected by a depressor. C, capitate; L, lunate; T, triquetrum. (*H*) The K-wires were driven across the intercarpal intervals into the lunate.

respectively. Correction of steps or rotational deformity of the intercarpal intervals could be obtained by a probe or depressor through midcarpal portal (see **Fig. 2**F, G). K-wires were then driven across the intercarpal intervals into the lunate (see **Fig. 2**H). In cases of gross instability and easily redislocated SL joint (4 of 5 PLDs in the authors' series), which meant both primary and secondary stabilizers of SL joint were incompetent, SL ligament was then reinforced by dorsal capsulodesis through a small incision. The 3-4 portal was extended transversely along the skin crease for 2 cm. The extensor tendons were retracted. Dorsal capsule was exposed but not opened. Two suture anchors were placed into scaphoid and lunate 1 cm away from the SL interval, respectively, under fluoroscopic guidance. After the SL joint was reduced and fixed with 2 wires, as described previously, sutures from 2 anchors were then tied together on the top of the dorsal capsule (**Fig. 3**).

Although PLDs are regarded as pure ligamentous injuries, the concomitant carpal bone fractures are not uncommonly seen. In the authors' 5 PLD patients, 2 had displaced intra-articular triquetral fractures, which required arthroscopic assisted percutaneous reduction and fixation (**Fig. 4**A–D).

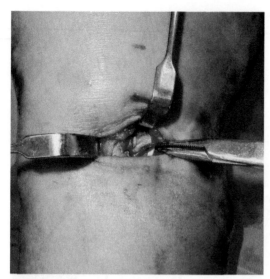

Fig. 3. Augmentation of the SL ligament through a minimally invasive approach.

One patient had associated TFCC combined large central tear and ulnar tear was treated with débridement of the central tear and repair of the ulnar tear.

Reduction and Fixation for Trans-scaphoid Perilunate Fracture Dislocations

A thorough examination and débridement of the radiocarpal and midcarpal joints were carried out, as previously described. Although there was no significant radiographic SL dissociation, almost all patients (25 of 26 patients) had hemorrhage and some attenuation of the SL ligament under arthroscopic examination, and 2 patients had concomitant SL ligament avulsion from the lunate (**Fig. 5**). Midcarpal joint arthroscopy revealed Geissler grade III injuries in these 2 wrists and SL pinning was required.

The scaphoid fractures were treated first. In trans-scaphoid PLFDs, the scaphoid fractures are usually significantly displaced with comminution (**Fig. 6**A, B). Close reduction was often unsatisfactory. The most critical and technically demanding step was arthroscopic-assisted reduction and percutaneous fixation of the scaphoid fracture. A guide wire was introduced along the axis of the distal fragment from scaphoid tubercle, not crossing the fracture line. In grossly unstable or comminuted fractures, 1 or 2 additional antirotation K-wires were inserted into the distal fragment as joysticks for manipulation and reduction. The authors found that 2 joysticks could efficiently correct the 3-D displacement of the fracture (see **Fig. 6**C). The fracture was visualized

at the ulnar midcarpal portal (see **Fig. 6**D). The fracture was reduced by manipulating the joysticks. Sometimes, additional leverage was required for reduction with a probe or a K-wire inserted over the proximal fragment as another joystick. Attention should be paid to correct the rotational and translational displacement in both sagittal and coronal planes. Some residual gap might be present, which could be reduced by a compression screw later. After the anatomic reduction was achieved, the assistant would drive the guide wire and antirotation K-wires across the fracture site toward the proximal fragment. The authors used cannulated headless screws for all scaphoid fracture fixations. Reaming and screw placement were performed with the traction released and the wrist put on the operation table. This facilitated screw compression and fluoroscopic screening. In 5 patients with proximal one-third scaphoid fractures, the cannulated screws were inserted antegrade from dorsal to volar. In these cases, the guide wire at the distal fragment was advanced out to the dorsal wrist with the wrist at flexion. Reaming and screw placement were conducted from a stab incision over dorsal wrist. In cases of significant fracture comminution or instability, 1 antirotation K-wire was left to enhance fracture stabilization. Reduction and fixation were confirmed both fluoroscopically and arthroscopically (see **Fig. 6**E, F).

Associated soft tissue injuries and carpal malalignment were addressed similarly, as previously described for PLDs. Three patients with TFCC injuries (2 large central tears with unstable flap and 1 partial dorsal tear) were treated with débridement.

POSTOPERATIVE MANAGEMENT

There were 4 patients (of 31 patients) with significant TFCC injuries. The wrists were immobilized in long arm thermoplastic casts with forearm at semisupination for 6 weeks and then in short arm splints for 2 more weeks. All other wrists were immobilized in short arm thermoplastic casts after the operation. The thumb was incorporated in the cast for trans-scaphoid PLFD. The K-wires and splint were removed at 8 weeks postoperatively, followed by active wrist motion exercise. Manual activities and sports could be started after the scaphoid united.

RESULTS

Arthroscopic-assisted reduction and percutaneous fixation were achieved in all 31 patients.

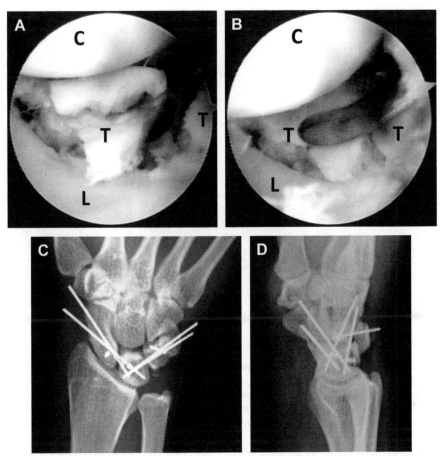

Fig. 4. (*A*) Midcarpal arthroscopy showed displaced triquetral fracture in a young golf player with PLD. C, capitate; L, lunate; T, triquetrum. (*B*) The triquetral fracture was reduced and fixed by percutaneous pinning. (*C*) Postoperative PA and (*D*) lateral radiographs. Note the triquetral fracture was reduced and fixed by a percutaneous wire.

The mean operation time was 155 minutes (range 90–300 minutes).

The normal carpal alignments were restored and maintained for all patients at the final evaluation; 25 of 26 scaphoid fractures healed at a mean time of 13 weeks (range 9–20 weeks). The only 1 patient with scaphoid nonunion declined further treatment at the final evaluation and he had minimal wrist pain and functionally problems.

Nine patients had median nerve symptoms, which resolved within 2 weeks after the surgery, and no patient required carpal tunnel release.

At the final follow-up, the mean flexion-extension arc was 115° (range 80°–150°), which was 86% of the contralateral wrist. The mean grip strength was 33 kg (range 8–48 kg), which was 83% of the contralateral wrist.

The mean Mayo wrist score was 87 (range 40–100), with excellent in 17 patients, good in 9, fair in 4, and poor in 1. The patient who had a poor result sustained associated central TFCC tear

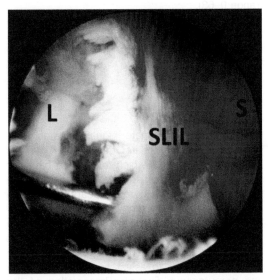

Fig. 5. SL ligament (SLIL) avulsion from the lunate in a patient who had trans-scaphoid PLFD. L, lunate; S, scaphoid.

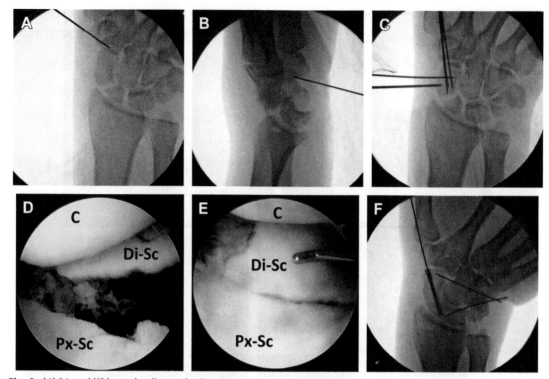

Fig. 6. (*A*) PA and (*B*) lateral radiographs showing a trans-scaphoid PLD. (*C*) Two joysticks were used to correct the 3-D displacement of the scaphoid fracture. (*D*) Midcarpal arthroscopy showing the displaced scaphoid fracture. C, capitate; Di-Sc, distal scaphoid; Px-Sc, proximal scaphoid. (*E*) Midcarpal arthroscopy showed accurate reduction of the scaphoid fracture. (*F*) Intro-operative fluoroscopy showed satisfactory reduction and fixation of the scaphoid fracture.

and complained of ulnar-sided wrist pain with gripping and forearm pronation-supination activities. The mean Disabilities of the Arm, Shoulder and Hand score was 7 (range 0–65) and Patient-Rated Wrist Evaluation score was 10 (range 0–63).

All 31 patients (15 were manual labor workers) could return to their preinjury occupations at a mean time of 4 months (range 1–12 months). Three labor workers returned to work with reduced workloads.

SUMMARY

Management of perilunate injuries remains challenging and controversial. Open surgery involves soft tissue dissection, which may led to capsular scarring, joint stiffness, and damage of the tenuous vascular supply to the scaphoid and the ligaments. Wrist arthroscopy allows direct visualization of the ligaments, joints, and carpal bone fractures. Combined with fluoroscopy, wrist arthroscopy gives a minimally invasive and more efficient approach to assist anatomic reduction and percutaneous fixation. Preservation of the vascularity of the scaphoid and torn ligaments facilitates the healing process. Although

arthroscopic management is technically demanding, the authors' series showed encouraging outcomes. This minimal invasive approach is a reliable and favorable alternative in the treatment of perilunate injuries.

REFERENCES

1. Mayfield JK, Johnson RP, Kilcoyne RK. Carpal dislocations: pathomechanics and progressive perilunar instability. J Hand Surg Am 1980;5:226–41.
2. Johnson RP. The acutely injured wrist and its residuals. Clin Orthop Relat Res 1980;149:33–44.
3. Herzberg G. Perilunate and axial carpal dislocations and fracture-dislocations. J Hand Surg Am 2008;33: 1659–68.
4. Weil WM, Slade JF, Trumble TE. Open and arthroscopic treatment of perilunate injuries. Clin Orthop 2006;445:120–33.
5. Cooney WP, Bussey R, Dobyns JH, et al. Difficult wrist fractures. Perilunate fracture-dislocations of the wrist. Clin Orthop Relat Res 1987;214:136–47.
6. Herzberg G, Forissier D. Acute dorsal trans-scaphoid perilunate fracture-dislocations: Medium-term results. J Hand Surg Br 2002;27:498–502.
7. Budoff JE. Treatment of acute lunate and perilunate dislocations. J Hand Surg Am 2008;33:1424–32.

8. Trumble TE, Verheyden J. Treatment of isolated perilunate and lunate dislocations with combined dorsal and volar approach and intraosseous cerclage wire. J Hand Surg Am 2004;29:412–7.

9. Knoll VD, Allan C, Trumble TE. Trans-scaphoid perilunate fracture dislocations: results of screw fixation of the scaphoid and luno-triquetral repair with a dorsal approach. J Hand Surg Am 2005;30:1145–52.

10. Souer JS, Rutgers M, Andermahr J, et al. Perilunate fracture-dislocations of the wrist: comparison of temporary screw versus K-wire fixation. J Hand Surg Am 2007;32:318–25.

11. Forli A, Courvoisier A, Wimsey S, et al. Perilunate dislocations and transscaphoid perilunate fracture-dislocations: a retrospective study with minimum ten-year follow-up. J Hand Surg Am 2010;35:62–8.

12. Kremer T, Wendt M, Riedel K, et al. Open reduction for perilunate injuries–clinical outcome and patient satisfaction. J Hand Surg Am 2010;35:1599–606.

13. Park MJ, Ahn JH. Arthroscopically assisted reduction and percutaneous fixation of dorsal perilunate dislocations and fracture-dislocations. Arthroscopy 2005;21:1153.

14. Wong TC, Yip TH. Minimally invasive management of trans-scaphoid perilunate fracture-dislocations. Hand Surg 2008;13:159–65.

15. Kim JP, Lee JS, Park MJ. Arthroscopic reduction and percutaneous fixation of perilunate dislocations and fracture-dislocations. Arthroscopy 2012;28:196–203.

16. Jeon IH, Kim HJ, Min WK, et al. Arthroscopically assisted percutaneous fixation for trans-scaphoid perilunate fracture dislocation. J Hand Surg Eur 2010;35:664–8.

17. Liu B, Chen SL, Zhu J, et al. Arthroscopically assisted mini-invasive management of perilunate dislocations. J Wrist Surg 2015;4:93–100.

18. Herzberg G, Burnier M, Marc A. The role of arthroscopy for treatment of perilunate injuries. J Wrist Surg 2015;4:101–9.

19. Kim JP, Lee JS, Park MJ. Arthroscopic treatment of perilunate dislocations and fracture dislocations. J Wrist Surg 2015;4:81–7.

Midcarpal Instability
The Role of Wrist Arthroscopy

Ryan P.C. Higgin, BM, BMedSci, MRCS (Eng), David G. Hargreaves, MBBS, FRCS (Tr & Orth)*

KEYWORDS

- Wrist arthroscopy • Midcarpal instability • Capsular shrinkage • Diagnosis • Treatment

KEY POINTS

- Diagnosis of midcarpal instability (MCI) is difficult and requires knowledge of the anterior midcarpal drawer test.
- Lack of proprioception is a factor in palmar MCI.
- Soft tissue reconstructions have failed in the past due to a tendency to stretch over time.
- Arthroscopy for MCI has a role for patients with mild dynamic symptoms.
- Partial wrist fusion will stabilize the carpus and is appropriate for patients with deformity or recurrent symptoms.

INTRODUCTION

There is poor consensus among surgeons in how to best treat patients with midcarpal instability (MCI). This is due to the lack of clarity concerning the initiating pathologic condition, the confusing nomenclature that has evolved over the last few decades, the lack of clear diagnostic investigations, the lack of evidence of the natural history of the condition, and the lack of evidence of comparative treatment options. The reason for this is the relative paucity of cases requiring treatment. For many years, surgeons failed to diagnose the condition correctly and opted for nonoperative treatments.

MCI is a condition that continues to be an area of significant controversy. In carpal instability, the concept of discreet anatomic abnormalities that cause pathologic pathways is well known. In MCI, the anatomy is often normal, but there is a dysfunction of the proprioception and subsequent biofeedback mechanisms that normally stabilize the wrist.

MCI is typically classified as being a nondissociative carpal instability. It is, therefore, presumed that there is instability between the carpal rows rather than within a row. The name suggests that it is the midcarpal (MC) joint that is the cause of the problem. Actually, it is both the MC and the radiocarpal (RC) joints that are functioning abnormally, causing a lack of normal control of the proximal carpal row. The dysfunction and instability typically occurs when the wrist is under load and pronated.

Although it is conventionally understood that joints become stiff with age, it may take decades before patients with MCI become stiff enough to be considered stable and asymptomatic. Many surgeons have previously considered that this is, therefore, a condition that does not require treatment. The literature does not contain any specific longitudinal studies on the natural history of MCI. There is evidence to suggest that patients may present with symptoms that have been present for as long as 10 years.[1] Some patients can start to become symptomatic in middle age instead of early adulthood, as is typically encountered.[1] There is no evidence to suggest that chronicity of MCI causes degenerative change.

Disclosure Statement: The authors did not receive any funding for this work and have no commercial or financial conflicts of interest to declare.
Department of Orthopaedics, University Hospital Southampton, Tremona Road, Southampton, SO16 6YD, UK
* Corresponding author.
E-mail address: DGHarg@aol.com

Hand Clin 33 (2017) 717–726
http://dx.doi.org/10.1016/j.hcl.2017.06.003

TYPES OF MIDCARPAL INSTABILITY

Despite MCI, and the so-called snapping wrist, being initially recognized in the literature in 1934, the concept of MCI as a recognized pathologic condition of the wrist was not fully accepted until the 1980s when Lichtman and other authors published work on the topic.[2–6] Originally describing and coining the term ulnar MCI, Lichtman was the first to publish a case series of subjects presenting the now typical MC clunk and pain when the wrist is ulnarly deviated while in pronation[2] and Johnson recognized that the MC subluxation could present in either a palmer or dorsal pattern.[3,4] The term ulnar MCI was then dropped in preference for palmar and dorsal, formally recognizing these patterns.[6] MCI now has 3 distinct subgroups caused by intrinsic ligamentous laxity: palmar, dorsal, and combined.

Palmar

Palmar MCI (PMCI) is by far the most common presentation of MCI. It is usually an intermittent palmar tilting of the proximal carpal row that occurs during the normal transition of wrist motion (from radial to ulnar deviation). Patients may occasionally have a static deformity, with a volar intercalated segmental instability (VISI) wrist deformity visible on a lateral radiograph. More recently, there has been a consensus that PMCI can predominate on either the radial or ulnar side of the wrist. Caputo and Watson have classified PMCI into 4 types.[7,8] Types 1 and 2 are ulnar based, and types 3 and 4 radial based.

Types 1 and 2 (ulnar)

It is currently understood that general laxity associated with some possible minor predisposing trauma leads to hypermobility of the proximal carpal row and the typical palmar sag.[9] Several studies have provided in vitro evidence to suggest the involvement of dorsal radiocapitate and palmar ulnar arcuate ligaments.[2,3,10]

This laxity allows abnormal kinematics when the wrist is moved from radial to ulnar deviation, and the patient can experience a typically painful clunk as the proximal carpal row moves from flexion to extension as the wrist is moving ulnarward. This sudden pain and clunk is colloquially referred to as a catch-up clunk.

Types 3 and 4 (radial)

Types 3 and 4 are much less common types of PMCI. They both involve rotation of the scaphoid. In type 3, there is laxity at the scapho-trapezio-trapezoid (STT) joint ligaments with the scapholunate ligament remaining intact. Type 4 involves rotatory subluxation due to scapholunate ligament disruption. Lichtman and Wroten[6] more recently suggested that historical failures of some surgically managed cases of PMCI may well be due to the lack of understanding of types 1 to 4 of PMCI, and their differing causes.

Dorsal

Dorsal MCI develops when there is ligamentous laxity that results in a dorsal subluxation at the MC joint. In capitolunate instability pattern (CLIP), Louis and colleagues[3] proposed that dynamic laxity of both the volar radiolunate and dorsal capitolunate ligament complex can lead to dorsal MCI. This was diagnosed by applying pressure on the scaphoid tuberosity with longitudinal traction and flexion of the wrist. Positive cases had fluoroscopic evidence of the dorsally subluxated proximal carpal row in addition to the capitate subluxating dorsally on the lunate.[3,10] In 1986, chronic capitolunate instability was described by Johnson and Carrera.[4] They documented normal carpal alignment aside from a patient with a static dorsal intercalated segmental collapse. Clinical diagnosis was made when pressure was placed on the capitate in a dorsal direction. Subjects became apprehensive and described a painful clunk as the lunate abruptly moved dorsally and ulnarly but then realigned itself. It was considered that trauma and laxity to the palmer radiocapitate ligament was the primary cause of this condition. Both these conditions are similar and, therefore, usefully termed as a single entity.

Combined

As the name suggests, patients with combined MCI have both palmar and dorsal subluxations. The subluxation can be seen at either RC or MC joints.[11] Combined MCI is a rare presentation and there is little evidence-based research or series specifically on this topic. It probably only occurs in the hyperlax individual, such as with Ehlers-Danlos syndrome.[12]

GRADING OF PALMAR MIDCARPAL INSTABILITY

Lichtman described a classification system based on the amount of palmar MC translation and whether this was under voluntary control. This system was at risk of poor interobserver correlation and did not include subjects with a static deformity. Hargreaves[11] has recently suggested a grading system that also includes the more severe end of the spectrum when a static VISI deformity may be present (**Table 1**).

The Beighton score is still the main assessment tool for grading patients with general hypermobility.[13] Validated upper limb functional scoring systems, such as the Disabilities of Arm, Shoulder, and Hand (DASH), modified Mayo wrist score, or Patient-Rated Wrist Evaluation score, are helpful in evaluating the degree of disability caused by the condition.[14–16] Although these scoring systems provide useful information with regard to general functional limitation, there are currently no wrist scoring systems that are specific for instability.

ASSESSMENT

In mild cases, there is no single sign, symptom, or radiological or arthroscopic finding that will reliably diagnose the condition. A combination of these is required, along with the exclusion of all other carpal instability patterns. The grade of PMCI does not seem to correlate with the level of pain.

History

A voluntary clunk with no pain and no inadvertent giving way can occur in normal, lax individuals. It is only clinically relevant when it is associated with pain or a painful clunk during use. Garcia-Elias[8] highlights the description of clunking as being principally important because it indicates either carpal subluxation or reduction. Specifically, knowing that this symptomatic, painful clunking habitually occurs in the pronated forearm, with the wrist flexing ulnarly and under load, is important to consider when obtaining a patient history.[1,2,11] Some patients may only have diffuse pain, without symptoms of giving way or clunking. Understanding this may help focus questions about particular movements or activities that may precipitate symptoms. Patients experiencing symptoms while writing or pouring water from a jug or kettle is common.[1] Symptoms often represent a significant loss of function for the individual.

Examination

Clinical examination requires the confirmation of PMCI with provocative tests and the exclusion of other unrelated pathologic conditions that may be causing the symptoms.

Anterior midcarpal drawer test

This is the most reliable clinical test. In the relaxed, pronated, forearm the examiner attempts to translate the midcarpus palmarward. Simply establishing the subluxating clunk does not represent a positive test. A positive test requires the reproduction of the patient's symptomatic pain or giving way associated with the clunk.

Midcarpal shift test

This involves the examiner placing a thumb over the dorsum of the capitate and applying a palmarward pressure as the pronated wrist is taken from radial to ulnar deviation. A positive test recreates the clunk of the proximal carpal row reducing. This is the catch-up clunk.

Dorsal midcarpal tests

These include tests to identify chronic capitolunate instability and a CLIP wrist (see previous discussion).

Asking the patient to try and voluntarily reproduce their symptoms and localize their pain is equally important. This may highlight other, unrelated, causes of their presentation, such as extensor carpi ulnaris subluxation or lunotriquetral instability.

Table 1
Hargreaves grading system for palmar midcarpal instability

Grade	Assessment	Description
0	Presymptomatic	Patient able to demonstrate voluntary subluxation and catch-up clunk but remains asymptomatic
1	Dynamic	Symptomatic instability with positive MC shift tests
2	Dynamic, voluntary	Symptomatic instability with voluntary subluxation and catch-up clunk
3	Static, reducible	Deformity reducible with manipulation and VISI deformity on lateral radiograph
4	Static, irreducible	Locked, irreducible deformity and VISI on lateral radiograph

From Hargreaves DG. Midcarpal instability. J Hand Surg Eur Vol 2016;41(1):89; with permission.

Imaging

Radiographs

In most cases of PMCI, plain radiographs are normal. However, it is important to obtain a series of standard wrist radiographs to exclude the more severe cases that have a static VISI deformity (**Fig. 1**). Other causes of wrist pain and instability need to be excluded with dynamic instability radiographs. Fluoroscopic imaging while performing MC provocative tests can be very helpful in confirming PMCI, as well as demonstrating the catch-up clunk and the direction of subluxation.

Computed tomography

Computed tomography scanning rarely provides more helpful information over plain radiographs.

MRI

MRI is able to show the integrity of the volar arcuate ligament and the intrinsic carpal ligaments.[17] MRI will also confirm normal STT joint alignment. Lunotriquetral ligament rupture must be excluded because it is among the main differential diagnoses and can easily be confused clinically.

Diagnostic Arthroscopy

Wrist arthroscopy rarely has any specific changes that confirm the diagnosis of PMCI. However,

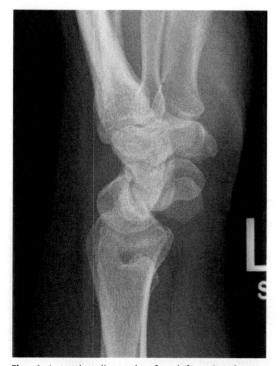

Fig. 1. Lateral radiograph of a left wrist demonstrating an extreme VISI deformity.

diffuse mild synovial hyperaemia is a common, nonspecific, observation. More important is the role of arthroscopy in excluding other pathologic conditions of the wrist that may present with similar features of PMCI. Pathologic conditions of intrinsic carpal ligaments, carpal Instability dissociative, and damage of the triangular fibrocartilage complex are all examples of diagnoses that must be excluded.

TREATMENT
Conservative

Individuals who demonstrate mild dynamic MCI symptoms are those most likely to benefit from conservative treatments. Although there remains a significant lack of published evidence specifically on nonoperative treatment, it is widely accepted from other cross-sectional studies that hand therapy can be helpful.[1,2,18,19] Therapies used for this treatment group range from basic hand therapy exercises to targeted muscle strengthening and proprioceptive awareness. Harwood and Turner[20] have recently published a review of the current evidence for the conservative management of MCI. There is general agreement that the role of splintage should be limited to patients who have severe pain and should only be used for short periods. The use of an ulnar boost splint is the most commonly advised orthosis.[21] If a splint is used for prolonged periods, the neuromuscular conditioning deteriorates and the wrist becomes less stable. The investigators only advise the use of such a splint to aid patients who have such severe pain that they are unable to perform useful proprioceptive exercises.

Garcia-Elias[8] has proposed the role for proprioception and neuromuscular rehabilitation as an important nonoperative management of these patients. Hagert has added to this, proposing that mechanoreceptors in ligaments and carpal joints play an important role in the sensorimotor reflex pathways.[22] This is particularly relevant to those patients with MCI. The investigators have, therefore, taken the view that isometric exercises and dynamic strengthening are advantageous, and that splinting with orthotics should be considered with caution. It seems that proprioceptive pathways play an important role in both the development and subsequent treatment of patients with MCI.

Soft Tissue Reconstruction

Over the last 4 decades, the surgical options in the treatment of PMCI were limited to either soft tissue tenodesis or bone fusion procedures. Soft tissue reconstructions have been used for the milder cases of MCI. Bone fusions are used predominantly for the more severe cases and for recurrences after surgery.

Lichtman initially used an Extensor carpi ulnaris rerouting technique to stabilize the triquetrohamate articulation, but at longer term follow-up all cases had subsequently failed.[9] Other recently described techniques have included dorsal capsular reefing, dorsal tendon transfers using extensor carpi radialis brevis as an active restraint, and the use of palmaris longus as a ligament graft.[9,19,23] Long-term follow-up is not available for any of these procedures, which all have shown some encouraging short-term success.

Bone Fusions

MC fusions are commonly performed for severe MCI. However, it is not clear which type of partial wrist fusion is best. Although most patients benefit from such procedures, many have suffered significant functional limitation and stiffness as a result.[22] Limited fusions, such as triquetrohamate fusion or capitolunate fusion, seem reasonable; however, Lichtman prefers a 4-corner fusion because it gives a more solid fusion mass.[9] It is well recognized that the loss of range of movement postoperatively following fusion is in the region of 40%.[24] Some lax patients continue to have radial side wrist pain after successful MC fusion because of the residual compensatory movements. Goldfarb and colleagues[22] have published the results of a study of 8 subjects following 4-corner arthrodesis to treat PMCI. Of these, 50% remained in mild to severe pain (such that they were unable to return to work) and the average arc of wrist motion decreased from 135° to 75°. The loss of the important dart-throwing axis leads to poor patient tolerance of such procedures. To address this, radiolunate arthrodesis has been suggested.[8] The control of the lunate tilting should prevent the instability, but long-term results in these MCI patients are still needed.

Arthroscopy

Since the initial use of arthroscopy in the wrist in the 1970s, the benefits of minimal access surgery has become more evident.[25] Initially, all surgical treatments were performed open; however, some surgeons started to use arthroscopy to assist in performing tenodesis procedures. Results of these hybrid-type procedures have not been published. Over the last 15 years, the progression to develop a purely arthroscopic technique seemed attractive. The use of thermal ablation in the wrist was already established.

Arthroscopic Thermal Capsular Shrinkage

Thermal capsular shrinkage was used initially in the shoulder and subsequently in the knee, ankle, and wrist. The concept of thermally reorganizing the collagen fibers within the capsule and extrinsic ligaments gave good early results in the shoulder, but midterm to late term results have highlighted a high rate of recurrence.[26,27] The initial enthusiasm for capsular shrinkage in the shoulder has, therefore, subsequently dwindled. Recent work in a rabbit model has shown that a 6-week period of immobilization after the thermal procedure is necessary to allow the collagen fibers to regenerate at the new, shortened, length despite being slightly weaker initially.[28]

Mobilization during this time is likely to cause the collagen fibrils to stretch out and lead to failure. Joints such as the shoulder are difficult to immobilize fully, but temporary immobilization of the wrist is relatively easy and is well tolerated. This makes the wrist joint a privileged site, being suitable for thermal capsular shrinkage. Studies have shown that the collagen fibrils can shorten by approximately 15% to 30% following thermal shrinkage.[29] For capsular shrinkage to be effective, this must be maintained. Postoperative immobilization is, therefore, essential and the lack of it was the probable cause of midterm recurrence in the shoulder joint.

Mason and Hargreaves[1] published early results of arthroscopic thermal shrinkage on a series of 15 wrists with PMCI. The technique involved thermal shrinkage to the extrinsic wrist ligaments that were assessable arthroscopically. This included the radial and ulnar limbs of the palmar arcuate ligament, as well as the dorsal capsule of both the RC and MC joints. In this series, 15 wrists in 13 subjects were treated with arthroscopic capsular shrinkage. Follow-up of 42 months revealed an improvement with regard to both stability and mean DASH scores in all cases. There was only a 10% loss of movement. The long-term (more than 10 years) follow-up of this series was recently presented. There were 80% excellent results with only mild recurrence of symptoms in a few subjects. There were no long-term complications. These results suggest that this treatment method is a useful alternative to other conventional soft tissue surgery.[1] Osterman[30] has recently presented a series of subjects with Ehlers-Danlos syndrome who underwent a similar arthroscopic capsular shrinkage. He presented a short-term follow-up with good results in a group of subjects who are recognized for being difficult to treat with a high risk of recurrence.[30] His published and long-term results are awaited.

With careful and selective electrothermal capsulorrhaphy the surgeon is able to shrink the wrist capsule, thereby providing stabilization, without significantly compromising wrist movement. Techniques used for performing capsular shrinkage have varied. The use of the activated wand as a paintbrush was initially suggested in the shoulder. In the wrist, Hargreaves[31] recommended a spotting-type technique. It is recognized that the risks of thermal burns need to be limited by the technique used. Prolonged activation of the wand will inevitably cause collateral damage to articular cartilage or neighboring extra-articular structures. The areas of the capsule that can be reached by a thermal probe using standard portals are limited. However, in all cases, the important dorsal RC ligaments and the palmar arcuate ligaments can be treated (**Figs. 2** and **3**).

As experience has grown, arthroscopic electrothermal shrinkage has subsequently been used for other conditions in the wrist. Mild scapholunate ligament instability and peripheral triangular fibrocartilage complex tears are examples.[31,32]

Arthroscopic capsular shrinkage has been shown to be suitable for patients with dynamic PMCI; Hargreaves grades 1 and 2 are shown in **Fig. 4**. It has allowed improved stability with no limitation of movement. The results have been adequately maintained over the long term. Despite this, Hagert raised concerns about the technique.[22] They suggest that the heat required for the shrinkage may damage the capsular mechanoreceptors and nervous terminal endings. This may ultimately effect the proprioception of the

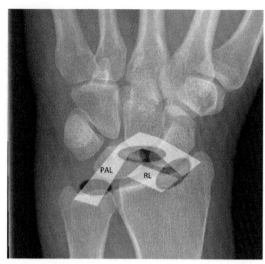

Fig. 3. Thermal ablation of the palmar capsule. Specific areas of the palmar capsule treated with thermal ablation. PAL, palmar arcuate ligament; RL, radiolunate ligament.

joint. From the authors' experience, it seems that the improved stability of the joint outweighs any potential loss of proprioception. Further published results from other centers and investigators would strengthen the case.

COMPLICATIONS OF ARTHROSCOPIC CAPSULAR SHRINKAGE

No significant complication was reported in the series by Mason and Hargreaves,[1] but it is clear that thermal wands can be associated with significant complications. Adjacent structures on the volar and dorsal surfaces are at risk of thermal injury. The authors are aware of cases of injury to skin, extensor tendons, and even the ulnar nerve. The incidence of such complications is difficult to quantify, but it is clear that care needs to be taken to avoid such.

Leclercq and colleagues[32] performed an international multicenter study of 10,107 subjects and identified a complication rate of 6% when performing all wrist arthroscopic procedures. They divided complications into those caused by subject positioning, portal insertion, and procedure. Their only documentation of thermal injury was of 3 subjects who received skin burns (0.03%). Chondral injury due to portal insertion and instrumentation is well documented with an incidence of 0.5%.[33] This is more common when the joint is tight and access is difficult.[33,34] The incidence of such chondral injuries is likely to be less in arthroscopy for PMCI because the joints are usually lax. This allows ease of instrumentation around the joint.

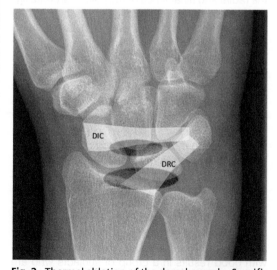

Fig. 2. Thermal ablation of the dorsal capsule. Specific areas of the dorsal capsule treated with thermal ablation. DIC, dorsal intercarpal ligament; DRC, dorsal RC ligament.

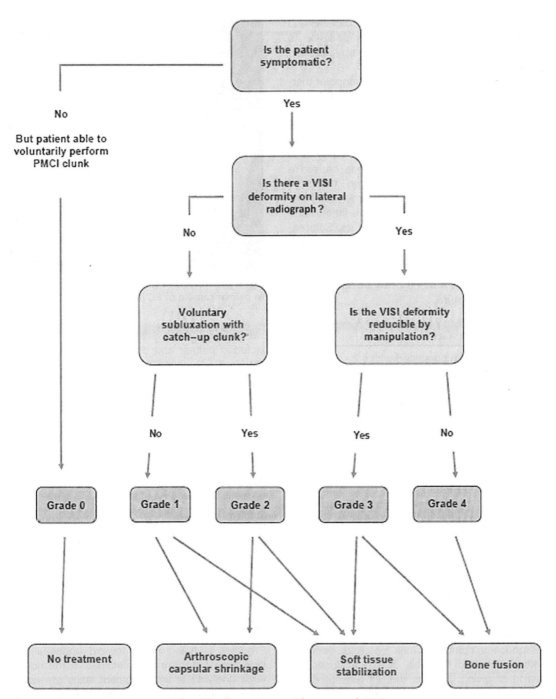

Fig. 4. Assessment and treatment algorithm for patients with suspected PMCI.

Cases of thermal injury have been documented following the use of thermal ablation. Pell and Uhl describe a series of 47 subjects, with 3 suffering significant complication directly caused by thermal ablation.[31] All 3 subjects sustained tendon ruptures with 1 also sustaining a full-thickness skin burn. It is not clear whether the injury in these cases was due to heat dissipating from the probe shaft or due to excessive use of the wand.

To minimize this risk of thermal injury it is, therefore, important to use thermal ablation selectively on specific areas only. The depth of heat penetration through specific tissues depends on their individual impedance. The wrist joint capsule and adjacent ligaments have a lower impedance to cartilage or bone and so thermal energy penetration is increased over a given time.[35]

In 2002, the use of bipolar and monopolar thermal wands was investigated in vitro by Edwards and colleagues.[36,37] They found that chondrocyte death was greater with higher thermal temperatures and that this could be directly related to poor fluid flow during arthroscopy. They also found that the use of bipolar wands caused a greater risk of chondrocyte death than did monopolar wards. Modern equipment is now thermoregulated and can give real-time monitoring of the irrigation fluid temperature. Sotereanos and colleagues[38] also investigated the fluid temperature during thermal wand use and advised using outflow portals to encourage increased flow as a mode of reducing the intra-articular temperature.

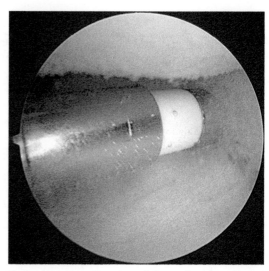

Fig. 5. Intraoperative view of thermal probe adjacent to palmar capsule of RC joint.

Recent Example Case

A 26-year-old man presented with a 2-year history of pain in the right dominant wrist. He presented following a minor injury while working as a steel fabricator. He had initially presented to his local hospital with symptoms of wrist pain, giving way, and weakness, which had developed gradually after his nonspecific injury. He was investigated with an initial working diagnosis of scapholunate ligament instability. Radiographs and MRI scans excluded any obvious ligament disruption. There was no MC malalignment. Physiotherapy had failed to improve his symptoms. He was referred for further specialist opinion. Examination showed some generalized joint laxity. The wrist had no deformity at rest. There was a full range of movement, but discomfort was reproduced at maximal extension. Specific instability tests were normal for scapholunate and lunotriquetral ruptures. A positive MC drawer test reproduced the feeling of giving way and pain. The patient was able to reproduce a catch-up clunk on ulnar deviation with a clenched fist. This also reproduced his feeling of giving way. On the left asymptomatic wrist, there was palmar MC laxity, but this did not reproduce pain nor a feeling of anxiety. A diagnosis of PMCI was made. He was advised to try a specific strengthening program, including proprioception and biofeedback. All exercises were performed in either supination or neutral rotation. He failed to made adequate progress over 6 months and so was offered the option of surgery. Surgical options were discussed and the patient chose an arthroscopic capsular shrinkage. The procedure was performed under general anesthetic. Passive

wrist motion was assessed fluoroscopically, this included palmar and dorsal stress views. Using standard arthroscopic portals, both the RC and MC joints were assessed to exclude any coexisting pathologic condition. A thermal capsular shrinkage was then performed on the palmar and dorsal capsule of both RC and MC joints (**Fig. 5**). A bulky wool and crepe bandage was applied postoperatively. This was reduced and changed to a removable wrist splint at 2 weeks. He was advised to stay in the splint continuously until 6 weeks postsurgery, at which point gentle mobilization was initiated. He was not referred for physiotherapy. At 4 months postsurgery, he had regained 80% of his wrist motion and an MC drawer test was negative. There was no palmar or dorsal MC laxity. His pain level was 1 out of 10 and he described his improvement as infinitely better.

SUMMARY

Progress is being made toward understanding how carpal stability is maintained in the normal wrist. Individuals with ligament laxity are reliant on proprioceptive reflexes for the stability in normal function. In PMCI, these reflexes fail to give adequate control, allowing the lax wrist to develop a VISI-type pattern while under load. The reason for the loss of proprioception is unknown, but many patients have a minor injury or a period of wrist immobilization as the initiating event. It is possible that the muscular responses to the reflexes are out of synchronization and possibly cause sensations that are interpreted as pain. It is probable that the dysfunctions of these proprioceptive reflexes are the cause for PMCI, rather than a single ligament failure.

The spectrum of PMCI has been documented by the grading system suggested by Hargreaves. This includes both the presymptomatic wrist and the more severe end of the spectrum with a fixed VISI deformity. This grading system guides treatment options. There is no single procedure that is appropriate for all grades of PMCI.

The treatment of PMCI continues to be controversial. Different new types of soft tissue tenodesis or tendon transfer techniques continue to be developed, but long-term results are not yet available. Wrist arthroscopy has a role in either assisting these particular soft tissue procedures or as a specific arthroscopic treatment (thermal capsular shrinkage). Arthroscopic capsular shrinkage is showing encouraging signs of longevity and has the advantage of maintaining almost full movement. Arthroscopic capsular shrinkage is only suitable for dynamic stages. In recurrent cases and static deformities, a more robust type of procedure is required. In these situations, a partial wrist fusion is advised. A radiolunate fusion is likely to be the bone procedure that will give the most normal wrist kinematics, but there are no published results of this in cases of PMCI. There may be a future for arthroscopic-assisted radiolunate fusion.

Long-term results and papers confirming replication from other centers are awaited for all techniques and treatments in PMCI. Comparative studies are unlikely due to the small numbers from each center, but, as confidence increases in diagnosis and treatment options, it is hoped that larger series will follow.

ACKNOWLEDGMENTS

The authors would like to thank their senior hand physiotherapist, Peter Belward, for providing his advice and experiences in the conservative management of PMCI.

REFERENCES

1. Mason WT, Hargreaves DG. Arthroscopic thermal capsulorrhaphy for palmar midcarpal instability. J Hand Surg Eur Vol 2007;32(4):411–6.
2. Lichtman DM, Schneider JR, Swafford AR, et al. Ulnar midcarpal instability-clinical and laboratory analysis. J Hand Surg Am 1981;6(5):515–23.
3. Louis DS, Hankin FM, Greene TL, et al. Central carpal instability-capitate lunate instability pattern: diagnosis by dynamic displacement. Orthopedics 1984;7(11):1693–6.
4. Johnson RP, Carrera GF. Chronic capitolunate instability. J Bone Joint Surg Am 1986;68(8):1164–76.
5. Lichtman DM, Bruckner JD, Culp RW, et al. Palmar midcarpal instability: results of surgical reconstruction. J Hand Surg Am 1993;18(2):307–15.
6. Lichtman DM, Wroten ES. Understanding midcarpal instability. J Hand Surg Am 2006;31(3):491–8.
7. Watson HK, Weinzweig J. The wrist. Philadelphia: Lippincott Williams & Wilkins; 2001.
8. Garcia-Elias M. The non-dissociative clunking wrist: a personal view. J Hand Surg Eur Vol 2008;33(6): 698–711.
9. Ming BW, Niacaris T, Lichtman DM. Surgical techniques for the management of midcarpal instability. J Wrist Surg 2014;3(3):171–4.
10. White SJ, Louis DS, Braunstein EM, et al. Capitate-lunate instability: recognition by manipulation under fluoroscopy. AJR Am J Roentgenol 1984;143(2): 361–4.
11. Hargreaves DG. Midcarpal instability. J Hand Surg Eur Vol 2016;41(1):86–93.
12. Woerdeman LAE, Ritt MJPF, Meijer B, et al. Wrist problems in patients with Ehlers-Danlos syndrome. Eur J Plast Surg 2000;23(4):208–10.
13. Beighton P, Horan F. Orthopaedic aspects of the Ehlers-Danlos syndrome. J Bone Joint Surg Br 1969;51(3):444–53.
14. Hudak PL, Amadio PC, Bombardier C. Development of an upper extremity outcome measure: the DASH (disabilities of the arm, shoulder and hand) [corrected]. The Upper Extremity Collaborative Group (UECG). Am J Ind Med 1996;29(6):602–8.
15. MacDermid JC, Turgeon T, Richards RS, et al. Patient rating of wrist pain and disability: a reliable and valid measurement tool. J Orthop Trauma 1998;12(8):577–86.
10. Cooney WP, Linscheld RL, Dobyns JH. Triangular fibrocartilage tears. J Hand Surg Am 1994;19(1): 143–54.
17. Chang W, Peduto AJ, Aguiar RO, et al. Arcuate ligament of the wrist: normal MR appearance and its relationship to palmar midcarpal instability: a cadaveric study. Skeletal Radiol 2007;36(7):641–5.
18. Ritt MJ, de Groot PJ. A new technique for the treatment of midcarpal instability. J Wrist Surg 2015;4(1): 71–4.
19. Wright TW, Dobyns JH, Linscheid RL, et al. Carpal instability non-dissociative. J Hand Surg Br 1994; 19(6):763–73.
20. Harwood C, Turner L. Conservative management of midcarpal instability. J Hand Surg Eur Vol 2016; 41(1):102–9.
21. Chinchalkar S, Yong SA. An ulnar boost splint for midcarpal instability. J Hand Ther 2004;17(3):377–9.
22. Hagert E, Lluch A, Rein S. The role of proprioception and neuromuscular stability in carpal instabilities. J Hand Surg Eur Vol 2016;41(1):94–101.
23. Chaudhry T, Shahid M, Wu F, et al. Soft tissue stabilization for palmar midcarpal instability using a

palmaris longus tendon graft. J Hand Surg Am 2015; 40(1):103–8.

24. Logan JS, Warwick D. The treatment of arthritis of the wrist. Bone Joint J 2015;97B(10):1303–8.

25. Chen YC. Arthroscopy of the wrist and finger joints. Orthop Clin North Am 1979;10(3):723–33.

26. de Vries JS, Krips R, Blankevoort L, et al. Arthroscopic capsular shrinkage for chronic ankle instability with thermal radiofrequency: prospective multicenter trial. Orthopedics 2008;31(7):655.

27. Toth AP, Warren RF, Petrigliano FA, et al. Thermal shrinkage for shoulder instability. HSS J 2011;7(2):108–14.

28. Demirhan M, Uysal M, Kilicoglu O, et al. Tensile strength of ligaments after thermal shrinkage depending on time and immobilization: in vivo study in the rabbit. J Shoulder Elbow Surg 2005;14(2):193–200.

29. Luke TA, Rovner AD, Karas SG, et al. Volumetric change in the shoulder capsule after open inferior capsular shift versus arthroscopic thermal capsular shrinkage: a cadaveric model. J Shoulder Elbow Surg 2004;13(2):146–9.

30. Osterman, L. Pre-Congress Seminar. Paper presented at: Federation for European Societies of Surgery of the Hand (FESSH). Santander Exhibition Centre, Santander (Spain), June 22nd–25th, 2016.

31. Pell RF, Uhl RL. Complications of thermal ablation in wrist arthroscopy. Arthroscopy 2004;20(Suppl 2):84–6.

32. Beredjiklian PK, Bozentka DJ, Leung YL, et al. Complications of wrist arthroscopy. J Hand Surg Am 2004;29(3):406–11.

33. Leclercq C, Mathoulin C, Member of EWAS. Complications of wrist arthroscopy: a multicenter study based on 10,107 arthroscopies. J Wrist Surg 2016;5(4):320–6.

34. El-Gazzar Y, Baker CL. Complications of elbow and wrist arthroscopy. Sports Med Arthrosc 2013;21(2):80–8.

35. Geissler W. Wrist and elbow arthroscopy: a practical surgical guide to techniques. 2nd edition. New York: Springer; 2015.

36. Edwards RB, Lu Y, Nho S, et al. Thermal chondroplasty of chondromalacic human cartilage. An ex vivo comparison of bipolar and monopolar radiofrequency devices. Am J Sports Med 2002;30(1):90–7.

37. Edwards RB, Lu Y, Rodriguez E, et al. Thermometric determination of cartilage matrix temperatures during thermal chondroplasty: comparison of bipolar and monopolar radiofrequency devices. Arthroscopy 2002;18(4):339–46.

38. Sotereanos DG, Darlis NA, Kokkalis ZT, et al. Effects of radiofrequency probe application on irrigation fluid temperature in the wrist joint. J Hand Surg Am 2009;34(10):1832–7.

The Role of Wrist Arthroscopy in Kienbock Disease

Simon B.M. MacLean, MBChB, FRCSEd, PGDipCE[a],
Karim Kantar, MBBS[a,*],
Gregory I. Bain, MBBS, FRACS, FA, PhD[a],
David M. Lichtman, MD[b,c]

KEYWORDS

- Kienbock disease • Avascular necrosis • Classification • Arthroscopy • Wrist

KEY POINTS

- Wrist arthroscopy is the "gold standard" for assessment of chondral surfaces of the lunate and wrist.
- Dry arthroscopy allows improved visualization and assessment of the wrist.
- The aim of surgical treatment is to bypass, fuse, or excise nonfunctional surfaces, and so reducing pain and maintaining functional wrist motion.
- Our new algorithm allows a patient-based and surgeon-based approach to disease management.

INTRODUCTION

Robert Kienbock, an Austrian radiologist, was the first to report on "Malacia of the Lunate," attributing a traumatic etiology to the disease.[1] Management of Kienbock disease (KD) has traditionally been based on radiologic findings as classified by Lichtman and colleagues.[2] Arthroscopy in KD has been previously described and has become a vital tool in the assessment and management of the disease.[3–6] Bain and colleagues[7–9] developed a pathoanatomical model of the disease, presenting a biomechanical and vascular theory for the development of KD. By correlating the osseous, vascular, and chondral status of the lunate and wrist, a new algorithm for treatment has been established.[7–9] This article highlights the diagnostic and therapeutic roles of wrist arthroscopy in the patient with KD.

WRIST PATHOANATOMY IN KIENBOCK DISEASE

Three columns, 2 carpal rows, and a wide joint surface constitute the wrist articulation. This accounts for a shared load transmission throughout the range of motion.

A collapsing lunate compromises the wrist as follows[7]:

1. Central column deformation, collapse, and proximal row instability

Lunate comminution or a coronal fracture (Fig. 1) allows proximal migration of the capitate. The scapholunate and lunotriquetral ligaments strain or tear as a result of lunate shortening and tilt. Loss of height of the central column results in shortening of the radial column as the scaphoid flexes. The lunate may flex or extend, depending

Conflicts of Interest: Nil.
[a] Department of Orthopaedic Surgery, Flinders University, Flinders Medical Centre, Adelaide, South Australia, Australia; [b] Uniformed Services University, Bethesda, MD, USA; [c] Department of Orthopaedic Surgery, University of North Texas, Health Science Center, Fort Worth, TX, USA
* Corresponding author. Department of Orthopaedics, Flinders University Hospital, Bedford Park, Adelaide South Australia 5042, Australia.
E-mail address: karimkantar@gmail.com

Hand Clin 33 (2017) 727–734
http://dx.doi.org/10.1016/j.hcl.2017.07.003

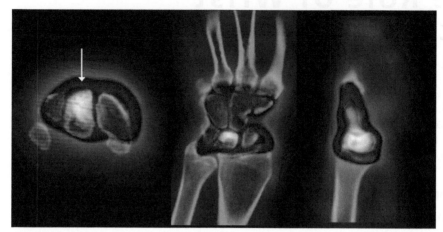

Fig. 1. Single-photon emission computed tomography (SPECT)-computed tomography (CT): a SPECT scan showing intense osteoclastic activity at the lunate. The anatomic detail provided by the CT scan shows a coronal fracture through the lunate on the axial section (*white arrow*). (© Gregory I. Bain.)

on the extent of osseous disruption and direction of force through the lunate.

2. Degenerative changes at the radiocarpal joint

Fractures of the lunate subchondral bone plate produce irregularity at the lunate fossa. Degenerative changes then progress in the radial direction; excessive scaphoid flexion leads to incongruence at the radioscaphoid articulation and degenerative changes at the scaphoid fossa.

3. Degenerative changes at the midcarpal joint and KD Advanced Collapse (KDAC)

Kissing lesions occur between the capitate and lunate facet and degenerative changes progress with further fragmentation of the lunate. Once there is significant involvement of both carpal rows and 2 or more columns, KDAC has occurred and a salvage procedure is now required.

WRIST ARTHROSCOPY IN KIENBOCK DISEASE

The arm is suspended with a traction tower and a 2.7-mm 30° arthroscope is used. We prefer to infiltrate the portal sites and the radiocarpal joint with 15 to 20 mL 1% lidocaine, 1:200,000 adrenaline mixture, 20 to 30 minutes before the procedure. A tourniquet is applied to the arm but not inflated. Standard portals used are 3 to 4, 6R, radial midcarpal portal, and ulnar midcarpal portal. Dry arthroscopy is then performed. This allows for better resolution of articular surfaces. Fluid insufflation compresses the capillaries within the joint and synovitis. As a result, tissue perfusion is better assessed dry.

Meticulous inspection of the articular surfaces of the lunate and surrounding carpus is then performed. Probe ballottement allows assessment of chondral integrity and the presence of a "floating" surface. A "floating" surface is created when a collapsed lunate is distracted on traction, creating a potential space between the intact articular surface and the collapsed subchondral bone. A concealed fracture of the lunate articular surface sometimes can be identified (**Fig. 2**). The state of the perilunate ligaments is assessed, and often found to be torn in more advanced cases. The "functional" status of the articular surfaces and the wrist is graded using the Bain and Begg classification (**Fig. 3**):

1. Inspect the lunate and perilunate surfaces for chondral damage or fracture
2. Probe the articular surface for softening, chondral flaps/defects, concealed lesions, and degeneration
3. Identify a "floating" lunate articular surface
4. Debride loose osteochondral fragments, flaps, and synovitis (see **Fig. 2**)

BAIN AND BEGG CLASSIFICATION

We have previously reported on the principles and pathology encountered at arthroscopy (**Box 1**) and have classified the articular surface into functional or nonfunctional based (see **Fig. 3**) on this evaluation[4]:

- Functional: Normal appearance, smooth and glistening
- Nonfunctional: Degenerative changes, including subchondral fracture

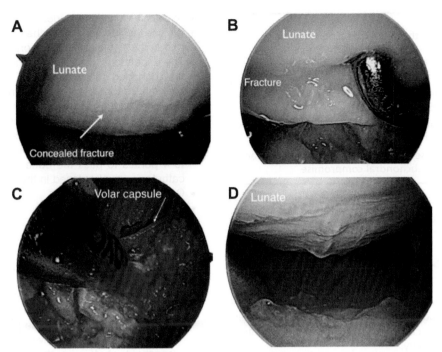

Fig. 2. (*A, B*) Wrist 1: arthroscopic images-probe ballottement under traction reveals the concealed fracture of the lunate. (*C*) Wrist 2: arthroscopic debridement of the radiocarpal joint. (*D*) Wrist 3: inspection reveals irregularity and softening of the lunate fossa of the radius and the proximal lunate. (© Gregory I. Bain.)

LICHTMAN AND BAIN CLASSIFICATION

Our new algorithm respects the vascular, chondral, and osseous changes in KD, combining clinical, radiologic, and arthroscopic findings to guide subsequent management[10–30] (**Box 2**). The algorithm also respects the skill set, training, and resources of the surgeon, as well as the age, functional demands, and comorbidities of the patient. We have made minor alterations to the algorithm since its original description to reflect the

Articular based classification

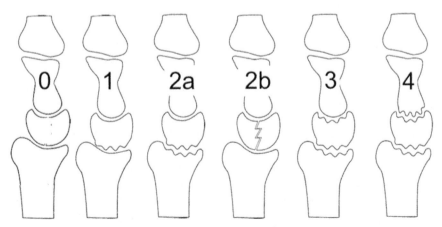

Fig. 3. The Bain and Begg arthroscopic classification for the treatment of KD. (*From* Bain GI, Durrant A. An articular-based approach to Kienbock avascular necrosis of the lunate. Tech Hand Up Extrem Surg 2011;15(1):41–7; with permission.)

Box 1
Tenets of arthroscopy in Kienbock disease

- Synovitis is always present and correlates with the grade of articular damage
- Articular damage is underestimated on plain imaging
- Findings on arthroscopy usually lead to a change in management plan
- Some cases have an intact chondral surface despite subchondral compromise

---

importance of carpal instability in the pathogenesis of the disease.

ARTHROSCOPIC SURGERY IN KIENBOCK DISEASE

Bain and colleagues[7] previously described the role of arthroscopy in the staging of KD; however, arthroscopy can be used to assist or substitute for open surgery.

Arthroscopic Forage

This is a compartment decompression procedure for the lunate (**Fig. 4**). This should be performed in cases in which there is no articular compromise and functional surfaces exist throughout the carpus (B1). An area of necrosis is perforated and a weep hole is created to decompress the venous hypertension. This then leads to reactive hyperemia and an acute inflammatory response within the lunate:

- The scope is introduced into the 6R portal and a 2.5-mm drill within a sheath through the 3 to 4 portal.
- The drill is positioned under arthroscopic control and confirmed to be satisfactory with fluoroscopy.
- The drill is then advanced onto the dorsal aspect of the lunate. The angle of the drill can be positioned to coincide with the area of necrosis.
- Once the drill is removed, morcellized bone graft can be tamped into the defect. Debris can then be removed arthroscopically from the joint.

Arthroscopic Radioscapholunate Fusion

For the arthroscopic radioscapholunate (RSL) procedure, it is vital to have a functional midcarpal articulation.[7] The procedure should therefore be performed only in patients with B2, C2a, and C2b disease if the midcarpal joint is intact:

- Assess for functional midcarpal articulation.
- We use the 4 to 5 portal for the scope with the burr in the 1 to 2 and 3 to 4 portals.
- The dependent radial styloid and fossae are first debrided followed by the overhanging proximal scaphoid and lunate surfaces.
- Bone grafting or substitutes may be required to address the incongruity between the scaphoid/lunate and its radial fossae.
- We use a 4.5-mm cannula via the 1 to 2 and 3 to 4 portals to pass the bone graft; a Foley catheter is usually placed in the 4 to 5 portal.
- Compact the graft.
- Under fluoroscopic guidance
  - A radiolunate "RL" guide pin is introduced 1 cm proximal to the dorsal rim of the radius and advanced percutaneously through the central column of the distal radius to the lunate aiming of the volar horn. This maximizes lunate purchase; however, care is required not to injure the medial nerve.
  - A radioscaphoid "RS" guide pin is passed from the radial column toward the proximal scaphoid at 45° on the anteroposterior view. On the lateral view, the pin is aimed along the mid axis of radial styloid and proximal scaphoid.
- Cannulated compression screws are then advanced.

Arthroscopic Scaphocapitate Fusion

The arthroscopic scaphocapitate (SC) fusion procedure is usually used for scaphoid nonunion using an open technique and has been reported in multiple series.[7,31–33] A functional radioscaphoid articulation is a prerequisite. It may relieve pain and the progression of KD by unloading the lunate through load transfer from central to radial column.[34,35]

It is indicated if the lunate is compromised (B2) or not reconstructable (B3) (**Fig. 5**). It is also indicated if carpal instability exists with intact articulations (C1) or if the radiolunate articulation is compromised (C2a).

The surfaces of the capitate and the waist and proximal scaphoid are resected as they face each other. SC fusion is more commonly undertaken than scapho-trapezium-trapezoidal (STT) fusion, as it is more accessible arthroscopically:

- Resect the surfaces of the capitate and the waist and proximal scaphoid as they face each other.
- Start inferiorly and work upward while debriding cartilage until there is punctate bleeding from subchondral bone; excessive bleeding masking the surgical field is thus minimized.

Box 2
A modified algorithm for the treatment of Kienbock disease

A. Patient's age?

    A1. *Younger than 15 years:* Nonoperative

    A2. *16 to 20 years:* Nonoperative first. Consider unloading procedure.

    A3. *Older than 70 years:* Nonoperative first. Consider synovectomy and/or follow algorithm below.

B. Stage of the lunate?

    B1. *Lunate intact* (Cortex and cartilage intact: Lichtman 0, I, II, Schmitt A, Bain 0)

        Protect/unload the lunate:

            Orthosis or cast first (trial for 2–3 months)

            Radial shortening osteotomy, capitate shortening for ulnar +ve (radial epiphysiodesis[a])

            (Alternatives: lunate decompression, vascularized bone graft,[a] lunate forage[a])

    B2. *Lunate compromised* (Localized lunate disease: Lichtman IIIA, Schmitt B, Bain 1)

        Lunate reconstruction: MFT,[a] lunate replacement,[a] PRC (RSL fusion, SC [or STT] fusion)

    B3. *Lunate not reconstructable* (Advanced lunate disease: Lichtman IIIC, Schmitt C, Bain 2b)

        Lunate salvage (excision): Lunate replacement,[a] capitate lengthening, PRC (SC fusion)

C. State of the wrist?

    C1. Carpal instability with intact articulations: Stabilize

        Typical scaphoid flexion, with RSA greater than 600 (Lichtman IIIB)

        Stabilize radial column (SC fusion)

    C2. Localized carpal degeneration: Reconstruct

        C2a. Radiolunate articulation compromised *(Lichtman IIIA, Bain 2a)*

            Bypass (SC fusion), reconstruct (MFT graft), or replace (lunate prosthesis), Fuse (RSL fusion)

        C2b. Radioscaphoid articulation compromised

            PRC if lunate facet intact, RSL fusion if lunate facet compromised and midcarpal joint Intact

    C3. KDAC, Advanced carpal collapse, and degeneration: Salvage

        Wrist not reconstructable (Advanced wrist disease: Lichtman IV, Bain 4)

        Salvage (fusion or arthroplasty)

Other options that can be considered have been placed in (parentheses). STT fusion is an alternative to SC fusion.
Abbreviations: KDAC, Kienbock disease advanced collapse; MFT, medial femoral trochlea; PRC, proximal row carpectomy; RSA, radial-scaphoid angle; RSL, radio-scapho-lunate; SC, scaphocapitate; STT, scapho-trapezium-trapezoidal.
[a] Alternate procedures, techniques that require specialized skills and therefore affect what the surgeon can offer. The classification determines the recommended treatment based on the patient's age (A), status of the lunate (B), and the status of the wrist (C). What the surgeon can offer (D) and what the patient wants (E) ultimately determine what is performed.

- The distal third of the scaphoid at the STT articulation is usually not debrided.
- Consider resecting a multifragmented lunate.
- Normal alignment should be checked on fluoroscopy; it is essential to maintain the height of the carpus so as to successfully transmit load through the scaphoid facet: scapholunate and scaphocapitate angle between 30° and 57°; the capitolunate angle should be 0° ± 15°.[36]
- Use a volar-directed force on the scaphoid tubercle to control its position.
- Insert 2 guide pins across the SC interval.
  - The first via the 1 to 2 portal; aim for a proximal and middle-third entry point on the scaphoid; direct the pin so that it is 60° to

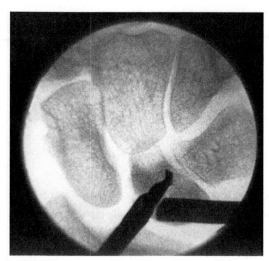

Fig. 4. Lunate forage fluoroscopic image of the wrist with the scope (6R portal) used to guide the drill within a sheath (3–4 portal) into the lunate. (*From* Bain GI, Durrant A. An articular-based approach to Kienbock avascular necrosis of the lunate. Tech Hand Up Extrem Surg 2011;15(1):41–7; with permission.)

the longitudinal axis of the wrist, and pass it through the center of both scaphoid and capitate on the lateral view.
  ○ The second is passed 5 mm distal and parallel to the first; a middle and distal third junction entry point is required.
• Use an over the guide wire technique to measure, drill, and place the screws using fluoroscopy.
• We do not routinely use bone graft.

POSTOPERATIVE MANAGEMENT: ARTHROSCOPIC PARTIAL CARPAL FUSIONS

A short-arm cast is placed for 6 to 8 weeks until union, then full active range of movement is encouraged.

Arthroscopic Proximal Row Carpectomy

• A functional articular surface of the proximal capitate and lunate fossa is required (B2 or 3, C2). The ideal patient would be of low demand and older than 45 years.[7,10]
• Start with a diagnostic arthroscopy, assess the articular surface, and perform a standard debridement.
• Remove the central osseous portion of the lunate, scaphoid, and triquetrum.
• Complete the lunate and triquetrum excision while preserving the scaphoid's distal one-third; this preserves the attachments of STT and the dorsal intercarpal ligaments.
• Iatrogenic injuries include radial artery compromise and thermal damage from the burr; these must be avoided by cautious surgical technique and continuous irrigation.
• The bipolar cautery and the pituitary rongeur (**Fig. 6**) are useful tools in releasing capsular attachments and removing joint fragments.

Postoperative Management of Proximal Row Carpectomy

• The wrist is placed in a wool and crepe bandage following surgery for 7 to 10 days.
• A removable brace is then given and a full range of active movement allowed.

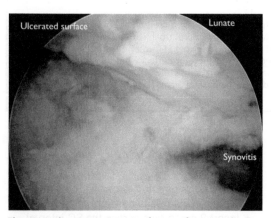

Fig. 5. Arthroscopic image of a nonfunctional proximal lunate articular surface with sclerosis and ulceration of the proximal articular surface. (© Gregory I. Bain.)

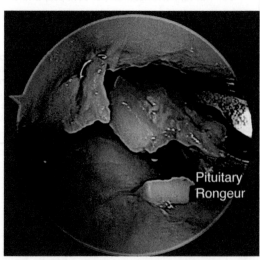

Fig. 6. Arthroscopic removal of necrotic bone from the proximal lunate using pituitary rongeurs. (© Gregory I. Bain.)

SUMMARY

Wrist arthroscopy is a vital tool in the management of patients with KD. As a diagnostic procedure and combined with medical imaging, it has allowed further staging and classification of the disease. We have outlined our current arthroscopic practice for the treatment of KD. With emerging technology, more therapeutic options will be available for patient care.

REFERENCES

1. R. K. Concerning traumatic malacia of the lunate and its consequences: joint degeneration and compression. Fortsch Geb Roentgen. 1910.

2. Lichtman DM, Mack GR, MacDonald RI, et al. Kienbock's disease: the role of silicone replacement arthroplasty. J Bone Joint Surg Am 1977;59(7): 899–908.

3. Schiltenwolf M, Martini AK, Mau HC, et al. Further investigations of the intraosseous pressure characteristics in necrotic lunates (Kienbock's disease). J Hand Surg Am 1996;21(5):754–8.

4. Bain GI, Yeo CJ, Morse LP. Kienbock disease: recent advances in the basic science, assessment and treatment. Hand Surg 2015;20(3):352–65.

5. Bain GI, Munt J, Turner PC. New advances in wrist arthroscopy. Arthroscopy 2008;24(3):355–67.

6. Bain GI, Begg M. Arthroscopic assessment and classification of Kienbock's disease. Tech Hand Up Extrem Surg 2006;10(1):8–13.

7. Bain GI, MacLean SB, Tse WL, et al. Kienbock disease and arthroscopy: assessment, classification, and treatment. J Wrist Surg 2010;5(4):255–60.

8. Bain GI, MacLean SB, Yeo CJ, et al. The etiology and pathogenesis of Kienbock disease. J Wrist Surg 2016;5(4):248–54.

9. Lichtman DM, Bain GI. Kienböck's disease: advances in diagnosis and treatment, vol. 1. Switzerland: Springer International Publishing; 2016.

10. Chim H, Moran SL. Long-term outcomes of proximal row carpectomy: a systematic review of the literature. J Wrist Surg 2012;1(2):141–8.

11. Pegoli L, Ghezzi A, Cavalli E, et al. Arthroscopic assisted bone grafting for early stages of Kienbock's disease. Hand Surg 2011;16(2):127–31.

12. Shin AY, Weinstein LP, Bishop AT. Kienbock's disease and gout. J Hand Surg Br 1999;24(3): 363–5.

13. Shin AY, Bishop AT, Berger RA. Vascularized pedicled bone grafts for disorders of the carpus. Tech Hand Up Extrem Surg 1998;2(2):94–109.

14. Sheetz KK, Bishop AT, Berger RA. The arterial blood supply of the distal radius and ulna and its potential use in vascularized pedicled bone grafts. J Hand Surg Am 1995;20(6):902–14.

15. Heymans R, Koebke J. The pedicled pisiform transposition in Kienbock's disease. An anatomical and functional analysis. Handchir Mikrochir Plast Chir 1993;25(4):199–203.

16. Heymans R, Adelmann E, Koebke J. Anatomical bases of the pediculated pisiform transplant and the intercarpal fusion by Graner in Kienbock's disease. Surg Radiol Anat 1992;14(3):195–201.

17. Brunelli F, Mathoulin C, Saffar P. Description of a vascularized bone graft taken from the head of the 2nd metacarpal bone. Ann Chir Main Memb Super 1992; 11(1):40–5 [in French].

18. Saffar P. Replacement of the semilunar bone by the pisiform. Description of a new technique for the treatment of Kienboeck's disease. Ann Chir Main 1982;1(3):276–9 [in French].

19. Fujiwara H, Oda R, Morisaki S, et al. Long-term results of vascularized bone graft for stage III Kienbock disease. J Hand Surg Am 2013;38(5): 904–8.

20. Doi K, Oda T, Soo-Heong T, et al. Free vascularized bone graft for nonunion of the scaphoid. J Hand Surg Am 2000;25(3):507–19.

21. Gabl M, Reinhart C, Lutz M, et al. Vascularized bone graft from the iliac crest for the treatment of nonunion of the proximal part of the scaphoid with an avascular fragment. J Bone Joint Surg Am 1999;81(10):1414–28.

22. Pechlaner S, Hussl H, Kunzel KH. Alternative surgical method in pseudarthroses of the scaphoid bone. Prospective study. Handchir Mikrochir Plast Chir 1987;19(6):302–5 [in German].

23. Lin HH, Stern PJ. "Salvage" procedures in the treatment of Kienbock's disease. Proximal row carpectomy and total wrist arthrodesis. Hand Clin 1993; 9(3):521–6.

24. Bain GI, Ondimu P, Hallam P, et al. Radioscapholunate arthrodesis—a prospective study. Hand Surg 2009;14(2–3):73–82.

25. Boyer JS, Adams B. Distal radius hemiarthroplasty combined with proximal row carpectomy: case report. Iowa Orthop J 2010;30:168–73.

26. Culp RW, Bachoura A, Gelman SE, et al. Proximal row carpectomy combined with wrist hemiarthroplasty. J Wrist Surg 2012;1(1):39–46.

27. Vance MC, Packer G, Tan D, et al. Midcarpal hemiarthroplasty for wrist arthritis: rationale and early results. J Wrist Surg 2012;1(1):61–8.

28. Buck-Gramcko D. Wrist denervation procedures in the treatment of Kienbock's disease. Hand Clin 1993;9(3):517–20.

29. Gaspar MP, Lou J, Kane PM, et al. Complications following partial and total wrist arthroplasty: a single-center retrospective review. J Hand Surg Am 2016;41(1):47–53.e4.

30. Sagerfors M, Gupta A, Brus O, et al. Total wrist arthroplasty: a single-center study of 219 cases

with 5-year follow-up. J Hand Surg Am 2015;40(12): 2380–7.

31. Sutro CJ. Treatment of nonunion of the carpal navicular bone. Surgery 1946;20:536–40.

32. Luegmair M, Saffar P. Scaphocapitate arthrodesis for treatment of late stage Kienbock disease. J Hand Surg Eur Vol 2014;39(4):416–22.

33. Pisano SM, Peimer CA, Wheeler DR, et al. Scaphocapitate intercarpal arthrodesis. J Hand Surg Am 1991;16(2):328–33.

34. Garcia-Elias M, Cooney WP, An KN, et al. Wrist kinematics after limited intercarpal arthrodesis. J Hand Surg Am 1989;14(5):791–9.

35. Horii E, Garcia-Elias M, Bishop AT, et al. Effect on force transmission across the carpus in procedures used to treat Kienbock's disease. J Hand Surg Am 1990;15(3):393–400.

36. Minamikawa Y, Peimer CA, Yamaguchi T, et al. Ideal scaphoid angle for intercarpal arthrodesis. J Hand Surg Am 1992;17(2):370–5.

Arthroscopic-Assisted Partial Wrist Arthrodesis

Eva-Maria Baur, MD

KEYWORDS

- Wrist arthroscopy • Partial wrist fusion • Partial wrist arthrodesis • Limited wrist fusion
- Arthroscopic assisted • SLAC • SNAC

KEY POINTS

- Osteoarthritis of the wrist is a common issue following trauma or occasionally following degenerative lesions. The most common form results from scapholunate lesions or scaphoid nonunion (scapholunate advanced collapse [SLAC] and scaphoid nonunion advanced collapse [SNAC]). It can also develop after distal radius fracture or other ligament lesions, and in degenerative conditions or systemic diseases.
- Partial wrist fusion or arthrodesis is a well-known procedure for these issues. The most common solution is four-corner fusion in wrists with SLAC and SNAC.
- Arthroscopic (assisted) partial wrist fusion has been described, but the established procedure is always performed as an open technique.
- The arthroscopic technique, results, pitfalls, and complications are described. Changes of the technique parallel an ongoing learning curve.
- Wrist arthroscopy is a helpful tool in these procedures. Better results are expected regarding range of motion and bony healing, but this technique still needs to be proved in randomized studies.

 Video content accompanies this article at www.hand.theclinics.com.

INTRODUCTION/NATURE OF PROBLEM

Partial wrist arthrodesis (PWA) is a salvage procedure designed to preserve joint motion, increase function, and reduce wrist pain.

Four-corner fusion (4CF) is probably the most frequently used and well-known procedure, primarily for scapholunate advanced collapse (SLAC) or scaphoid nonunion advanced collapse (SNAC). Watson described degenerative wrist disorders, the SLAC wrist and PWA in the early 1980.[1–3] Treatment mostly consisted of 4CF with or without silicone replacement of the scaphoid. In other publications there are results and technical points described for only 2 or 3 bone fusions.[4–7] However, the first publication of PWA was by Thornton[8] in 1924.

These are the treatment goals in order to achieve good results:

Solid fusion: if no stable fusion is achieved (at least a very solid fibrotic union), the results are mostly bad. In the literature there are varying results, with 0% to 63% of absent bony healing and nonunion.

Good function and grip strength: objective (range of motion [ROM], Jamar, radiographs) and subjective measurements (visual analog scale [VAS], patient's satisfaction) and scores are used to determine the maximal wrist function.

The postoperative satisfaction depends on:

1. Preoperative ROM. If the patient has less ROM, compared with very good preoperative

Conflict of interest: The author has no conflict of interest.
Practice for Plastic and Hand Surgery, James-Loeb-Str. 13, Murnau D-82418, Germany
E-mail address: baur@baur-fromberg.de

mobility, satisfaction will not be good compared with somebody with the same preoperative and postoperative ROM. However, with time patients adapt to it. In general, wrist extension is more important than flexion.[1,2,6] In 1985, Palmer and colleagues[9] showed that a functional wrist needs: 30° of extension, 5° of flexion, 15° of radial duction, and 10° of ulnar duction.

2. Preoperative pain and strain. If there is only occasional pain and restriction of work or hobbies, it is better to refuse the salvage procedure and ask the patient to come back when the patient feels the need for some help.

3. Any pseudarthrosis/nonunion and/or hardware problems, which are often caused by intraoperative technical errors[10] like bad reduction and/or insufficient osteosynthesis.

Correct indications: example of bad indication; for example, SLAC 4 (**Fig. 1**). Systemic diseases like pseudogout or gout. Because of disease progression, the results are not comparable with posttraumatic cases.

Motion-preserving procedures include PWA or resection arthroplasty like proximal row carpectomy (PRC). The most frequent complications of PWA are lack of bone healing and/or hardware problems.

After PWA, the expected ROMs are 50% extension/flexion, 40% radial/ulnar abduction, and the expected grip strength is 70% of the opposite side.[6] Pain can be reduced on average to VAS 2 at rest and 4 with load, compared with 8 to 10 preoperatively.

In comparisons of PRC with 4CF, the authors get mostly similar results. Some differences are[11] that PRC gives a better ROM, has no hardware problem, and is an easier procedure, but it remains restricted for cases of SLAC/SNAC 1 to 2. 4CF gives better patient satisfaction and grip strength, but has more complications. A bias could be that

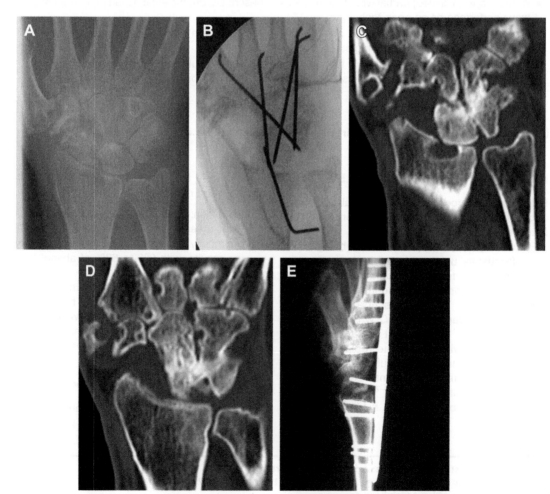

Fig. 1. (*A*) Preoperative radiograph (no rheumatoid arthritis). (*B*) Postoperative, bony healing after 6 weeks with Kirschner wires. (*C, D*) Wrong indication SLAC 4°. (*E*) Total wrist arthrodesis. Case 24 in **Table 1**.

the group of 4CF mostly consists of SLAC/SNAC 3, so the preoperative ROM, function, and pain are worse.

WHY DO IT AS AN ARTHROSCOPIC PROCEDURE: INDICATIONS AND CONSIDERATIONS

Cons: the procedure is more time consuming. It is a difficult and challenging operation.

Pros: better bone healing and ROM are expected because of less scarring, better blood supply, and less damage to ligaments and capsular structures (**Fig. 2**).

Early publications from Ho[12] in 2008 and del Piñal and colleagues[13] and Piñal and Tandioy-Delgado[14] in 2012 and 2014 described the advantages and problems.

There are still open questions concerning arthroscopic procedures:

- The theory of better bone healing and ROM has not yet been proved. Ho[12] described 3 nonunions (2 stable fibrotic) out of 12 patients, with the need for 1 revision operation. del Piñal had no nonunion in their 4 cases.[13,14]
- The fusion rate is assessed in 2 radiographic planes, which is not sufficient to prove bone union.[15]

My Personal Thoughts

- Clinicians can expect better bone healing (see **Figs. 1** and **2**), ROM, and function, and more postoperative comfort because of less scarring, less swelling, and an earlier rehabilitation. If the general surgical and orthopedic

rules of good reduction and stable osteosynthesis are respected, clinicians can expect better bone healing because of better blood supply and less damage to soft tissues.

- Clinicians should check all patients with computed tomography (CT) scan for bone healing at postoperative weeks 6 to 8 or earlier if there is any doubt about hardware position.

INDICATIONS/CONTRAINDICATIONS FOR PARTIAL WRIST ARTHRODESIS

In order to determine stage 2 or 3 of SLAC/SNAC, clinicians can perform wrist arthroscopy before PWA.

The most common indications are advanced osteoarthritis (OA) like SLAC 2/3, SNAC 2/3, malunited fractures with secondary OA, mostly distal radius fracture, scaphoid-trapezium-trapezoid (STT) OA, isolated midcarpal (MC) OA (**Fig. 3**), Kienbock disease, and severe carpal instability. Inflammatory diseases like rheumatoid arthritis (RA) and gout/pseudogout could also be an indication. It is important to optimize the medical treatments of the underlying diseases to achieve the best operative result.

Contraindications are progressive inflammatory diseases, acute infection, or osteomyelitis. Patients asking for a final solution are not contraindicated for PWA because total wrist fusion (TWF) is not a guarantee of the absence of pain and good function. A study by Krimmer and colleagues[16] in 2000 showed that MC fusion is superior to TWF with respect to function and satisfaction.

Is smoking a contraindication? The authors do not refuse smokers for PWA but explain that they

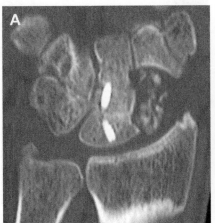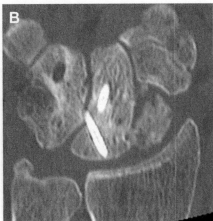

Fig. 2. Neoscaphoid, originated from the removed scaphoid. Arthroscopic surgery preserved vascularity. Bone debris left behind reformed a neoscaphoid. (*A*) Six weeks postoperative. (*B*) Six months postoperative. Case 19 in **Table 1**.

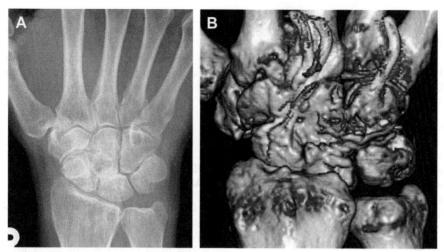

Fig. 3. (*A, B*) Isolated midcarpal OA. Case 35 in **Table 1**.

have a higher risk of inferior or slower bone healing.

Insufficient surgeon experience in arthroscopic operations may be a contraindication because there is a high demand on experience and skills.

Are long-standing carpal collapse and joint contracture contraindications? It is not more difficult to perform arthroscopic compared with open resection and address the most palmar portion of the MC joint.

Very advanced OA is a contraindication, such as SLAC 4 (see **Fig. 1**; **Fig. 4**), and the authors perform a TWF or total wrist arthroplasty.

SURGICAL TECHNIQUE/PROCEDURE
Preoperative Planning

Conventional radiographs, with the option of a CT scan and/or MRI, are required to plan the treatment. Arthroscopic staging of SLAC or SNAC 2 or 3 (or 4) is necessary.

To decide whether to plan for a 2-corner fusion (2CF), 3-corner fusion (3CF), or 4CF, arthroscopy helps clinicians look at the type of lunate according to Viegas.[17] If it is planned to do only a 2CF or 3CF, I choose a 3-bone fusion in a type 2 lunate.

If there is a positive ulnar variance or other signs of an ulnar and/or hamate impaction syndrome, it

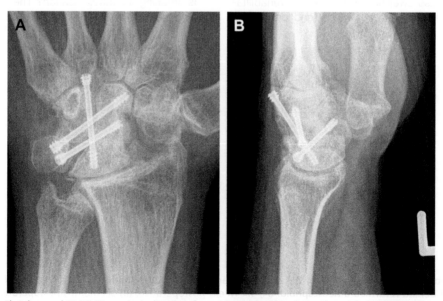

Fig. 4. (*A, B*) Advanced SLAC 4°: contraindication for midcarpal arthrodesis. Case 4 in **Table 1**.

is better to choose a 4CF or resect the tip of the hamate.

Preparation of the Operation Room, Patient Positioning, and Surgical Approach

The patient is in a supine position. The arm is put on a hand table. The hand is suspended in a traction device with 3 to 4 kg (**Fig. 5**). The operation is usually done under general anesthesia, optionally with an additional nerve block for pain reduction intraoperatively and postoperatively.

Setup and Instrumentation

A tourniquet is applied at least for the initial steps of the operation, depending on the expected operation duration.

Usually it is sufficient to use the tourniquet for steps 1 to 6 (discussed later) only, so there is no need to use a tourniquet for the remainder of the operation.

Instruments

- A small joint scope 2.4-mm or 2.7-mm diameter with 30° angulation
- A burr with a bigger tip; for example, 3.5 to 4.5 mm

Tip: a bigger oval burr (eg, from Arthrex) removes bone more efficiently and faster.

- A full-radius shaver or an aggressive cutter to address the soft tissues
- A radiofrequency probe

Dry conditions are best for diagnostic arthroscopy and semidry arthroscopy for resection. No pump is required, just the help of gravity (**Fig. 6**).

Tip: saline solution 30 cm above the hand level is enough to avoid fluid extravasation and compartment syndrome, especially in long operations.

- Special instruments from the maxillofacial or ear, nose, and throat (ENT) departments can be useful (**Fig. 7**)
- Suction pump
- Kirschner wires (K-wires), and small cannulated (headless) bone screws
- C-arm fluoroscopy (**Fig. 8**)
- Option to harvest bone graft if necessary (bone substitute is also possible [the author has no personal experience])

Arthroscopic Diagnostic View

The author uses the standard portals 3/4 and 6R for the radiocarpal joint, and ulnar midcarpal (UMC) and radial midcarpal (RMC) for the MC joint.

Use the outflow via a 2-valve trocar cannula (**Fig. 9**).

For diagnostic procedures, use dry conditions; for resection and so forth, semidry conditions

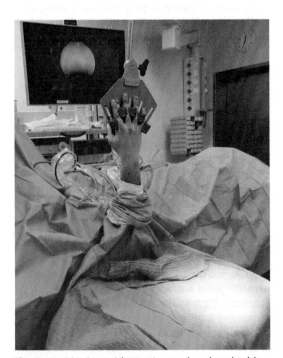

Fig. 5. Positioning with traction and on hand table.

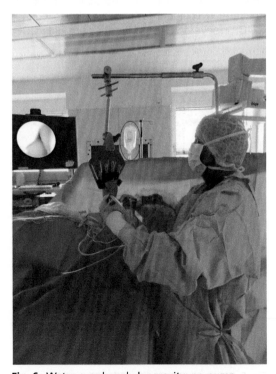

Fig. 6. Water supply only by gravity; no pump.

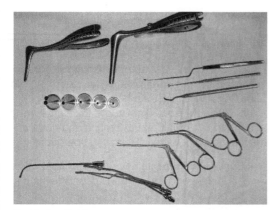

Fig. 7. Special instruments.

(wash out through 2 valves) (Videos 1–3). Confirm the correct diagnosis and the correct procedure in dry conditions. Check the cartilage; for example, dorsal rim of scaphoid if scaphoid-capitate (SC) or scaphoid-capitate-lunate (SCL) fusion is planned. Turn the lens 30° up and down. Repeatedly perform synovectomy as needed.

Swap and change portals if needed. Also check whether debridement of triangular fibrocartilage complex (TFCC) and synovectomy in the ulnocarpal joint are necessary.

For the MC joint, starting with the UMC portal (very ulnar for later resection of MC joint), view through the RMC portal (more radial for 4CF; check cartilage, check scapholunate and lunotriquetral [LT] ligament lesions in order to change to 4CF in severe LT instabilities and not just a 2CF).

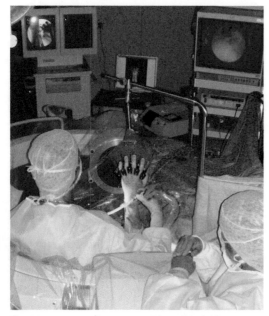

Fig. 8. Intraoperative setup with radiograph.

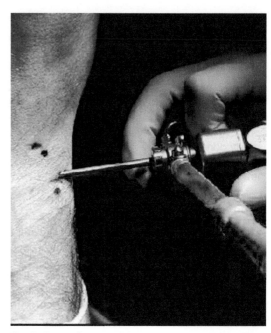

Fig. 9. Two-valve trocar.

Additional portals in the radiocarpal joint are 1/2; 6U; and, in the MC joint, hamate-triquetral or 6UMC/UUMC (new portal; – discussed later) (**Fig. 10**). The ulnar and radial STT portals are used if needed for STT procedures.

Surgical Procedure in Scapholunate Advanced Collapse or Scaphoid Nonunion Advanced Collapse: 4-Corner Fusion

Step 1: arthroscopic cleaning, synovectomy, and debridement

Check the structures confirming that in the radiocarpal area there is no or limited OA. Use the following portals: 3/4, 6R, RMC (enlarging later for bone grafting), UUMC or UMC, and 6UMC (new portal distal to 6U, ulnar to extensor carpi ulnaris [ECU] tendon between hamate and triquetrum).

Tip: make portals larger than normal.

Tip: the 6UMC portal ulnar to the ECU tendon is very tight, and is only an option in very lax wrists or wrists to be fused. This portal is helpful in 4CF (see **Fig. 10**).

Step 2: midcarpal arthroscopic resection of arthritic joint surfaces

Repeatedly clean the joint as needed. Resect the remaining cartilage and sclerotic bone surfaces, especially in advanced OA, until punctate bleeding is seen. With suction, this is visible even with the tourniquet inflated (**Fig. 11**). Smooth and

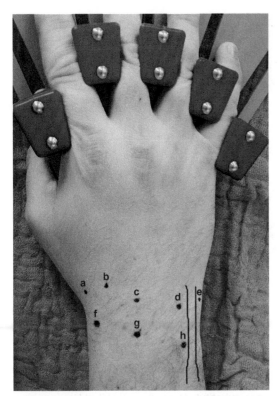

Fig. 10. Portals. a, STT radial; b, STT ulnar; c, RMC; d, UUMC; e, 6UMC; f, 1/2; g, 3/4; h, 6R.

well-matching opposing bony surfaces should be achieved.

Tip: resect as much as needed and as little as possible in order to maintain as much carpal height as possible.

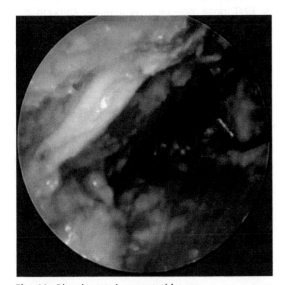

Fig. 11. Blood spots in resected bone.

Tip: there is risk of damage to the adjacent cartilage and the lens when the burr slips over the hard sclerotic bone. To avoid slipping, burr the bone surface at one end and proceed from this point, and avoid burring into the soft subsclerotic bone.

Tip: during burring, suction and irrigate intermittently to clean the burr and cool down the small joint. The heat production can damage the remaining adjacent cartilage and bone surface, which affects subsequent bone healing.

Tip: semidry/dry arthroscopy is useful to ensure that there is no bubble and no "growing" synovitis during the operation. However, beware of heat.[18]

Tip: resect the joint surfaces first rather than resecting the scaphoid. If the MC joint surfaces are very sclerotic, they are hard to remove if the support from the adjacent scaphoid is lost. This finding is in contrary to those of del Piñal and Ho.[12]

Step 3: resection (of part) of the scaphoid in a miniopen approach

The resected scaphoid bone can occasionally be used for bone grafting. Take the hand down from the traction device. A small radiopalmar zig-zag-incision is made. STT ligaments are released. Use a carpal stick (KLS Martin) to remove the scaphoid completely (**Fig. 12**).

Step 4: correction of dorsal intercalated segment instability or other deformities or malalignments

Temporarily transfix the radiolunate (RL) joint at wrist flexion and ulnar duction. More lunate flexion allows more wrist extension. Overall functional range of 60° is better with an extension/flexion 40°/20°, than 20°/40°.[9] Make a small skin incision, bluntly dissect with scissors onto the radius, and use a drill protector to avoid injury to the fourth extensor compartment. A 1.4-mm K-wire (European wrists are probably stronger than Asian wrists because Ho[12] proposed a 1.1-mm K-wire) is then inserted from the radius to the lunate. Be careful not to enter the MC joint. The K-wire position is verified fluoroscopically. Avoid putting the K-wire in the center of the lunate in order to leave more lunate bone substance for future screw placement/osteosynthesis.

If reduction is difficult in severe carpal collapse, leave the RL K-wire for 3 weeks (**Fig. 13**).

Step 5: temporary osteosynthesis after aligning the carpal bones under image intensifier

Transfix the capitolunate (CL) joint with a 1.4-mm K-wire from distal to proximal. Withdraw the K-wire from the lunate before bone grafting and advance it afterward. The K-wires can be used as a final osteosynthesis with additional K-wires or screws or be replaced by screws.

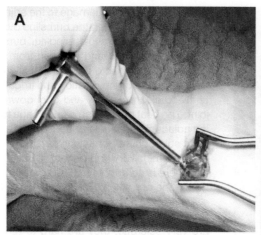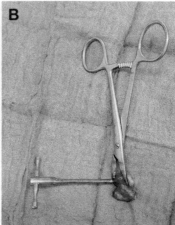

Fig. 12. (*A*) Scaphoid excision with help of (*B*) carpal stick. (*Courtesy of* [*B*] KLS Martin, Tuttlingen, Germany.)

Tip: advance the K-wire into the lunate after bone grafting without traction.

Tip: when reducing the MC joint, respect the lunate type. Do not overcorrect the ulnar translation in type II lunates.

Step 6: arthroscopic bone graft
Put the hand back under arthroscopic traction. Fill up the gap of the fusion site with bone graft. This step is perhaps not necessary because some

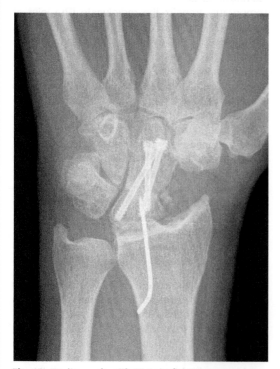

Fig. 13. Radiograph with RL transfixation at postoperative week 3.

investigators do not bone graft the gap. I do it anyway and use mostly bone chips from the resected scaphoid, if available. Iliac crest, distal radius, or other typical donor sites for bone grafting are the other options. The superior bone quality with enclosed bone marrow/stem cells still makes the iliac crest the first bone graft choice. Artificial bone substitute is an alternative, but I have no personal experience.

A urinary catheter can be inserted into the scaphoid or other defects to prevent spillage of the bone graft, as proposed by Ho.[12] A 10-French children's catheter with guidewire is easier to introduce (**Fig. 14**; see **Fig. 2**). The author recommends dry arthroscopy or as little fluid inflow as possible to avoid bone graft being flushed to elsewhere in the joint.

A second arthroscopic trocar or ENT ear funnel or ENT nose speculum is inserted through the arthroscopic portal into the fusion site. Bone chips crushed to very small pieces are introduced through the funnel and impacted by a switching stick or blunt obturator into the joint under dry arthroscopic control (**Fig. 15**). Continue bone grafting until sufficient grafting is achieved. If in doubt, check with the image intensifier. Deliver a small number of bone graft pieces each time to avoid blocking the cannula. If the joint/space is large enough, a bigger trocar or cannula of a bigger burr, ENT funnel, or speculum can be used. The author needs the help of 1, or preferably 2, assistants in the process of bone grafting.

Step 7: final osteosynthesis
Readvance the prepositioned K-wire in the capitate into the lunate. The tourniquet can be released and there is no undue need for the tourniquet in the final osteosynthesis.

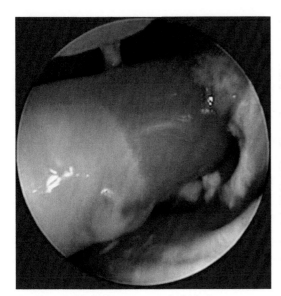

Fig. 14. Urinary catheter in scaphoid hole.

Release the hand from the arthroscopic traction and place it on a hand table. Insert more K-wires, from distal to proximal, to fix the carpal bones, or replace the K-wires with cannulated headless screws.

Tip: if the bone is hard, insertion of the cannulated screw guide pin might be difficult.

Insert a 1.4-mm K-wire and replace it with the smaller cannulated screw guide pin (0.9 mm or 1.1 mm). Smaller K-wires are easily bent on sclerotic bones.

Tip: if the neck of the capitate is too curved, the K-wire will be too dorsal to engage into the lunate. This problem can be solved by going through the bases of the metacarpal bone, carpometacarpal joint III or IV, as described by Ozyurekoglu and Turker[19] (**Fig. 16**). First drill through the metacarpal bone to allow measurement of the exact length of the screw necessary to sit inside the capitate. Take care with regard to the order of screw placement to avoid compressing the joint interval in which another screw is already in place (**Fig. 17**). Check all planes with the image intensifier. Keep in mind the arch shape of the carpus and avoid inserting hardware into the carpal tunnel (**Fig. 18**).

Tip: K-wires tend to glide on the dorsal side in sclerotic bone and are not suitable for screw guidance. If the K-wire is stable and in a good position, it is better to leave the K-wire as the final osteosynthesis.

Tip: check the pisotriquetral joint ensure there is no hardware protrusion. This step is done with an lateral view with 20 to 30° of supination.

Step 8: wound closure
Use stitches if needed, and Steri-Strips. Apply the final dressing and a palmar splint.

Postoperative Treatment

Keep the splint or orthosis for 6 weeks. Start active motion out of the splint several times a day after 3 weeks. Perform a CT scan after 6 weeks to assess bone healing, or earlier if in doubt about hardware position.

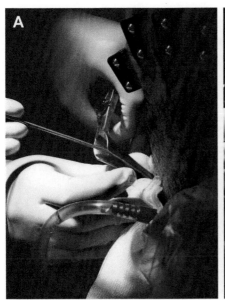
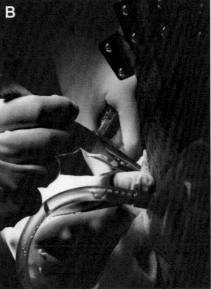

Fig. 15. (*A*, *B*) Arthroscopic bone grafting.

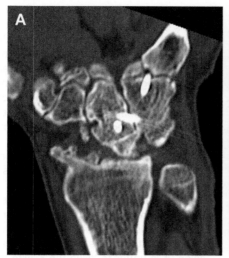
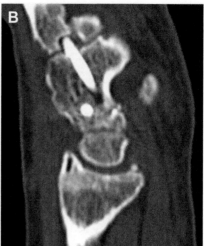

Fig. 16. (*A*, *B*) Screwing through the bases of MC bones.

Return to work depending on the job: after 8 weeks (white collar) to 16 weeks (blue collar).

OTHER ARTHROSCOPIC PARTIAL WRIST ARTHRODESIS

The surgical steps and postoperative treatment are similar to those described earlier. The specific varying points are listed.

Scaphoid-Trapezium-Trapezoid Arthrodesis

Indications
Kienbock disease (2 patients in this series), severe STT OA.

Assess the scapholunate in patients with STT OA. An advanced carpal collapse can also occur in pantrapezial OA and scapholunate instability.

- The author uses modified RMC (more radial) and UMC (more radial) as well as STT radial and ulnar.
- During arthroscopic burring of the STT joint, keep in mind the distal curved shape of the scaphoid (**Fig. 19**).
- If necessary, an adjunctive arthroscopic radial styloid resection can be performed.
- Give a scaphoid splint (**Fig. 20**) after the operation, supporting up to the thumb interphalangeal joint.

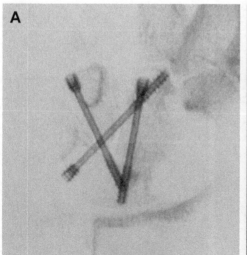
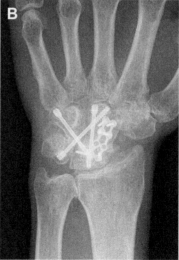

Fig. 17. (*A*, *B*) Broken screw: revision with plate (the screw was bent). Case 6 in **Table 1**.

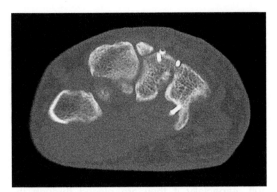

Fig. 18. Protrusion of screw in carpal tunnel.

Scaphoid-Capitate/Scaphoid-Capitate-Lunate Arthrodesis

Indications
Kienbock disease, scaphoid-capitate-lunate OA, severe instability; for example, carpal collapse after trapezectomy.

The author has 4 patients in one series: 1 patient with Kienbock disease and 3 patients with isolated MC OA.

- Use portals 3 to 4, 6R, RMC (enlarged later for bony grafting), and UMC ulnar.
- Resect the distal scaphoid through a mini-open approach at the radiopalmar wound as in 4CF. Identify the resection line in the scaphoid with the help of the intensifier and cut with an osteotome. Use carpal stick (KLS Martin) to stabilize the scaphoid. Cut the adjacent ligaments and take the resected scaphoid out.

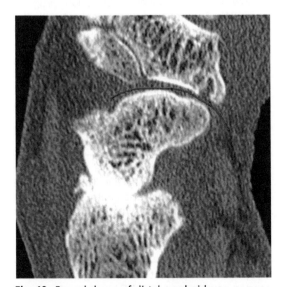

Fig. 19. Round shape of distal scaphoid.

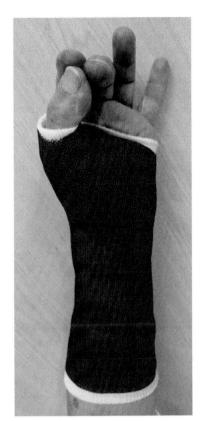

Fig. 20. Scaphoid cast.

- Harvest bone graft from the distal scaphoid. If this is insufficient, harvest from the iliac crest or from the distal radius, ideally simultaneously by another surgeon to reduce the operation time.
- Perform the reduction and temporary osteosynthesis using the image intensifier with the scaphoid and wrist in neutral position. This method may be easier with the hand in traction, especially when severe instability complicates matters.
- Arthroscopically check again whether hardware has protruded into the radiocarpal joint.
- Apply a scaphoid splint (see **Fig. 20**) after the operation, supporting up to the thumb interphalangeal joint.

Radioscapholunate Arthrodesis

Indications
Severe radiocarpal OA, posttraumatic OA from distal radius fracture, early stages of SLAC/SNAC 1 to 2, and instability after severe scapholunate or LT trauma.

The author has 2 patients in a series with radiocarpal OA after distal radius fracture, and 1 with severe ligament lesions.

- Check the MC joint arthroscopically to prove that there is no OA there.
- Use portals 1/2, 3/4, and 4/5 or 6R for the radiocarpal and RMC and UMC for the MC joint.
- Resect the distal scaphoid as in SC/SCL arthrodesis.
- In cases of dorsal intercalated segment instability (DISI) deformity, RL transfixation is necessary with wrist flexion (Linscheid maneuver).
- In cases of ulnar-plus variance, more bone graft is needed to maintain the carpal height. A small corticocancellous bone graft from the iliac crest is necessary and is introduced through an enlarged 3/4 portal.
- In severe ulnar-plus variance, ulnar shortening, or arthroscopic wafer procedure (if associated Palmer IID to IIE TFCC lesion) may be needed.
- Final arthroscopy to check MC joint again in case hardware protrudes.
- No removal of triquetrum is necessary in order to preserve ligament stability and proprioceptive functions.[20,21]

Radiolunate Arthrodesis

Indications

- RA with ulnar translation, ulnar translation after severe ligament lesions or pseudogout.
- No personal experience.
- The technique is similar to radioscapholunate (RSL) arthrodesis, except there is no removal of the distal part of the scaphoid.

Lunotriquetral Arthrodesis

Indications

- Severe LT instability.
- No personal experience.
- High nonunion rate (up to 57% in open procedures) and poor outcome were reported following open procedures. 4CF may be a more reliable and secure procedure for severe LT instability.[6]
- The technique consists of an arthroscopic resection of the LT joint and bone grafting from the MC joint.

COMPLICATIONS AND MANAGEMENT
Screw Malposition and Hardware Problems

The curvature of the dorsal aspect of the capitate, and sclerotic bone in advanced OA, especially in male patients, make perfect hardware placement difficult. The arch shape of the carpus also risks hardware protrusion into the carpal tunnel. The author had a case of protrusion of the screw tip into the carpal tunnel that needed removal, bone grafting, reosteosynthesis, and suture of partial flexor tendon lesions (see **Fig. 18**, case 3 in **Table 1**).

The author had to (partially) remove hardware in 7 cases. Postoperative CT scan showed that the cannulated screws were too long or not in perfect positions to control bone healing. There were 13 cases of planned removal of hardware (K-wires).

Removal of K-wires is quick and easy. Removal of screws can be very time consuming and difficult, especially if they are placed through the base of the metacarpal bones, where the screw tracks are occluded with healed bone. Correct measurement of screw length is important to avoid possible screw removal in the future.

There was 1 broken screw, which was replaced with a dorsal plate in an open procedure (see **Fig. 17**, case 6 in **Table 1**). The screw failed and another screw was then inserted to compress the bone in another direction. The order of screw placement is important.

Nonunion and Delayed Bone Healing

Using plain radiographs, bone healing is often impossible to prove. The author always performs CT scan after 6 weeks. In delayed bone healing, the author repeats this after another 4 or 6 weeks. If hardware position is in doubt, the author obtains the CT scan much earlier.

The author had partial nonunion in 4 cases requiring reoperation and bone graft (2 from distal radius, 2 from iliac crest) (cases 8 and 10 in **Table 1**). One of these patients has a history of drug abuse and chronic hepatitis C infection, and is now in a methadone substitution program (case 31). Another was not compliant with the rehabilitation and did not turn up regularly because of long holidays with his camping vehicle (case 27).

One complete nonunion of the STT joint was reoperated in another clinic and lost to follow-up.

One patient was not satisfied with the result despite complete bone union and he did not turn up for follow-up.

New Intra-articular Bone

One patient needed removal of a so-called neoscaphoid (see **Fig. 2**, case 19 in **Table 1**) formed from the bone graft slipped into the scaphoid defect. Blocking the gap with a urinary catheter is helpful to avoid the loosening of bone graft.

Wrong Indication

One patient with perfect bone healing after 6 weeks needed conversion to a TWF because of a wrong

Table 1
Outcomes of the operations

								Lunate (Type			RL			Fusion/	
Patient Number	Age (y)	Sex	Diagnosis	Secondary Diagnosis	Side	Operation Date	Operation Time (min)	1 or 2)	Joints (Fused)	Osteosynthesis	Transfix	Reoperation	Reoperation	Pseudarthrosis	Clinic
1	52	M	SLAC 2°–3°	—	L	November 2011	184	1	4CF	2 S	—	—	—	Fusion	Good
2	46	M	SNAC 3°	—	R	April 2011	128	1	4CF	2 S	—	—	—	Fusion	Good
3	45	M	SNAC 2°	Pseudogout	R	May 2011	130	1	4CF	4 S	—	HR S, part. Flexor tendon reconstruction	HR KW	Fusion after revision	—
4	52	M	SNAC 3°	—	L	June 2011	136	1	4CF	3 S	—	—	—	Fusion	Bad/persistent problems (SLAC 4)
5	62	F	SLAC 3°	—	R	December 2011	204	1	4CF	3 S	—	—	—	Fusion	Good
6	57	M	SLAC 3°	—	L	March 12	120	1	4CF	3 S	—	HR S, broken screw, plating, iliac crest bone graft	—	Fusion after revision	Good
7	50	F	SLAC 3°	—	R	June 2012	155	1	4CF	2 S/1 KW	—	HR KW	—	Fusion	Good
8	63	M	SLAC 2°–3°	—	R	June 2012	195	1	4CF	4 S	—	HR S, radius bone graft partial NU	—	Fusion after revision	Good
9	71	M	SLAC 2°–3°	Pseudogout	R	October 2012	196	1	4CF	3 S	—	—	—	Fusion	Good
10	64	M	SLAC 2°–3°	—	R	February 2012	228	1	4CF	3 S	—	HR S, radius bone graft partial NU	—	Fusion after revision	Good
11	59	F	SLAC 2°	—	R	December 2012	150	1	4CF	3 S	—	—	—	Fusion	Good
12	28	F	Kienbock 3A	—	R	April 2013	249	—	STT	3 KW	—	HR KW	—	Fusion	Good
13	78	F	SLAC 3°	Pseudogout	R	May 2013	246	2	4CF	2 S/1 KW	—	HR KW	—	Pseudarthrosis ongoing destruction pseudogout	Bad/persistent problems
14	58	M	SLAC 3°	—	R	June 2013	218	2	4CF	3 S	—	HR S	—	Fusion	Good

(continued on next page)

Table 1
(continued)

									Arthroscopic Partial Wrist Arthrodesis						
Patient Number	Age (y)	Sex	Diagnosis	Secondary Diagnosis	Side	Operation Date	Operation Time (min)	Lunate (Type 1 or 2)	Joints (Fused)	Osteosynthesis	RL Transfix	Reoperation	Reoperation	Fusion/ Pseudarthrosis	Clinic
15	50	M	SLAC 3°	—	R	September 2013	181	1	4CF	3 S/1 KW	RL	HR KW/S	—	Fusion	Good
16	52	M	SLAC 3°	—	L	October 2015	190	1	CL + resection of tip of hamate	3 S	—	HR S	—	Fusion	Bad/persistent problems (tip of hamate)
17	70	M	SLAC 3°	Pseudogout	L	October 2013	223	1	4CF	3 S	—	—	—	Fusion	Good
18	72	M	SLAC 3°	—	R	November 2015	180	1	3CF	3 S	—	—	—	Fusion/ pseudarthrosis (delayed union)	Bad/persistent problems
19	65	M	SLAC 3°	—	L	November 2013	244	1	4CF	3 S	—	HR S, resection of neoscaphoid	—	Fusion revision	Bad/persistent problems
20	55	M	Kienböck 3B	—	L	November 2013	158	—	STT	3 KW	—	HR KW	—	Pseudarthrosis	Bad/persistent problems (lost to FU)
21	48	M	SLAC 2°–3°	—	L	February 2014	170	1	4CF	4 KW, 1 KW RL	RL	HR KW	—	Fusion	Good
22	50	M	SLAC 3°–4°	—	L	February 2014	137	1	4CF	1 S, 3 KW, 1 RL	RL	HR KW	—	Fusion	Bad/persistent problems (lost to FU)
23	44	M	SLAC 2°	—	R	February 2014	188	1	4CF	4 KW, 1 RL	RL	HR KW	—	Fusion	Good
24	56	F	SLAC 3°–4°	Suspected RA	L	March 2014	139	2	4CF	4 KW, 1 RL	RL	HR KW	TWF	Fusion	Bad/persistent problems (SLAC 4)

25	50	M	SLAC 2°–3°	—	R	September 2014	194	1	4CF	3 S	—	HR S	—	Fusion	Good
26	63	F	SLAC 2°–3°	—	R	January 2015	175	1	4CF	2 S	—	—	—	Fusion	Good
27	70	M	SLAC 3°	Bad compliance	R	May 2015	180	2	CL	1 S/2 KW	—	HR KW, iliac crest bone graft	—	Pseudarthrosis	Bad/persistent problems
28	54	M	SLAC 2°–3°	—	L	May 2015	199	1	CL	2 S	—	—	—	Fusion	Good
29	21	F	Kienbock 3B	—	R	July 2015	216	—	SC	3 S	—	HR S	—	Fusion	Good
30	35	F	Mediocarpal OA	—	R	January 2016	151	1	SCL + iliac crest	2 S	—	HR S	—	Fusion	Good
31	46	M	SNAC 3°	Hepatitis .C., methadone substitution	L	September 2015	180	1	CL	2 S	—	HR S, iliac crest bone graft	—	Fusion after revision	Good
32	53	M	SLAC 3°	Pseudogout	L	October 2015	165	1	CL	3 S	—	—	—	Fusion	Good
33	51	M	SNAC 3°–4°	—	L	January16	185	2	CL	1 S/2 KW	—	HR KW	—	Fusion	Good
34	56	M	SLAC 2°	—	L	November 2016	194	1	4CF	3 S/2 KW	—	—	—	Fusion	Good
35	56	M	Mediocarpal OA	—	R	November 2016	194	2	SCLH	4 KW	—	HR KW	—	Fusion	Good
36	55	F	Radiocarpal OA	—	L	December 2016	142	—	RSL	2 S	—	—	—	Ongoing	—
37	54	M	SLAC 3°	—	R	April 2015	180	—	CL	2 S	—	—	—	Fusion	Good
38	58	M	Radiocarpal OA	—	L	June 2015	145	—	RSL	4 KW	—	—	—	Fusion	Good
39	54	M	Mediocarpal OA	—	R	February 2014	148	—	SCL	2 S/2 KW	—	HR KW	—	Fusion	Good

Abbreviations: F, female; FU, follow-up; HR, hardware removal; KW, K-wire; L, left; M, male; NU, nonunion; R, right; RL, radiolunate; S, screw.

indication with an SLAC 4 (case 24 in **Table 1**). Another patient with a SLAC 4 wrist also has problems and probably needs to be converted (see **Figs. 1** and **4**).

Infections

There were no deep infections. Two patients had some of the K-wires removed because of superficial infections/irritations.

Chronic Regional Pain Syndrome

None. This finding may be caused by less postoperative swelling and pain.

PROS AND CONS OF KIRSCHNER WIRES VERSUS SCREWS

K-wire
+: Easier to place
+/−: Placement does not have to be perfect
+/−: Removal necessary, but easy
−: Postoperative rehabilitation is potentially slower
+: Low costs (but there are costs of removal, depending on the local conditions in different countries)
Screws
+: Stable fixation
+: With compression if perfectly placed
−: Screw loosening later if fibrous healing
−: Higher price

PROS AND CONS OF OPEN VERSUS ARTHROSCOPIC TECHNIQUE

Cons of arthroscopic technique:
- Highly demanding, even for surgeons well trained in arthroscopic procedures.
- Operation time is much longer than in open procedures. In my cases it takes almost 3 hours on average, ranging from 120 to 249 minutes.
- Percutaneous osteosynthesis is more difficult based only on radiograph control of the hardware placement.

Pros of arthroscopic technique:
- Better healing (see **Figs. 1** and **2**), as shown in the case of the neoscaphoid, and also in the case of SLAC 4 later converted to TWF (see **Fig. 1**).
- Better ROM, because of less scarring and damage to the ligaments and capsule.

However, clinicians need to respect all surgical and orthopedic rules regarding reduction, hardware placement, and postoperative rehabilitation in order to get good union and ROM.

There is a steep learning curve with many possible mistakes in arthroscopic PWA (A-PWA). The problems and mistakes addressed in this article should not undermine clinicians' motivation but should prevent them from making the same mistakes.

Outcomes

From March 2011 to December 2016, my institution treated 39 patients with A-PWA. Two patients were lost to follow-up. There were 29 male and 10 female patients with a mean age of 54 years. We performed different A-PWAs, as described earlier: 23 4CF, 7 2CF (CL), 2 RSL, 4 SCL/SC/SCLH, 2 STT, and 1 3CF. Details are given in **Table 1**.

There were 8 revision cases: 4 partial nonunions, 1 case with protrusion of the screw tip into the carpal tunnel, 1 case with a broken screw, 1 case of re-SLAC with a neoscaphoid, and 1 case with a wrong indication that was converted to TWF. Two patients were lost to follow-up. Apart from the last 2 cases, all A-PWAs healed with satisfying results after revision.

With more experience, the technical problems and mistakes are fewer. The first 5 revision cases were in the group of the first 20 patients.

DISCUSSION

There were 7 cases of unplanned removal of screws. Pseudoarthrosis happened in 3 out of 26 screw fixations, 1 out of 6 combined screws/K-wires, and 1 out of 7 K-wire fixations. Arthrodesis with K-wire fixation did not produce more pseudarthrosis. We try to maintain solid screw fixation and also accept a good stabilization by K-wires or combinations if screw fixation is difficult. We try to prevent removal of screws.

Rodgers and colleagues[22] showed that equivalent results could be obtained using a circular plate and K-wires when equivalent bone graft sources and fusion techniques were used.

Whether compression is needed for osteosynthesis is an ongoing discussion; for example, in scaphoid nonunion. Probably a good blood supply and less damage to the soft tissue is at least as important. A-PWA probably does not need fusion site compression, at least as shown in our small series. If the bone quality is poor, as in some systemic diseases or postmenopausal women, K-wires would be better, because they allow sintering during healing, depending on the positioning of the wires (see **Fig. 1**).

Long-term results after 4CF by Trail and colleagues[23] showed that there was 31% nonunion, especially on the ulnar column. We also see more nonunion on the ulnar side. Using screws for CL and K-wires for the ulnar column could be an option. If using K-wires on the ulnar side and if there is fibrotic nonunion, the K-wires can be taken out; however, if screws are used instead, they can become loose, migrate, and cause pain.

Previous studies have shown that the nonunion rate varies from 25% to 33%.[24–27] In our series, the overall revision rate was 20%, and the partial nonunion rate was 10%.

Screw placement from distal to proximal can be difficult. This placement can be facilitated by penetrating through the metacarpal base. There are disadvantages of placement from proximal to distal because the screw head is close to the remaining healthy joint surface. The danger of screw proximal migration can also arise, as described by Wolfe[28] in 4 out of 107 patients with screw placement from proximal do distal.

Because of the undisturbed capsule and ligaments, earlier motion can be allowed from 3 weeks onward and the splint kept for 6 weeks only; unless insufficient bone healing is shown in the CT scan, it is kept for 3 to 4 weeks more. Some investigators maintain a cast for 12 to 16 weeks for open PWA.[27,29]

There is an ongoing discussion about the indication for 2-bone, 3-bone (with or without removal of the triquetrum), or 4-bone fusion in SLAC/SNAC.[4–7]

In our series, we changed our indications with respect to how many carpal bones were to be fused in SLAC and SNAC. We performed 4CF in the initial 23 cases. One 3CF was done without excision of the triquetrum. Seven 2CFs were done with 2 resections of the hamate tip, in which 1 had residual hamate tip impaction, probably caused by insufficient hamate resection (**Fig. 21**).

An optional indication for 2CF is a type 1 lunate, ulnar neutral/negative variance, absence of ulnar/hamate impaction, or an additional wafer and/or hamate tip resection, although type 2 lunate is indicated. If the indication is in doubt, we still prefer a 4CF.

In the literature the 4CF was described as being potentially more solid and producing less nonunion, but our results did not support this.

Fusing 2 columns is more time consuming. Clinicians need to take care not to damage the joint surfaces of the ulnar column and to address the ulnar variance. I do not perform triquetral removal, which is described by Bain and McGuire[6] as producing better results.

We use CT scan routinely at 6 weeks to assess bone healing. However, Henry[15] recommended CT scan after 8 weeks because he thought 6 weeks was too early to diagnose bone healing.

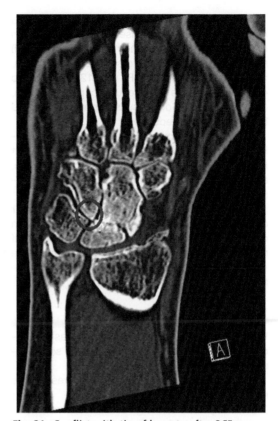

Fig. 21. Conflict with tip of hamate after 2CF.

Maintain the original contour of carpal bones and radius as far as possible in order to fit them together more easily, and to minimize carpal malalignment and the need for bone graft. I do bone grafting, mostly from the scaphoid, so there is no donor site morbidity. Some colleagues do not do it. A bone substitute, proposed by Ho,[12] could be an alternative.

Correct and effective reduction of malalignment is important. Potentially overcorrecting the DISI deformity to get more wrist extension than flexion might produce a better outcome.[9]

Arthroscopic procedures have long operation times. The tourniquet is released after bone grafting and temporary osteosynthesis. There is no need for a tourniquet in the remaining operation.

It is important to pay attention to the amount of fluid and potential compartment syndrome in wet arthroscopy. Do not use a pressure pump, or use it at a very low pressure setting. I recommend dry and semidry arthroscopy (semidry means only flushing the joint from time to time; Videos 1–3). Use a 2-valve trocar for intermittent fluid and air inflow. There is no problem with excess fluid, "growing" synovitis, or bubbles obscuring the operation field, especially with enlarged portals.

Some investigators have postulated that good results in 4CF are only caused by the denervation effect from the posterior interosseous nerve (PIN) resection in open procedures. In our small series, we compared 13 open 4CFs with 12 arthroscopic 4CFs. Both had the same results for pain, function, and satisfaction. Good results depended on good bone healing and reduction.

Hagert and Persson[20] and Hagert and colleagues[21] showed the importance of an intact PIN to preserve innervation and proprioception, although it is not clear whether this is also necessary in a destroyed wrist.

Enhancing ROM, especially in radial and ulnar duction, is possible with radial styloid resection during PWA or as a secondary procedure if needed. Similarly, to enhance extension of the wrist, resection of the dorsal rim and/or osteophytes may be helpful (see **Fig. 4**).

SUMMARY

With training, A-PWA is a reliable and feasible procedure. The learning curve is steep and so the results are better with training.

The type of hardware (screws or K-wires) seems not to be important.

More important is the good correction of malalignment and stable osteosynthesis, as in open procedures.

If all surgical and orthopedic rules are respected, better function and ROM can be expected because there will be less scarring and damage of the soft tissues. However, arthroscopic procedures cannot be expected to heal everything and overcome technical mistakes.

Less postoperative swelling and pain and also high satisfaction rates were detected and no chronic regional pain syndrome was found.

ACKNOWLEDGMENTS

Special thanks to my plastic and hand surgery team for collecting the data and supporting me.

SUPPLEMENTARY DATA

Supplementary data related to this article can be found online at http://dx.doi.org/10.1016/j.hcl.2017.07.013.

REFERENCES

1. Watson HK, Ballet FL. The SLAC wrist: scapholunate advanced collapse pattern of degenerative arthritis. J Hand Surg Am 1984;9(3):358–65.
2. Watson HK, Ryu J. Degenerative disorders of the carpus. Orthop Clin North Am 1984;15:337–53.
3. Watson HK. Limited wrist arthrodesis. Clin Orthop Relat Res 1980;149:126–36.
4. Singh HP, Dias JJ, Phadnis J, et al. Comparison of the clinical and functional outcomes following 3- and 4-corner fusions. J Hand Surg Am 2015;40(6):1117–23.
5. van Riet RP, Bain G. Three-corner wrist fusion using memory staples. Tech Hand Up Extrem Surg 2006;10(4):259–64.
6. Bain GI, McGuire DT. Decision making for partial carpal fusions. J Wrist Surg 2012;1(2):103–14.
7. Yao YC, Wang JP, Huang TF, et al. Lunocapitate fusion with scaphoid excision for the treatment of scaphoid nonunion advanced collapse or scapholunate advanced collapse wrist. J Chin Med Assoc 2017;80(2):117–20.
8. Thornton L. Old dislocation of os magnum: open reduction and stabilization. South Med J 1924;17:430.
9. Palmer AK, Werner FW, Murphy D, et al. Functional wrist motion: a biomechanical study. J Hand Surg Am 1985;10(1):39–46.
10. Tünnerhoff H-G, Haußmann P. Complications after midcarpal arthrodesis - attempt to analyse the pitfalls. Handchir Mikrochir Plast Chir 2003;35:288–98.
11. Mulford JS, Ceulemans LJ, Nam D, et al. Proximal row carpectomy vs four corner fusion for scapholunate (SLAC) or scaphoid nonunion advanced collapse (SNAC) wrists: a systematic review of outcomes [Review]. J Hand Surg Eur Vol 2009;34(2):256–63.
12. Ho PC. Arthroscopic partial wrist fusion. Tech Hand Up Extrem Surg 2008;12(4):242–65.
13. del Piñal F, Klausmeyer M, Thams C, et al. Early experience with (dry) arthroscopic 4-corner arthrodesis: from a 4-hour operation to a tourniquet time. J Hand Surg Am 2012;37(11):2389–99.
14. del Piñal F, Tandioy-Delgado F. (Dry) arthroscopic partial wrist arthrodesis: tips and tricks [Review]. Handchir Mikrochir Plast Chir 2014;46(5):300–6.
15. Henry M. Reliability of the 8 week time point for single assessment of midcarpal fusion by CT scan. J Hand Microsurg 2011;3(1):1–5.
16. Krimmer H, Wiemer P, Kalb K. Comparative outcome assessment of the wrist joint–mediocarpal partial arthrodesis and total arthrodesis. Handchir Mikrochir Plast Chir 2000;32(6):369–74 [in German].
17. Viegas SF, Wagner K, Patterson R, et al. Medial (hamate) facet of the lunate. J Hand Surg Am 1990;15(4):564–71.
18. Huber M, Loibl M, Eder C, et al. Effects on the distal radioulnar joint of ablation of triangular fibrocartilage complex tears with radiofrequency energy. J Hand Surg Am 2016;41(11):1080–6.
19. Ozyurekoglu T, Turker T. Results of a method of 4-corner arthrodesis using headless compression screws. J Hand Surg Am 2012;37(3):486–92.

20. Hagert E, Persson JK. Desensitizing the posterior interosseous nerve alters wrist proprioceptive reflexes. J Hand Surg Am 2010;35(7):1059–66.

21. Hagert E, Ferreres A, Garcia-Elias M. Nerve-sparing dorsal and volar approaches to the radiocarpal joint [Review]. J Hand Surg Am 2010;35(7):1070–4.

22. Rodgers JA, Holt G, Finnerty EP, et al. Scaphoid excision and limited wrist fusion: a comparison of K-wire and circular plate fixation. Hand (N Y) 2008; 3(3):276–81.

23. Trail IA, Murali R, Stanley JK, et al. The long-term outcome of four-corner fusion. J Wrist Surg 2015; 4(2):128–33.

24. Shindle MK, Burton KJ, Weiland AJ, et al. Complications of circular plate fixation for four-corner arthrodesis. J Hand Surg Eur 2007;32:50–3.

25. Vance MC, Hernandez JD, Didonna ML, et al. Complications and outcome of four-corner arthrodesis:

26. Wyrick JD, Stern PJ, Kiefhaber TR. Motion-preserving procedures in the treatment of scapholunate advanced collapse wrist: proximal row carpectomy versus four-corner arthrodesis. J Hand Surg Am 1995;20:965–70.

27. Kirschenbaum D, Schneider LH, Kirkpatrick WH, et al. Scaphoid excision and capitolunate arthrodesis for radioscaphoid arthritis. J Hand Surg Am 1993;18:780–5.

28. Shifflett GD, Athanasian EA, Lee SK, et al. Proximal migration of hardware in patients undergoing midcarpal fusion with headless compression screws. J Wrist Surg 2014;3(4):250–61.

29. El-Mowafi H, El-Hadidi M, Boghdady GW, et al. Functional outcome of four-corner arthrodesis for treatment of grade IV scaphoid non-union. Acta Orthop Belg 2007;73:604–11.

circular plate fixation versus traditional techniques. J Hand Surg Am 2005;30:1122–7.

Arthroscopic Transplantation of Osteochondral Autograft for Treatment of Cartilage Defects in the Wrist

Pak-cheong Ho, MBBS, FRCS (Edinburg), FHKCOS, FHKAM (Orth Surg)[a],*,
Wing-lim Tse, MBChB, MRCS, FRCSEd (Orth), FHKAM (Orth Surg), FHKCOS[b],
Clara Wing-yee Wong, MBChB, MRCS, FRCSEd (Orth), FHKAM (Orth Surg), FHKCOS[c]

KEYWORDS

- Wrist arthroscopy • Osteochondral graft • Radiocarpal joint • Wrist surgery • Cartilage defect
- Chondral lesion

KEY POINTS

- Focal chondral lesions are a common cause of chronic wrist pain. The best treatment remains unknown, especially for larger lesions greater than 5 mm in size.
- Wrist arthroscopy enables more accurate and early diagnosis of chondral lesion in the wrist and helps define the treatment strategy based on size, severity, and location.
- Restoration of the normal hyaline cartilage is the goal of treatment to relieve pain, restore function, and halt the progression of arthritis.
- Arthroscopic transplantation of osteochondral autograft from knee joint is an effective treatment in symptomatic focal osteochondral lesion of the wrist to restore normal articular environment.

INTRODUCTION

Focal chondral lesions are a common cause of chronic pain in the wrist, especially after trauma.[1] The incidence remains uncertain due to the difficulty in making proper diagnosis in this small and complex joint.[2] With a wider use of wrist arthroscopy, diagnosis becomes more accurate and accessible. Cartilage has poor regeneration potential due to the lack of intrinsic blood supply and the very high proportion of matrix to cellular components. Focal disruption of cartilage can lead to secondary osteoarthritis. Restoration of the normal hyaline cartilage is, therefore, the goal of treatment to relieve pain, restore function, and halt the progression of arthritis. In the lower extremity on the major weight-bearing joints, various

Disclosure Statement: Nil.
[a] Division of Hand and Microsurgery, Department of Orthopaedics and Traumatology, Prince of Wales Hospital, Chinese University of Hong Kong, 5/F, Lui Che Woo Clinical Sciences Building, 30-32 Ngan Shing Street, Shatin, NT, Hong Kong SAR; [b] Division of Hand and Microsurgery, Department of Orthopaedics and Traumatology, Prince of Wales Hospital, Chinese University of Hong Kong, Room 09A31, Main Clinical Block and Trauma Centre, 30-32 Ngan Shing Street, Shatin, NT, Hong Kong SAR; [c] Division of Hand and Microsurgery, Department of Orthopaedics and Traumatology, Prince of Wales Hospital, Chinese University of Hong Kong, The Club Lusitano, 16/F, 16 Ice House Street, Central, Hong Kong SAR
* Corresponding author.
E-mail address: pcho@ort.cuhk.edu.hk

techniques have been developed to repair cartilage defects, including open or arthroscopic abrasion chondroplasty, microfracture, osteochondral autograft transfer, osteochondral allograft, and autologous chondrocyte implantation (ACI), with variable success. There are, however, few reports in the wrist. Whipple[3] considered arthroscopic drilling chondroplasty an effective treatment of small chondral defects of less than 5 mm. For larger lesions, the best treatment method is unknown. The authors have reported 4 consecutive cases of restoration of focal chondral defect in the articular surface of the distal radius using arthroscopic implantation of osteochondral autograft from the knee joint with satisfactory clinical results.

PATIENT SERIES

Between December 2006 and December 2010, the authors operated on 4 patients with posttraumatic localized osteochondral lesion over the lunate fossa of the distal radius. There were 3 male patients and 1 female patient of average age 31 (range 24–41). The affected sides were the dominant right wrists. They all presented with chronic wrist pain and loss of motion after injury episode. The average duration of symptom was 28.3 months (range 11–71 months). All patients had preoperative imaging, including CT scan and/or MRI. The definite diagnoses were confirmed by arthroscopy. The authors performed arthroscopic transplantation of autogenous osteochondral graft taken from the knee. In 2 patients, there were concomitant procedures to deal with other associated pathology in the wrist. All patients were assessed by an occupational therapist before the index procedures, during and at final follow-up. The range of motion of the wrist, grip power, wrist functional performance scores, pain score, and return-to-work status were charted. The wrist functional performance score was developed by the authors' hospital based on a study by Nelson.[4] It consists of 10 common standardized tasks of activities of daily living to be performed by the patient under the scrutiny of an occupational therapist.[5,6] The performance on each task was rated by a therapist according to a 4-point scale, with a maximum total of 40 for a normal performance of the complete test. A pain score on a 3-point scale was rated by the patients according to the pain level perceived during the performance of each activity of daily living task. The total score ranged from zero to a maximum pain level of 20 points. Postoperative CT scan or MRI was performed to assess incorporation of the osteochondral graft. Serial radiograph was checked for degenerative change. In 3 patients, second-look arthroscopy was performed to directly evaluate the status of the chondral graft. Biopsy was performed in one case.

SURGICAL TECHNIQUE

The authors performed diagnostic arthroscopy under portal site local anesthesia in all patients prior to the index procedures to evaluate the cause of the chronic wrist pain and to confirm the location and extent of the osteochondral lesions.[7]

The osteochondral graft transplantation operation was performed under general anesthesia. Patients were put in the supine position while the operated arm was supported on a hand table. A tourniquet was applied to the arm but was not inflated most of the time. A vertical traction force of 10 lb to 12 lb was applied through plastic finger trap devices fitted to the middle 3 fingers on a wrist traction tower. The authors used continuous saline irrigation with a 3-L bag of normal saline instilled under gravity.

Arthroscopic examination and intervention was confined to the radiocarpal joint. To minimize bleeding, the authors routinely injected a 1:200,000 adrenaline solution mixed with 2% lidocaine through a 25G needle into the various standard portal sites just down to the level of capsule. The authors performed routine inspection of radiocarpal joint with a 1.9-mm or 2.7-mm arthroscope introduced through the 3-4 portal. Fluid outflow was maintained with an 18G needle inserted at the 6U portal. The synovitis around the dorsal rim of the lunate fossa was débrided with a 2.0-mm shaver and radiofrequency miniprobe inserted from the 4-5 portal. This uncovered the underlying osteochondral lesion. The cartilage debris was cleaned until the subchondral bone was reached. The true extent of the lesion was determined using the probe for measurement. The proximal side of the articular surface of the lunate should be evaluated. A well-developed kissing chondral lesion might preclude the choice of osteochondral graft as a treatment option.

The arthroscope was then inserted to the joint through the 4-5 portal. The authors used the Osteochondral Autograft Transfer System (OATS) (Arthrex, Naples, Florida) to carry out the harvest and transfer process. The 3-4 portal was gently dilated with a small hemostat, and a 6-mm recipient harvester with an obturator from the OATS was inserted into the joint with extreme care to avoid damage to the healthy cartilage (**Fig. 1**). The harvester was directed toward the osteochondral lesion at the dorsal aspect of the lunate fossa. At this junction, the wrist was passively flexed to approximately 50° while it was still maintained by

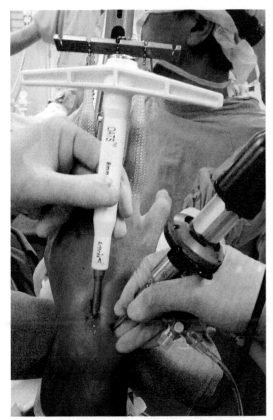

Fig. 1. A 6-mm trephine of OATS was inserted into the osteochondral defect through the 3-4 portal. (*Courtesy of* Arthrex, Naples, FL; with permission.)

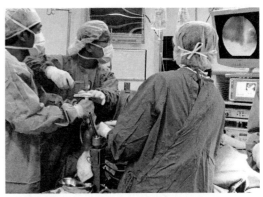

Fig. 2. The wrist is flexed to allow easy passage of the trephine. The arthroscope is placed at 4-5 portal to monitor the process. With the harvester positioned vertically and perpendicular to the articular surface of the lunate fossa just over the osteochondral lesion, the harvester is manually impacted to drive the trephine into the bone.

digital traction (**Fig. 2**). This maneuver moved the dorsal horn of the lunate palmarward and opened up the space between the lunate and the lunate fossa to accommodate the harvester. With the harvester positioned vertically and perpendicular to the articular surface of the lunate fossa just over the osteochondral lesion, the harvester was manually impacted to drive the trephine into the bone to a depth of approximately 10 mm to 12 mm, which was monitored through observing the gauge of the trephine (**Fig. 3**). The tendency to direct the harvester dorsally and obliquely should be avoided as far as possible, to prevent the iatrogenic fracture of the dorsal rim of the distal radius. An intact articular margin of at least 2-mm should be maintained dorsally. By removing the harvester, the cylindrical plug of bone containing the osteochondral defect was removed from the joint.

The osteochondral graft was harvested by a second team of surgeons from the knee of the nondominant leg according to the technique described by Hangody and colleagues.[8] A tourniquet was applied to the thigh. A small incision was made over the lateral aspect of the knee at the lateral femoral condyle. A 6-mm donor harvester was inserted to the sulcus terminalis of the lateral femoral condyle to a depth slightly deeper than that in the wrist (**Fig. 4**). The osteochondral plug was removed and delivered to the wrist. The defect in the knee was refilled partially by packing in the cancellous bone obtained from the recipient site (**Fig. 5**).

A short transparent plastic delivery tube was attached to the tip of the donor harvester containing the osteochondral plug. It was then gently inserted into the defect through the 3-4 portal with the aid of a rotating dial (**Fig. 6**). Graft insertion was monitored through the plastic sheath. The harvester was removed when the graft was flushed with the surrounding articular surface. A plastic

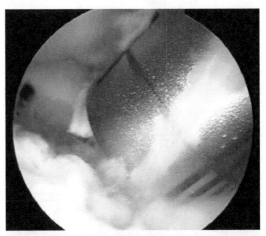

Fig. 3. Arthroscopic view of the trephine over the osteochondral defect at the dorsal lunate fossa.

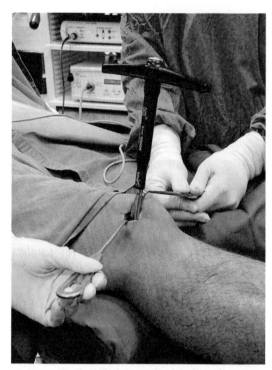

Fig. 4. A 6-mm OATS harvester was inserted to the lateral femoral condyle to harvest the osteochondral graft. (*Courtesy of* Arthrex, Naples, FL; with permission.)

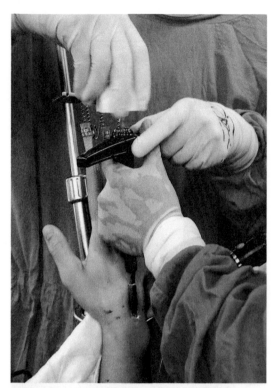

Fig. 6. The 6-mm OATS harvester with the osteochondral graft on was inserted into the wrist joint through the 3-4 portal. The graft was delivered into the defect with the dialed pusher. (*Courtesy of* Arthrex, Naples, FL; with permission.)

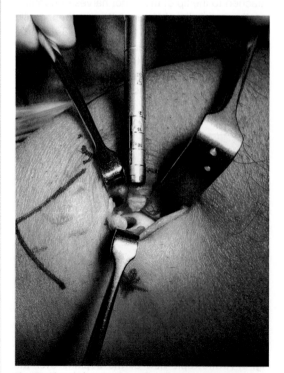

Fig. 5. The defect in the donor knee.

tam was used to tap the plug to obtain the best press-fit effect. When there was mismatch noted at the junction of the articular cartilage, the redundant cartilage was excised using an arthroscopic banana knife. Because the articular cartilage of the knee was generally thicker than that of the wrist, this shaving maneuver did not result in significant loss of articular cartilage. The graft was stable after press-fitting so no internal fixation was required. The stability of the graft and the smoothness of articulation were tested by passively moving the wrist.

The harvester was removed and the wound was closed by adhesive skin closure strips, followed by bulky compressive dressing (**Fig. 7**). A wrist splint was prescribed for 2 weeks to 4 weeks and patients were instructed to perform gentle active wrist motion from day 3 onward. Passive motion exercise was initiated by 4 weeks to 6 weeks. Active use of the hand in self-care and daily activities was allowed, but load bearing of the wrist was discouraged for the first 6 weeks to allow incorporation of the graft. Follow-up MRI scan and radiograph were arranged to monitor the incorporation.

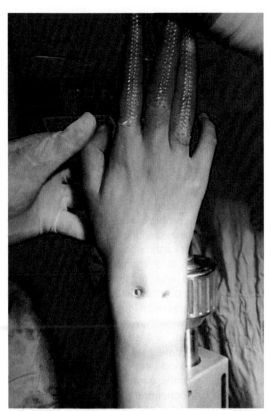

Fig. 7. Small wound access at completion of surgery.

RESULT

In all cases, the osteochondral grafts were healed and incorporated to the host bone 3 months to 4 months after the operation as confirmed by CT scan or MRI. A second-look arthroscopy at 6 months to 9 months postoperation in 3 patients confirmed the preservation of normal articular cartilage in the grafted area. There was a 1-mm to 2-mm rim defect between the graft and the host cartilage. In 1 patient, a third-look arthroscopy at 29 months postoperation showed complete coverage of the junction defect by cartilage. A biopsy of the grafted area in 1 patient confirmed viable hyaline cartilage.

At the final follow-up of average 70.5 months (range 24–116 months), all patients showed an improvement in the wrist performance score (preoperative 27.5 ± 6.4 and postoperative 38.5 ± 2.6 out of a 40-point scale) and pain score (preoperative 9.5 ± 2.2 and postoperative 0.5 ± 0.9 out of a 20-point scale). Grip strength improved from 62.6% ± 9.0% to 91.1 ± 2.6% of the contralateral side. Wrist motion improved from a flexion/extension arc of 115.5% ± 28.8° to 131%.3 ± 21.3°. Three patients returned to their previous occupations although 1 could not do so because of the

pisotriquetral instability problem. They were all satisfied with the procedure. The surgical scars were inconspicuous. Follow-up radiograph showed good graft incorporation, with no joint space narrowing or other sign of degeneration. There was no complication of infection, tendon, or nerve injury in this series.

CASE REPORT 1

A 24-year-old female professional dancer developed right dorsal central wrist pain after manual activities 16 months before. Radiograph showed no abnormality. Diagnostic arthroscopy revealed a 6-mm × 4-mm osteochondral defect over the dorsal lunate fossa, Outerbridge grade 1 to 2 chondral lesion over dorsal ulnar lunate, and minor tear of the scapholunate ligament (**Fig. 8**). The grip power was 22 kilogram-force, or 75.3% of the unaffected side. The combined extension/flexion range of the wrist was 150°. Her wrist performance score was 31/40 and pain score was 10/20. In July 2008, arthroscopic transplant of an osteochondral autograft of 6-mm diameter and 12-mm long harvested from the left knee lateral femoral condyle was performed to repair the osteochondral defect (**Fig. 9**). Postoperation she was allowed to assume immediate full range-of-motion exercise for her right wrist. CT scan and MRI of her right wrist at 3 months and 6 months postoperation, respectively, revealed good incorporation of the graft (**Fig. 10**). A second-look arthroscopy at 7 months revealed stable osteochondral graft with preserved hyaline cartilage. Biopsy of the grafted area demonstrated normal hyaline cartilage. There was narrow rim of cartilage defect of less than 1 mm at the junction. She developed a second

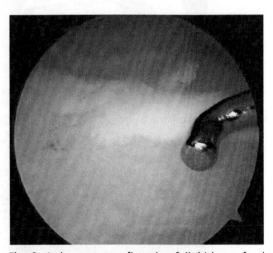

Fig. 8. Arthroscopy confirmed a full-thickness focal osteochondral lesion of size 6 mm × 4 mm over the dorsal lunate fossa.

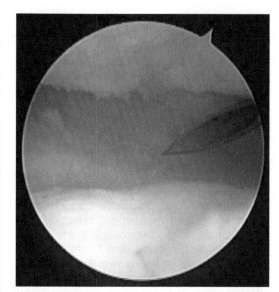

Fig. 9. Osteochondral autograft of 6-mm diameter and 12-mm long was implanted into the osteochondral defect at the lunate fossa.

problem of symptomatic pisotriquetral instability since June 2010 with significant ulnar wrist pain on the same wrist. Another arthroscopic evaluation at 29 months postoperation showed a completely incorporated hyaline cartilage with minimal junctional change (**Fig. 11**). At 44 months postoperative follow-up, she had no pain or

tenderness in the dorsal central wrist and the left knee. Wrist examination did not reveal any joint crepitus or pain at extreme of flexion and extension. Grip power was 21 kilogram-force or 87.5% of the unaffected side. The combined extension/flexion range of the wrist was 160°. Radiograph showed no arthrosis. Surgical scar was inconspicuous (**Fig. 12**).

CASE REPORT 2

A 31-year-old man injured his right dominant wrist during a fall 11 months before. MRI of his right wrist showed a suspected injury to the triangular fibrocartilage complex. Radiograph showed no fracture and ulnar variance was 2 mm positive (**Fig. 13**). Wrist arthroscopy was performed in another center at 2 months postinjury. It was said that there was no triangular fibrocartilage complex lesion but the distal radioulnar joint was subluxed. He received a long arm cast for 6 weeks afterward. The wrist, however, persisted and progressed. Repeat MRI showed a new lesion of osteochondral defect at the lunate fossa. He received a second arthroscopy in the authors' center at 8 months postinjury and confirmed an iatrogenic osteochondral defect of 7 mm × 5 mm at the dorsal part of the lunate fossa. There was another 5 mm × 2 mm chondral lesion on the ulnar aspect of the dorsal lunate, more compatible with change associated with ulnar impaction

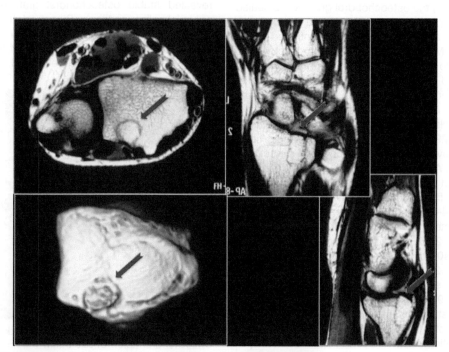

Fig. 10. CT scan and MRI showed good incorporation of the graft (*arrows*).

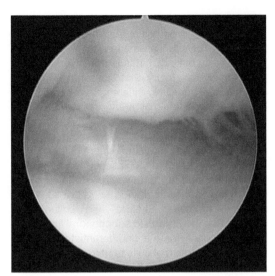

Fig. 11. A third-look arthroscopic evaluation at 29 months postoperative showed a completely incorporated hyaline cartilage with minimal junctional change.

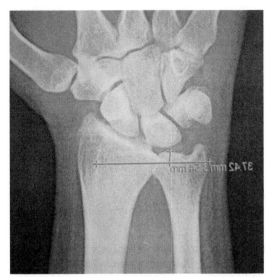

Fig. 13. Radiograph showed no fracture and ulnar variance was 2 mm positive.

syndrome. There was also a concomitant split tear of the ulnocarpal ligament (**Fig. 14**). His pain persisted despite joint débridement. Finally in December 2010, arthroscopic transplant of osteochondral autograft was performed. The lesion had increased in size to 12 mm × 5 mm and extended to a more central location in the lunate fossa. Two osteochondral plugs, each 6 mm × 12 mm in size, were harvested from the left knee (**Fig.15**). The grafts were transplanted to the defect through the 3-4 portal (**Fig. 16**) and the 4-5 portal (**Fig. 17**), respectively, and sequentially to fill up the defect as far as possible. The cartilaginous surface of the grafts was shaped and rounded off by arthroscopic knife (**Fig.18**). Concomitant procedures included arthroscopic repair of the split tear in the ulnocarpal ligament using epidural needle

technique as well as an ulnar shortening osteotomy of 4 mm with plating of the ulna (**Fig. 19**). The repair was protected with wrist splint for 4 weeks. At 2 years postoperative follow-up, he had no knee pain and minimal wrist pain. Wrist examination did not reveal any joint tenderness, joint crepitus, or pain on grinding test. He had resumed

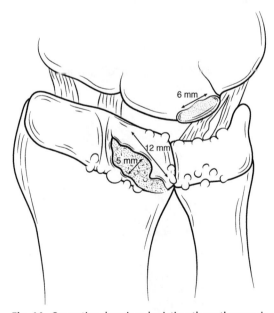

Fig. 14. Operative drawing depicting the arthroscopic lesions: an osteochondral defect of 12-mm × 5-mm extended from the dorsal part to a more central location in the lunate fossa; a 6-mm × 2-mm chondral lesion on the ulnar aspect of the dorsal lunate compatible with ulnar impaction syndrome; and a concomitant split tear of the ulnocarpal ligament.

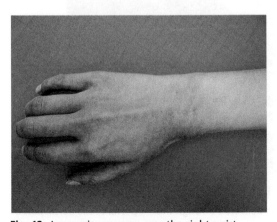

Fig. 12. Inconspicuous scar over the right wrist.

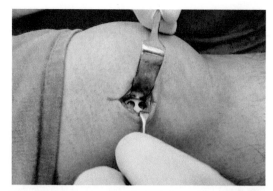

Fig. 15. Two osteochondral plugs, each of 6 mm × 12 mm in size, were harvested from the left knee.

his normal work at 3 months. The combined extension/flexion range of the wrist was 145° (**Fig. 20**). Radiograph showed normal joint space at radiolunate joint and ulnar minus 2-mm negative. CT scan showed good incorporation of the grafts (**Fig. 21**).

DISCUSSION

For decades, healing a cartilage defect has continued to be a clinical challenge for orthopedic surgeon. Articular cartilage is an avascular and aneural soft tissue. The cellular components contribute to less than 10% of the tissue volume. Given the lack of an undifferentiated cell pool within the cartilage substance and the low mitotic activity of chondrocytes in the physiologic status, the healing of even a small cartilage lesion can be extremely difficult.[9] This is particularly true for partial-thickness injury that does not reach the subchondral bone. No inflammatory response or influx of mesenchymal stem cells and potent cellular mediators is feasible to initiate the healing. Even in full-thickness injury, including osteochondral fractures and defects where inflammatory response is present at the vascularized and innervated subchondral bone level, restoration of the defect with normal cartilage is rarely seen and seldom complete. Shapiro and colleagues[10] showed that the breached subchondral area could provide access for the undifferentiated spindle-shaped mesenchymal cells to migrate to the injury site. They secrete type I collagen in restoring the matrix components initially. Within a few weeks, a greater proportion of the mesenchymal cells gradually transform into chondrocyte-like cells, secreting type II collagen and proteoglycans. Within 6 weeks to 8 weeks, most of the repair tissue, however, exhibits fibrocartilagenous or fibrous property instead of hyaline cartilage-like property. By 12 weeks to 24 weeks, there is superficial cartilage degeneration with fibrillation, decreased proteoglycan content, and loss of cellularity. The transformation of a majority of the chondrocyte-like cells to fibroblast-like cells is

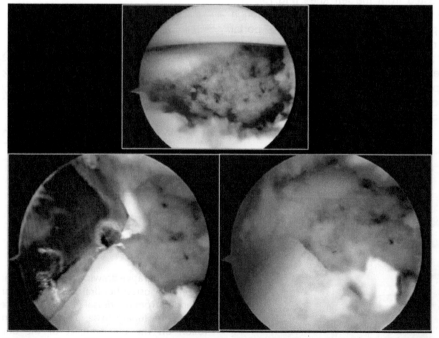

Fig. 16. Arthroscopic view of the osteochondral graft being delivered through the 3-4 portal to the dorsal part of the lunate fossa.

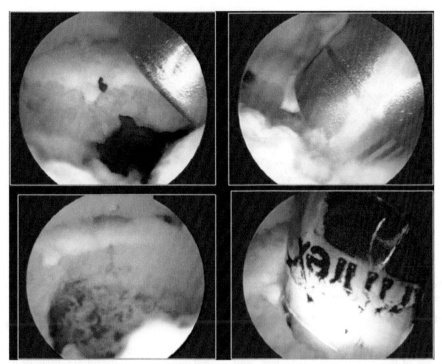

Fig. 17. Arthroscopic view showing sequence of the resection of the osteochondral defect and delivery of the osteochondral graft through the 4-5 portal to the central part of the lunate fossa.

usually evident at 1 year.[11] Depletion of matrix proteoglycan and further fibrillation, as well as fissuring and thinning of the chondral tissue, follows. Regeneration of cartilage is never complete or perfect. Cartilage defects gradually lead to degeneration of the articular cartilage and osteoarthritis.

Various surgical strategies have been developed trying to overcome this biological hurdle. The techniques were mainly used in the large joints, such as knee and ankle, and embraced either the encouragement of mesenchymal stem cells pouring into the cartilage injury zone or introduction of exogenous chondral tissue into the defect aiming at incorporation with host tissue. The former includes Pridie drilling,[12] abrasion arthroplasty, and Steadman microfracture oonocpt,[13] with an aim of producing blood clots at the subchondral bone, which in turn induce fibrous tissue production locally to promote fibrocartilagenous regeneration. The clinical outcomes of these methods vary with the unpredictable composition of the tissue filling the defect and the age and activity level of the patients. The second strategy includes periosteal/perichondral grafts,[12,13] osteochondral autograft transplantation,[8] osteochondral allograft transfer,[14] and ACI.[15] The American Academy of Orthopaedic Surgeons has recommendations for treating chondral defects in the knee joint.[16] They suggest the use of osteochondral autograft for small defects of less than 2 cm^2, microfracture for defects between 2 cm^2 and 4 cm^2, and ACI or osteochondral allograft for defects greater than 2 cm^2 to 4 cm^2. In small defects associated with bone loss, osteochondral graft transfer was associated with a quicker return to sport for athletes compared with microfracture (93% vs 52%).[17] Osteochondral autograft transplantation can be associated, however, with complications, such as harvest

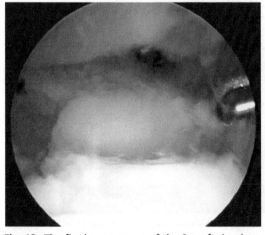

Fig. 18. The final appearance of the 2 grafts in place.

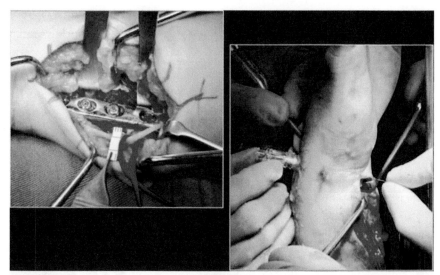

Fig. 19. The concomitant procedures of arthroscopic repair of the split tear in the ulnocarpal ligament using epidural needle technique (*right*) as well as an ulnar shortening osteotomy of 4 mm with plating of the ulna (*left*).

morbidity, degeneration of the surrounding cartilage, necrosis of the transplanted cylinders, and a lack of integration of the cartilage into the surrounding innate cartilage.

The optimal treatment of chondral lesion in the wrist is controversial. It has been recognized, however, as a common cause of wrist pain. It may result from osteochondral fractures, chronic carpal instability, or chondromatosis or it may occur idiopathically.[18] Araf and Moattar[19] noted an incidence of 33% articular cartilage injury larger than 3 mm in 30 patients of ages between 20 and 50 years old with distal radius fracture of group B and group C according to AO/ASIF classification.

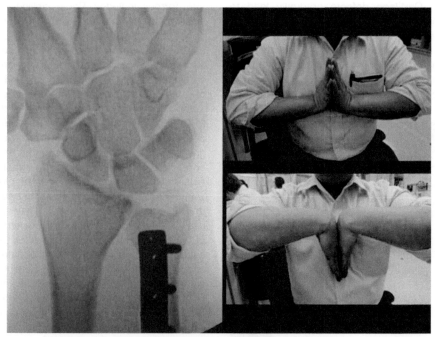

Fig. 20. The patient has good combined extension/flexion range of the wrist of 145° with no pain. Radiograph showed no progressive arthrosis change at 2 years.

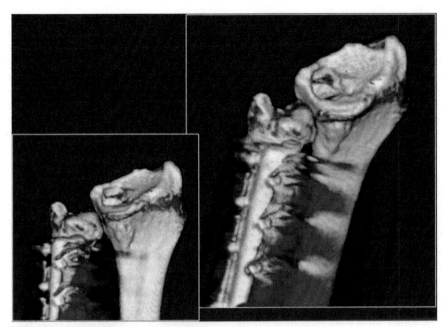

Fig. 21. CT scan showed a good incorporation of the graft.

Cheng and colleagues,[5] in reviewing the surgical treatment on 22 patients with chronic pain post–distal radius fracture treatment, noted a high incidence of 63.6% of chondral lesions responsible for the pain; 50% of them occurred at the distal radius side either on the scaphoid or lunate fossa. Culp and colleagues[20] have modified the Outerbridge classification for chondral lesion in the wrist as grade I representing softening of hyaline cartilage, grade II consisting of fibrillation and fissuring, grade III representing a fibrillated lesion of varying depth in the articular surface, and grade IV having a full-thickness defect down to bone. It has been recommended to have débridement and synovectomy for grades I to III lesions. Grade IV lesions can be treated with abrasion chondroplasty and subchondral drilling. Roth and Poehling[21] noted improvement in 83% of patients treated with debridement alone. Whipple[3] reported significant relief of symptom by abrasion chondroplasty if the defect is smaller than 5 mm in size. There were few studies, however, on treatment of larger chondral lesion in the wrist.

Periosteum has chondrogenic potential during development, attributed by the presence of chondrocyte precursor cells in the cambial layer. Perichondral graft was first used successfully to resurface cartilage loss in the arthritic wrist and finger joint by Engkvist and Johansson[22] in late 1980s. It was applicable, however, only to a limited indication in which the damage was confined to cartilage and the underlying bone was healthy with uniform surface.[23] Clinical experiences with

periosteal grafts have been disappointing in the longer term, because complete restoration of the hyaline cartilage layer and the long-term stability of the repair tissue were not achieved. There was also technical difficulty in fixing the graft securely to the defect.

Small osteochodral autografts have been used for articular defects in the hand and the wrist. Boulas and colleagues[24] first reported the use of osteochondral metatarsophalangeal autografts for traumatic articular metacarpophalangeal defects in 5 patients in 1993. Gaul[25] used free partial toe joint osteochondral autografts to replace the destroyed condyle of the proximal interphalangeal joints in 5 patients in 1998. In 2003, Lo and Chang[26] used graft from radial styloid to replace a defect at the base of proximal phalanx at the metacarpophalangeal joint. Ozyurekoglu[27] used multiple cyclindrical osteochondral grafts to replace defect at the proximal interphalangeal joint in 2010, using the small joint OATS to harvest the graft from the hamate and transferred to the finger joint through an open approach. Follow-up radiological study at 4 years showed no degenerative changes.

In the wrist, Mehin and colleagues[28] reported 2 cases of autogenous osteochondral graft transfer from the proximal tibiofibular joint to resurface the distal radius in 2000. Merrell and colleagues[29] described a technique of using the scaphoid facet of the same wrist as a neovascularized osteochondral graft to reconstruct the sigmoid fossa in 1 patient in 2002. del Piñal and colleagues[30] reported in 2005 the use of a free vascularized osteochondral auto graft from the base of the third metatarsal to reconstruct the scaphoid facet of the distal radius, in which 70% was destroyed after a severe comminuted fracture of the distal radius. Lee and colleagues[31] reported a case of osteo-chondritis dissecans of the scaphoid treated with osteochondral autograft in 2011. They used OATS to harvest a graft of 6-mm diameter from the lateral femoral condyle and performed press-fit insertion.

The authors developed an arthroscopic technique and approach to enable transfer of the auto-graft without violating the soft tissue envelope of the wrist and hence achieved the advantages of minimally invasive surgery. In the authors' series, the indication for autogenous osteochondral graft was the highly localized osteochondral defect at the lunate fossa. This provided a favorable location to enable the graft to be delivered arthroscopically. Extreme caution had to be exercised to avoid iat-rogenic injury to the unaffected articular surface. In the authors' series, there were no complications due to technical problems. Difficulty of inserting a harvester larger than 6 mm in smaller patients or to other locations in the wrist was anticipated. For le-sions larger than 7 mm to 8 mm, as in case report 2, 2 osteochondral plugs are preferred. It is recom-mended that the harvesting of the osteochondral plug in the wrist should be perpendicular to the surface of the joint so that the cartilage surface can be aligned to that of the unaffected part. Thus, if the lesion is located in the central or volar part of the wrist, access to the arthroscopy instru-ment may become difficult or it may be impossible to obtain a perpendicular direction. Using an open approach may be needed. The technique is also contraindicated in diffuse or progressive cartilage disease and in the presence of active sepsis. In the authors' series, there was no major complaint about pain at the donor site over the knee. This is probably due to the small size and number of the graft, in contrast to the experience in knee or ankle, where multiple plugs are generally required.

For rehabilitation of isolated osteochondral graft transfer, because the graft fixation by press-fit is generally stable, immobilization of the wrist is un-necessary after the operation. Early active and gentle passive motion exercise should be encour-aged. Load bearing, however, should be avoided until clinical and radiological signs of graft incorpo-ration are ascertained, usually by 2 months to 4 months postoperative.

SUMMARY

Arthroscopic transplantation of osteochondral autograft is an effective treatment option in symptomatic focal osteochondral lesion of the distal radius articular surface to restore the normal hyaline cartilage and the articular environment. Due to limitation by the current instrumentation, the size of the osteochondral plug is restricted to 6 mm. In the future, more patients can benefit if the instrument can be downsized so that multiple grafting is made possible. A larger patient sample and longer-term follow-up will further establish the value of this surgical procedure.

REFERENCES

1. Koman H, Poehling GG, Toby EB, et al. Chronic wrist pain: indications for wrist arthroscopy. Arthroscopy 1990;6:116–9.
2. Haim HA, Moore AE, Schweitzer ME, et al. MRI in the diagnosis of cartilage Injury in the wrist. AJR Am J Roentgenol 2004;182:1267–70.
3. Whipple TL. Chronic wrist pain. Instr Course Lect 1995;44:129–37.
4. Nelson DL. Function wrist motion. Hand Clin 1997; 13(1):83–92.
5. Cheng HS, Hung LK, Ho PC, et al. An analysis of causes and treatment outcome of chronic wrist pain after distal radius fractures. Hand Surg 2008; 13(1):1–10.
6. Estrella EP, Hung LK, Ho PC, et al. Arthroscopic repair of triangular fibrocartilage complex tear. Arthroscopy 2007;23(7):729–37.
7. Ong TY, Ho PC, Wong WYC, et al. Wrist arthroscopy under portal site local anaesthesia (PSLA) without tourniquet. J Wrist Surg 2012;1:149–52.
8. Hangody L, Rathonyi GK, Duska Z, et al. Autoge-nous osteochondral mosaicplasty. Surgical tech-nique. J Bone Joint Surg Am 2004;86A(Suppl 1): 65–72.
9. Buckwalter J. Articular cartilage: injuries and poten-tial for healing. J Orthop Sports Phys Ther 1998;28: 192–202.
10. Shapiro F, Koide S, Glimcher MJ. Cell origin and dif-ferentiation in the repair of full-thickness defects of articular cartilage. J Bone Joint Surg Am 1977;75: 532–53.
11. Furukawa T, Eyre DR, Koide S, et al. Biochemical studies on repair cartilage resurfacing experimental defects in the rabbit knee. J Bone Joint Surg Am 1980;62:79–89.
12. Pridie EA. A method of resurfacing osteoarthritic knee joints. J Bone Joint Surg Am 1959;41:618.
13. Steadman R. Chondral defects in athletes. The 5th Annual Panther Sports Medicine Symposium. Pitts-burgh (PA): 1992.
14. Czitrom AA, Keating S, Gross AE. The viability of articular cartilage in fresh osteochondral allografts after clinical transplantation. J Bone Joint Surg Am 1990;72:574–81.

15. Micheli L, Curtis C, Shervin N. Articular cartilage repair in the adolescent athlete: Is autogenous chondrocyte implantation the answer? Clin J Sport Med 2006;16:465–70.

16. Gomoll AH, Far J, Gillogly SD, et al. Surgical management of articular cartilage defects of the knee. J Bone Joint Surg Am 2010;92:2470–90.

17. Gudas R, Kalesinskas RJ, Kimtys V, et al. A prospective randomized clinical study of mosaic osteochondral autologous transplantation versus microfracture for the treatment of osteochondral defects in the knee joint of young athletes. Arthroscopy 2005;21:1066–75.

18. Slutsky D, Nagle DJ. Wrist arthroscopy: current concepts. J Hand Surg 2008;33A:1228–44.

19. Araf M, Moattar R Jr. Arthroscopic study of injuries in articular fractures of distal radius extremity. Acta Ortop Bras 2014;22(3):144–50.

20. Culp R, Osterman AL, Kaufmann RA. Wrist arthroscopy: operative procedures. In: Green DP, Hotchkiss RN, Pederson WC, et al, editors. Operative hand surgery. 5th edition. New York: Churchill Livingstone; 2005. p. 781–803.

21. Roth JH, Poehling GG. Arthroscopic "ectomy" surgery of the wrist. Arthroscopy 1990;6:141–7.

22. Engkvist O, Johansson SH. Perichondrial arthroplasty: a clinical study in twenty-six patients. Scand J Plast Reconstr Surg 1980;14:71–87.

23. Seradge H, Kutz JA, Kleinert HE, et al. Perichondral resurfacing arthroplasty in the hand. J Hand Surg 1984;9A:880–6.

24. Boulas HJ, Herren A, Buchler U. Osteochondral metatarsophalangeal autografts for traumatic articular metacarpophalangeal defects: a preliminary report. J Hand Surg 1993;18A:1086–92.

25. Gaul JS Jr. Articular fractures of the proximal interphalangeal joint with missing elements: repair with partial toe joint osteochondral autografts. J Hand Surg 1999;24A:78–85.

26. Lo CY, Chang YP. Osteochondral grafting of the metacarpophalangeal joint in rheumatoid arthritis. J Hand Surg 2003;28B:94–7.

27. Ozyurekoglu T. Multiple osteochondral autograft transfer to the proximal interphalangeal joint: case report. J Hand Surg 2010;35A:931–5.

28. Mehin R, Giachino AA, Backman D, et al. Autologous osteoarticular transfer from proximal tibiofibular joint to the scaphoid and lunate facets in the treatment of severe distal radius fractures: a report of two cases. J Hand Surg 2003;28A:332–41.

29. Merrell GA, Barrie KA, Wolfe SW. Sigmoid notch reconstruction using osteoarticular graft in a severely comminuted distal radius fracture: a case report. J Hand Surg 2002;27A:729–34.

30. Del Piñal F, Garcia-Bernal FJ, Delgado J, et al. Reconstruction of the distal radius facet by a free vascularised osteochondral autograft: anatomic study and report of a patient. J Hand Surg 2005;30A:1200.e1-14.

31. Lee YK, Lee M, Lee JM. Osteochondral autograft transplantation for osteochondritis dissecans of the scaphoid: case report. J Hand Surg 2011;36A:820–3.

Arthroscopic Management of Dorsal and Volar Wrist Ganglion

Christophe Mathoulin, MD, FMH*, Mathilde Gras, MD

KEYWORDS

- Dorsal ganglion • Volar ganglion • Wrist arthroscopy • Treatment

KEY POINTS

- Dorsal and volar wrist ganglia are benign tumors that can disappear spontaneously.
- Conservative treatment is the best primary treatment of dorsal or volar wrist ganglia owing to the benign character and the frequency of its spontaneous disappearance.
- Arthroscopic resection is a simple technique, which is minimally invasive and avoids the complications of open excision, especially unsightly scarring and joint stiffness.
- The patient must be informed of the recurrence rate, similar to that after open surgery.
- Scapholunate instability can be associated with a dorsal wrist ganglion, should not be missed, and should be treated with arthroscopy.

INTRODUCTION: NATURE OF THE PROBLEM

Dorsal and volar wrist ganglia are benign tumors that can disappear spontaneously, and most of them are asymptomatic. Surgery is reserved for the rare painful ganglia, or more often for cosmetic concern.

Even in painful wrist ganglia, range of motion and function are usually well preserved, and those tumors are benign. In effect, the treatment has to be safe, with a low complication rate and good preservation of wrist motion. Arthroscopic resection fills those criteria and is simple and reliable.[1]

For dorsal wrist ganglia, recent cadaveric studies has allowed the precise understanding that the dorsal scapholunate (SL) region is a complex composed of 3 distinct elements[2]:

- The dorsal segment of the SL ligament
- The dorsal intercarpal ligament (DIC)

- The dorsal capsuloscapholunate septum (DCSS), which unites the SL ligament to the DIC and contributes to the stabilization of the SL bony interval (**Fig. 1**).

The hypothesis of its origin is a mucoid dysplasia associated with intracapsular and extra-synovial ganglia, which occurs at the level of this dorsal SL complex. Medially, the dysplasia herniates into the wrist joints, usually into the midcarpal joint. Laterally, the dysplasia is extended by a pedicle between the DIC and the radio lunotrique-tral (LRLT) ligament, or either distally beneath the DIC or laterally toward the radial border of the radiocarpal compartment. Dorsal ganglia are more common (70%). The incidence in men and boys is 25/100,000 and in women and girls is 43/100,000. Conservative treatment is probably the best primary treatment for dorsal wrist ganglia owing to the benign character and the high

Disclosure Statement: The authors declare no relationship with a commercial company that has a direct financial interest in subject matter or materials discussed in article or with a company making a competing product.
Institut de la Main, Clinique BIZET, 23 Rue Georges BIZET, Paris 75116, France
* Corresponding author.
E-mail address: cmathoulin@orange.fr

Hand Clin 33 (2017) 769–777
http://dx.doi.org/10.1016/j.hcl.2017.07.012
0749-0712/17/© 2017 Elsevier Inc. All rights reserved.

hand.theclinics.com

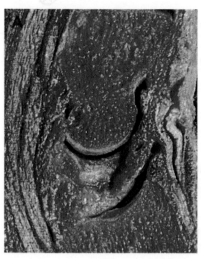

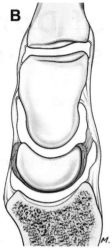

Fig. 1. (*A*) Sagittal cut of the wrist passing through the lunate and showing the dorsal SL complex. (*B*) The 3 components of the dorsal SL complex: the dorsal portion of the SL ligament in brown, the dorsal capsuloligamentous septum, DCSS, in blue, and the DIC, the integrating part of the dorsal capsule, in white.

frequency of spontaneous disappearance by 6 months. Arthroscopic resection is a simple and minimally invasive technique. The patient must be informed of the recurrence rate of 11%,[3] similar to that following open surgery. Arthroscopic resection avoids the complications of open excision, especially unsightly scarring and joint stiffness.

An SL instability can be associated with a dorsal wrist ganglion and should not be missed. Arthroscopic treatment allows assessment and repair to the SL ligament if necessary.

Volar wrist ganglia are less common (20%). They occur mainly in the radiocarpal joint, and rarely in the midcarpal joint, and in scapho-trapezio-trapezoid (STT) osteoarthritis. They are due to capsule destruction at the volar insertion of the SL ligament in the midcarpal joint. Like dorsal ganglia, these are benign tumors. The operative risks are related to the proximity of the cyst with the radial artery and nerve, especially in the open procedure. Arthroscopic resection is a simple and reliable procedure as long as the surgical technique is performed correctly, given that the intracapsular origin of the ganglion is far from tendons, ligaments, and muscles.

Surgical treatment is indicated only in cases whereby the ganglion causes pain or is unsightly. Its recurrence rate is similar to open resection, but without the risk of injuring tendons, ligaments, nerves, and muscles. Arthroscopic resection involves less scarring, minimal time away from work, and faster functional recovery.

INDICATIONS/CONTRAINDICATIONS

Conservative treatment is probably the best primary treatment for dorsal and volar wrist ganglia, as mentioned before.

In the case of persistence of ganglion, aspiration is a current treatment. However, the recurrence rate is high: 59% with a low rate of complication (3%) according to a systematic review and metaanalysis.[4] Steroid injection after aspiration has been proposed but does not give better results.[5]

Open surgical excision offers significantly lower chance of recurrence with a rate of 21% but a higher rate of complications of 14%.[5]

According to this same review, arthroscopic excision has yielded promising outcomes with a 6% recurrence rate and 4% complication rate. However, the data from comparative clinical trials are limited and have not demonstrated the superiority of the arthroscopic approach. In another study with 114 dorsal wrist ganglia at a minimum of 2 years follow-up, the recurrence rate was 11%.[3] Arthroscopic treatment of ganglion cyst seems to be at least as good with fewer complications.

An SL instability can be also associated with a dorsal wrist ganglion and should not be missed. Arthroscopic SL ligament assessment and repair are necessary during the same procedure.

Arthroscopic resection of volar ganglion is also an effective method for well-selected ganglia arising from the radiocarpal joint.[6] The risk is related to the proximity of the cyst with the radial artery and nerve.

There is no contraindication of arthroscopic ganglion excision.

SURGICAL TECHNIQUE/PROCEDURE
Preoperative Planning

MRI assists in the diagnosis and identification of the pedicle of the ganglion in order to plan the procedure (**Fig. 2**). The resection of the ganglion must be performed at the origin of the pedicle.

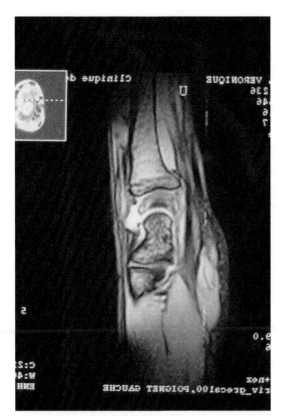

Fig. 2. Lateral view of MRI showing a small painful ganglion in midcarpal position.

Preparation and Patient Positioning

The surgery is performed as a day surgery, under regional anesthesia. The tourniquet is placed on the arm near the elbow to minimize the leverage during upward traction. Countertraction is applied on the tourniquet. After exsanguinating and placing an upper limb sterile drape, traction is applied using a traction system or tower. The required traction of 5 to 7 kg is applied using Chinese finger traps. The patient lies supine with the shoulder at 90° abduction. The surgeon is positioned at the head of the patient, and the assistant is positioned on the palmar side of the wrist. The arthroscopy column may be on the other side of the patient facing the surgeon or sometimes facing the arm table (**Fig. 3**).

Dorsal wrist ganglion

Surgical approach The scope is inserted through the ulnar midcarpal portal (MCU). A blunt trocar is introduced and then the scope. Midcarpal exploration usually reveals a dorsal synovial bulge at the SL interval corresponding to the intra-articular portion of the ganglion. Associated SL instability must be looked for and excluded.

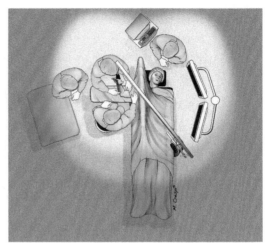

Fig. 3. Position of the patient and the operators. The surgeon is at the head of the patient.

Surgical procedure

Step 1: resection of the dorsal mucoid dysplasia at the midcarpal interval through a transcystic approach A needle is introduced through the ganglion into the midcarpal joint by the radial midcarpal portal (MCR). A direct transcystic MCR approach is performed and a shaver is introduced through the ganglion into the joint (**Fig. 4**). The shaver resects the dorsal pathologic capsule, which represents the mucoid dysplasia herniated into the midcarpal joint, under direct arthroscopic vision. The DCSS and the continuity of the DIC must be preserved. Electrocoagulation should be avoided because of the risk of cartilage and extensor tendon lesions.

Step 2: resection of the ganglion wall The scope follows along the shaver, from the MCU portal, over the ganglion, toward the MCU portal, and into the joint, in order to see the cyst wall.

The shaver is always in the MCR position but is extraarticular. This part of the procedure is more of an endoscopy than an arthroscopy (**Fig. 5**). Caution is required at this stage to avoid extensor tendon injury. The walls of the cyst can be resected by moving the scope and the shaver from top to bottom to obtain a cosmetically perfect final result. The resection is performed step by step by the shaver until the extensor tendons are visible at the end (**Fig. 6**).

Step 3: treating the scapholunate instability or dorsal capsuloscapholunate septum lesion if any A radiocarpal control is performed with the scope in the 6R portal, and the probe in 3-4 portal. Arthroscopic shaving can be performed as previously mentioned if necessary. Then, the SL ligament is checked as well as the DCSS. In the

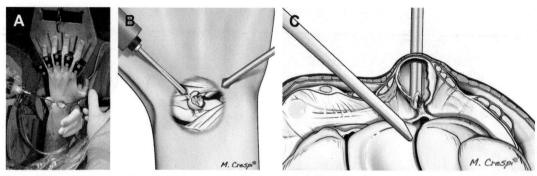

Fig. 4. (*A*) Operative view showing the scope in MCU portal and the shaver in MCR portal, through a transcystic approach. (*B*) Scope and shaver positions. (*C*) The transcystic position of the shaver.

case of SL instability or DCSS lesion, a capsuloligamentous repair is performed. Two needles with absorbable suture are passed through the 3-4 portal, through the capsule and the SL ligament, toward the midcarpal joint. Then, the scope is placed through the MCU portal, and the 2 sutures are grasped with a grasper through the MCR portal. The 2 sutures are tied together, and a knot is formed. The 2 suture remnants at the 3-4 portal are pulled and the knot is anchored onto the SL ligament. After releasing the traction, with wrist at extension, another knot is made by tying the 2 suture remnants at the 3-4 portal. This other knot is applied onto the capsule, closing the DCSS space (**Fig. 7**).

Step 4: wound closure and postoperative care Skin suture is not necessary. Immediate active range-of-motion exercise is allowed without any passive motion for 3 weeks. In the case of SL or DCSS repair, a splint is placed for 6 weeks, and then rehabilitation is started.

Volar wrist ganglion
Surgical approach The surgical approach is through the radiocarpal joint. The blunt trocar is introduced through the 3-4 portal and then the scope. The shaver is inserted through the 1-2 portal.

Surgical procedure
Step 1: location of the ganglion The surgeon presses on the ganglion outside the wrist while the arthroscope is in the radiocarpal joint to confirm that the origin of the pedicle situates between the radio scaphocapitate ligament (RSC) and the long radiolunate ligament (LRL) (**Fig. 8**). Sometimes a mass of inflammatory tissue can be seen in between the 2 ligaments.

Step 2: ganglion resection The shaver is passed through between the RSC and the LRL ligament under arthroscopic control to resect the pedicle of the ganglion (**Fig. 9**). When the ganglion is open to the joint, the ganglion mucus flows into the joint. The resection is performed cautiously, from inside the joint and continuing carefully deeper toward the volar side. It is not necessary to remove all the cyst walls. The shaver should not resect outside the joint because of the risk of damaging the radial artery and the median nerve. In some case, flexor pollicis longus can be seen through the resection (**Fig. 10**). The resection can be completed by exchanging the scope and the shaver by placing the scope in the 6R or 4-5 portal, and the shaver through the 3-4 portal.

Step 3: closing and postoperative care The arthroscopy portal incisions do not need to be

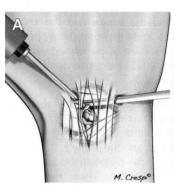
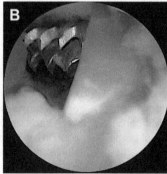

Fig. 5. (*A*) The scope position passing through the MCU portal and exiting through the MCR portal to control the resection of the ganglion walls extraarticularly. (*B*) Arthroscopic view through the MCR portal with the scope in MCU portal, showing the shaver resecting the ganglion walls from inside out while the extensor tendons are protected.

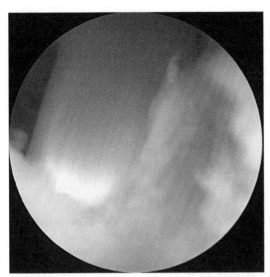

Fig. 6. Arthroscopic view through the MCR portal from inside out with the scope in MCU, showing the extensor tendons after the resection of the cyst wall.

sutured, but only covered with dressing. Wrist motion is allowed immediately.

COMPLICATIONS AND MANAGEMENT

Arthroscopic resection avoids the complications of open excision, especially unsightly scarring and joint stiffness. The various complications described after arthroscopic surgery for wrist

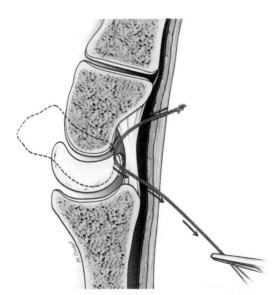

Fig. 7. The SL repair: 2 needles are passed through the 3-4 portal, through the capsule, and the SL ligament; a knot is made through the MCR portal, and the knot is pulled onto the SL ligament, closing the DCSS space.

ganglia were injuries to the sensory branches of the median nerve or the radial nerve (neurapraxia), radial artery or its branches, and tendons, and hematoma formation.[7–11]

The complication rate varies from 0% to 12.3% (**Table 1**). For Fernandes and colleagues,[12] the average rate of complications for the volar wrist ganglia was 6.8%.

In dorsal ganglion, complications are very rare; a few have been reported, as follows:

- Some degreeof loss of wrist flexion (which is still less than with open surgery)
- Neurapraxia
- Extensor tenosynovitis
- Complex regional pain syndrome[7]

In volar ganglion, the risks are related to the proximity of the cyst with the radial artery and nerve, as follows:

- Radial artery injuries with hematoma and 1 pseudoaneurysm[8]
- Neuropraxia of dorsal radial nerve
- Partial lesion of median nerve

A systematic review of arthroscopic resection of volar ganglion reported 6.89% of complications.[9]

No postoperative infection has been described in the literature. Similarly, no complications related to the scar were identified (sensitivity, aesthetics).

POSTOPERATIVE CARE

In cases of ligament repair, a splint is placed for 6 weeks; then rehabilitation is started. In other cases, immediate mobilization of the wrist is allowed.

OUTCOMES
Recurrence

The recurrence rate of arthroscopic removal of wrist ganglia varies from 0% to 26%[1,3,7,10,11,13–17] (**Table 2**). In 2014, Fernandes[12] showed an average recurrence rate of 6% for volar ganglia treated by arthroscopy in his review of the literature.

Objective and Subjective Clinical Results

Pain
Many investigators highlighted an improvement in pain after arthroscopic resection of the ganglion.[14,17,18] In 2010, Gallego and Mathoulin[3] described a complete disappearance of pain in 44% of patients. Kang and colleagues[8] in 2013 showed a decrease in visual analogue scale of pain to 2.4 preoperatively and to 0.6 2 years after surgery.

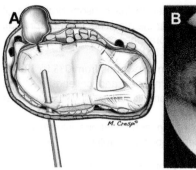

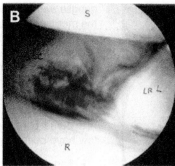

Fig. 8. (*A*) The scope is inserted in the 3-4 portal to locate the pedicle of the ganglion between the RSC and LRL ligaments. (*B*) Intra-articular view of the ganglion's stalk between the RSC and LRL ligaments. LRL; long radio lunate ligament; R, radius; RSC, radio scapho capitate ligament; S, scaphoid.

Postoperative range of motion and strength

Mobility and wrist strength seemed preserved or even improved postoperatively in most cases[3,8,9,14,17] (**Table 3**).

In his review of literature on the volar ganglia operated arthroscopically, Fernandes[12] did not describe any loss of postoperative mobility.

Functional scores and patient satisfaction

Edwards and Johansen[9] demonstrated an improvement in the Disabilities of the Arm, Shoulder, and Hand score from 14 to 1.7 stable at 2 years postoperative follow-up. Similarly, Kang and colleagues[8] showed an improvement of Mayo Wrist Score from 74 to 91.

For Mathoulin and colleagues,[3] more than 96% of patients were satisfied with arthroscopic surgery.

Return to work and daily activity

Postoperative time off from work is on average 10 to 14 days.[3,7,17] Mathoulin and colleagues[3] described an immediate return to work in 37% of patients. Similarly, Aslani and colleagues[17] described 36% of patients returned to work immediately.

Comparison Between Open Surgery and Arthroscopic Removal of Wrist Ganglia

Indications

All ganglia of the wrist are not easily treated arthroscopically. Indeed, several investigators described a technical difficulty in midcarpal wrist ganglia.[5,14,18] In a comparative study in 2008, Rocchi and colleagues[7] showed better results with arthroscopic treatment of radiocarpal volar ganglia and better outcomes with open surgery for midcarpal volar ganglia. They therefore recommended open surgery for these midcarpal volar ganglia. For Ho and colleagues,[1] the ganglion of the STT joint is not a good indication of arthroscopic surgery.

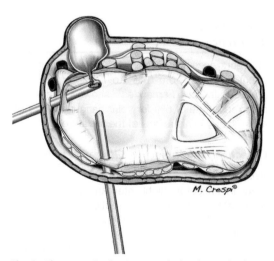

Fig. 9. The scope in the 3-4 portal; the shaver in the 1-2 portal is used to start resecting the pedicle of the ganglion cyst.

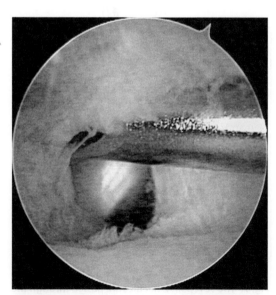

Fig. 10. Intra-articular view of the flexor pollicis longus tendon after the cyst has been resected; the RSC and LRL ligaments remain intact.

Table 1
Complication rate of arthroscopic resection

Authors	Ganglion Location	Rate of Complications (%)	Details
Osterman & Raphael,[14] 1995	Dorsal	0	
Luchetti et al,[15] 2000	Dorsal	0	
Ho et al,[1] 2001	Dorsal	0	
	Volar	0	
Mathoulin et al,[11] 2004	Dorsal	0	
	Volar	3.1	1 hematoma
Rocchi et al,[10] 2006	Dorsal & volar	8.5	1 radial artery lesion, 1 hematoma, 2 axonotmesis
Kang et al,[13] 2008	Dorsal	2.1	1 neurapraxia
Rocchi et al,[7] 2008	Volar	8	1 neurapraxia, 1 radial artery lesion
Edwards & Johansen,[9] 2009	Dorsal	5.5	3 tenosynovitis of extensors
Mathoulin et al,[3] 2010	Dorsal	12.3	1 neurapraxia of radial nerve, 1 synovitis extensor pollicis longus tendon, 1 tendinitis extensor communis digitis tendon, 2 hematomas

Recurrence and complications

The recurrence rate of a ganglion after arthroscopic surgery looks identical to that of open surgery.[3,7,13]

In 2008, Kang and colleagues[13] carried out a prospective randomized study comparing the recurrence rate between open surgery and arthroscopy in 72 patients with a dorsal ganglion. No significant difference was found on the recurrence rate at 1 year of follow-up.

Similarly, Rocchi and colleagues[7] performed a randomized study comparing open surgery with arthroscopy for the treatment of volar ganglia. They did not find any significant difference in the recurrence rate.

However, they showed that arthroscopy provided better results in the treatment of radiocarpal ganglia without major complications. Similarly, functional recovery seemed faster with shorter time off work with arthroscopic surgery.

Table 2
Recurrence rate of arthroscopic removal of wrist ganglia

Authors	Ganglion Location	Follow-up (mo)	Number of Ganglia	Rate of Recurrences (%)
Osterman & Raphael,[14] 1995	Dorsal	—	18	0
Luchetti et al,[15] 2000	Dorsal	16	34	5.9
Ho et al,[1] 2001	Dorsal	25	19	26
	Volar	16	5	0
Rizzo et al,[16] 2004	Dorsal	47	41	4.9
Mathoulin et al,[11] 2004	Dorsal	34	96	4.2
	Volar	26	32	0
Rocchi et al,[10] 2006	Dorsal & volar	15	47	4.3
Kang et al,[13] 2008	Dorsal	12	28	7.1
Rocchi et al,[7] 2008	Volar	24	25	12
Edwards & Johansen,[9] 2009	Dorsal	Minimum 24	55	0
Mathoulin et al,[3] 2010	Dorsal	42	114	12.3
Aslani et al,[17] 2012	Dorsal	39	52	17.3
Kang et al,[8] 2013	Dorsal	39	41	7.3

Table 3
Postoperative range of motion and wrist strength

Authors	Range of Motion	Strength
Osterman et al,[14] 1995	↗ in 94% of patients	↗ until 90% of comparative side in 27% patients
Rizzo et al,[16] 2004	↘ in 21% of patients	
Edwards et al,[9] 2009	↘ of 13° flexion at 6 wk ↘ 5° maximum after 2 y	↗ of 5.9 kg
Mathoulin et al,[3] 2010	↗ 15° of flexion ↗11° of extension	↗ from 22 to 31 kgf (jamar)
Aslani et al,[17] 2012	↗ flexion & extension	↗
Kang et al,[8] 2013	= same as preoperative	↗ from 28 to 36 kgf after 2 y

Abbreviations: kgf, kilogram force; Jamar, jamar dynamometer.

Aesthetics

Most requests for removal of a wrist ganglion are for aesthetic discomfort. The appearance of postoperative scar is therefore essential. However, the assessment of scarring cannot be found in the literature.

After open surgery on wrist ganglia, Dias and colleagues[18] mentioned 4 sensitive scars and keloid. Similarly, Lidder and colleagues[19] described scar sensitivity in 32% of patients, which was severe in 13% of patients. They also described an unsightly scar in 3.4% of the cases. Rocchi and colleagues[7] found 4 cases of sensitive scars, and painful or scar hypertrophy was found in 25 patients operated by the open approach.

No complication related to the scar has been described in the literature during ganglion surgery done arthroscopically.[3,7,10,12,14] It is another significant advantage of arthroscopy over open surgery in the treatment of wrist ganglia.

SUMMARY

Various conservative treatments of wrist ganglia exist, such as aspiration with or without injection of anti-inflammatory medications,[18,20,21] hyaluronidase injection,[22] or simple immobilization.[21] Therapeutic abstinence may also be proposed because spontaneous resolution of ganglion is 40% to 58%.[1,5]

Nevertheless, several investigators[21,22] have demonstrated superiority of surgery compared with medical therapy based on the risk of recurrence and major complications. In 2007, Dias and colleagues[18] highlighted a recurrence rate of 39% after ganglion surgery against 58% with aspiration. Similarly, in 2011, Khan and Hayat[20] compared the treatment of steroid injection with surgical excision of the ganglion in 36 patients in a randomized controlled study. The recurrence rate was statistically lower in surgery (<6%) compared with medical therapy (39%).

Surgical treatment allows a lower risk of recurrence, but complications occur more frequently. Dias and colleagues[18] showed a complication rate of 20% with surgery against 5% with suction. The rate of secondary complication from an open surgery was 0% to 28%.[7,13,22] In 1995, Osterman and Raphael[14] performed arthroscopic resection of dorsal ganglion in 18 patients without any complications.

The goal of arthroscopic surgery for ganglion is to have a low risk of recurrence, fewer surgical complications than open surgery, and satisfactory cosmetic appearance of scars. Indeed, the aesthetic side is important because it represents most of the indications of ganglion excision.[3,23] Arthroscopy also has the advantage of performing an assessment of potential associated damage inside the wrists[14] and treats the "hidden" ganglion, which is not visible or palpable on physical examination but is symptomatic.[7]

REFERENCES

1. Ho PC, Griffiths J, Lo WN, et al. Current treatment of ganglion of the wrist. Hand Surg 2001;6(1):49–58.
2. Overstraeten LV, Camus EJ, Wahegaonkar A, et al. Anatomical description of the dorsal capsuloscapholunate septum (DCSS). Arthroscopic staging of scapholunate instability after DCSS sectioning. J Wrist Surg 2013;2(2):149–54.
3. Gallego S, Mathoulin C. Arthroscopic resection of dorsal wrist ganglia: 114 cases with minimum follow-up of 2 years. Arthroscopy 2010;26(12): 1675–82.
4. Head L, Gencarelli JR, Allen M, et al. Wrist ganglion treatment: systematic review and meta-analysis. J Hand Surg 2015;40(3):546–53.e8.

5. Richman JA, Gelberman RH, Engber WD, et al. Ganglions of the wrist and digits: results of treatment by aspiration and cyst wall puncture. J Hand Surg 1987;12(6):1041–3.

6. Ho PC, Lo WN, Hung LK. Arthroscopic resection of volar ganglion of the wrist: a new technique. Arthroscopy 2003;19(2):218–21.

7. Rocchi L, Canal A, Fanfani F, et al. Articular ganglia of the volar aspect of the wrist: arthroscopic resection compared with open excision. A prospective randomised study. Scand J Plast Reconstr Surg Hand Surg 2008;42(5):253–9.

8. Kang HJ, Koh IH, Kim JS, et al. Coexisting intraarticular disorders are unrelated to outcomes after arthroscopic resection of dorsal wrist ganglions. Clin Orthop 2013;471(7):2212–8.

9. Edwards SG, Johansen JA. Prospective outcomes and associations of wrist ganglion cysts resected arthroscopically. J Hand Surg 2009;34(3):395–400.

10. Rocchi L, Canal A, Pelaez J, et al. Results and complications in dorsal and volar wrist ganglia arthroscopic resection. Hand Surg 2006;11(1–2):21–6.

11. Mathoulin C, Hoyos A, Pelaez J. Arthroscopic resection of wrist ganglia. Hand Surg 2004;9(2):159–64.

12. Fernandes CH, Miranda CDO, Dos Santos JBG, et al. A systematic review of complications and recurrence rate of arthroscopic resection of volar wrist ganglion. Hand Surg 2014;19(3):475–80.

13. Kang L, Akelman E, Weiss A-PC. Arthroscopic versus open dorsal ganglion excision: a prospective, randomized comparison of rates of recurrence and of residual pain. J Hand Surg Am 2008;33(4):471–5.

14. Osterman AL, Raphael J. Arthroscopic resection of dorsal ganglion of the wrist. Hand Clin 1995;11(1):7–12.

15. Luchetti R, Badia A, Alfarano M, et al. Arthroscopic resection of dorsal wrist ganglia and treatment of recurrences. J Hand Surg Br 2000;25(1):38–40.

16. Rizzo M, Berger RA, Steinmann SP, et al. Arthroscopic resection in the management of dorsal wrist ganglions: results with a minimum 2-year follow-up period. J Hand Surg Am 2004;29(1):59–62.

17. Aslani H, Najafi A, Zaaferani Z. Prospective outcomes of arthroscopic treatment of dorsal wrist ganglia. Orthopedics 2012;35(3):e365–70.

18. Dias JJ, Dhukaram V, Kumar P. The natural history of untreated dorsal wrist ganglia and patient reported outcome 6 years after intervention. J Hand Surg Eur Vol 2007;32(5):502–8.

19. Lidder S, Ranawat V, Ahrens P. Surgical excision of wrist ganglia; literature review and nine-year retrospective study of recurrence and patient satisfaction. Orthop Rev (Pavia) 2009;1(1):e5.

20. Khan PS, Hayat H. Surgical excision versus aspiration combined with intralesional triamcinolone acetonide injection plus wrist immobilization therapy in the treatment of dorsal wrist ganglion; a randomized controlled trial. J Hand Microsurg 2011;3(2):55–7.

21. Limpaphayom N, Wilairatana V. Randomized controlled trial between surgery and aspiration combined with methylprednisolone acetate injection plus wrist immobilization in the treatment of dorsal carpal ganglion. J Med Assoc Thai 2004;87(12):1513–7.

22. Jagers Op Akkerhuis M, Van Der Heijden M, Brink PRG. Hyaluronidase versus surgical excision of ganglia: a prospective, randomized clinical trial. J Hand Surg Br 2002;27(3):256–8.

23. Westbrook AP, Stephen AB, Oni J, et al. Ganglia: the patient's perception. J Hand Surg Br 2000;25(6):566–7.

Arthroscopic Synovectomy of Wrist in Rheumatoid Arthritis

Jae Woo Shim, MD, Min Jong Park, MD*

KEYWORDS

• Rheumatoid arthritis • Rheumatoid wrist • Arthroscopy • Synovectomy

KEY POINTS

• Arthroscopic synovectomy of the rheumatoid wrist can reduce pain and improve function.
• Arthroscopic synovectomy is a safe and minimally invasive procedure.
• Long-term control rate of synovitis after arthroscopic synovectomy is approximately 75%.

INTRODUCTION

Rheumatoid arthritis (RA) is a systemic inflammatory disorder affecting multiple joints. The etiology is unclear. It is probably related to a T-lymphocyte–mediated immune response to autoantigens mediated by activation at the HLA-II locus.[1] Growth factors and cytokines, such as tumor necrosis factor and interleukin-1, play important roles during the initiation and progression of RA.[2] RA has an incidence of 0.5% to 1.0% of the population.[3] RA occurs 3 times more frequently in women than in men.[4] It has a peak onset of 40 to 60 years old.[4] Wrist involvement in RA is common, affecting up to 50% of patients within the first 2 years after the onset of the disease, and more than 90% of patients after 10 years.[5] Initial treatment for RA is medical treatment, including disease-modifying antirheumatic drugs and biologic agents.[6] In cases of failed medical treatment, surgical procedures may be necessary to relieve pain and preserve joint function. Surgical treatment options include joint-preserving techniques, such as synovectomy, and joint-salvage techniques, such as arthrodesis.[7] Synovectomy is usually considered unless the articular cartilage is severely damaged. Arthroscopic synovectomy was introduced in the 1990s with results similar to those of conventional open surgical synovectomy.[8–10] Arthroscopic synovectomy has several advantages, including minimal postoperative pain with small incision and early rehabilitation.

DIAGNOSIS AND CLASSIFICATION

Synovitis is the major clinical feature of RA. Rheumatoid wrist begins with reversible pain, swelling, and tenderness of the dorsal wrist for weeks to months. Range of motion, grip strength, and function may be affected. Deformity occurs in advanced stages. Ligaments become attenuated, triangular fibrocartilage complex is progressively destroyed, and tenosynovitis occurs. Typical deformity includes scapholunate dissociation, carpal supination, translocation of the carpus in an ulnar and volar direction, radial deviation of the carpus, and dorsal subluxation of the ulna. These deformities cause carpal collapse, ultimately leading to pan-carpal arthritis.[11]

Disclosure statement: The authors have no conflict of interest to declare.
Department of Orthopaedic Surgery, Samsung Medical Center, Sungkyunkwan University School of Medicine, Gangnam-gu, Seoul 06351, Republic of Korea
* Corresponding author. Department of Orthopaedic Surgery, Samsung Medical Center, Sungkyunkwan University School of Medicine, 81 Irwon-ro, Gangnam-gu, Seoul 06351, Republic of Korea.
E-mail address: mjp3506@skku.edu

Abnormal findings are rarely seen at the initial stage on simple radiographic examination. When the disease progresses, radiologic changes will occur, including narrowing of the joint space, multiple subchondral bone cysts, and periarticular osteoporosis. There are various scoring systems for RA, such as the Larsen classification (**Table 1**).[12] The Wrightington classification has been introduced as a radiographic means to evaluate RA of the wrist (**Table 2**).[13] The Simmen classification represents a prognostic typing for RA wrists (**Table 3**).[14]

TREATMENT

The goal of treatment for RA is to alleviate pain and preserve joint function by preventing articular cartilage damage. Treatment is based on antirheumatic drugs, including disease-modifying antirheumatic drugs and biological agents. The development of medical treatments, especially biological agents, has reduced the necessity for surgical treatment.[15] However, surgical treatment is sometimes required because not all patients can achieve treatment goals with medical treatments alone. Surgical treatments for rheumatoid wrist generally include synovectomy, tenosynovectomy, tendon repair/reconstruction, treatment for arthritic distal radioulnar joint, partial and complete arthrodesis of the radiocarpal joint, and wrist arthroplasty.[7,16–18]

SYNOVECTOMY

Synovectomy means surgical resection of the hypertrophied synovium of the joint.[7,18] Synovectomy in the rheumatoid wrist has been reported to be an effective procedure for relieving pain and preventing further destruction of the tendons

and joint by several investigators.[19–26] Open synovectomy is usually performed with tenosynovectomy, tendon repair or transfer, and distal ulnar surgery.[20,22,23,25] Synovectomy also can reduce sensory innervation of synovial tissues, thus reducing pain with improved mobility.[27] However, open synovectomy might be associated with decreased range of motion (ROM) and increased

---

Table 1
Definition of Larsen's grading system

Score	Definition
0	Normal
1	Soft tissue swelling and/or joint space narrowing/subchondral osteoporosis
2	Erosion with destruction of the joint space (DJS) of <25%
3	DJS: 26% ∼50%
4	DJS: 51% ∼75%
5	DJS >75%

From Rau R, Herborn G. A modified version of Larsen's scoring method to assess radiologic changes in rheumatoid arthritis. J Rheumatol 1995;22(10):1977; with permission.

Table 2
The Wrightington classification for rheumatoid arthritis of the wrist

Grade	Definition
Grade I	Wrist architecture preserved, mild rotatory instability of the scaphoid, periarticular osteoporosis, early cyst formation
Grade II	Ulnar translocation, lunate volar flexed, flexed scaphoid, radiolunate destruction (radio-scaphoid and midcarpal preserved)
Grade III	Intercarpal joints arthritic, radio-scaphoid eroded, volar subluxation of carpus (gross bony architecture preserved)
Grade IV	Loss of large amount of bone stock from distal radius, gross erosion of ulnar side of radius

From Hodgson SP, Stanley JK, Muirhead A. The Wrightington classification of rheumatoid wrist X-rays: a guide to surgical management. J Hand Surg Br 1989;14(4):452; with permission.

Table 3
The Simmen classification for rheumatoid arthritis of the wrist

Type	Definition
Type I (ankylosis)	Spontaneous tendency to fuse, stable pattern
Type II (arthrosis)	Articular loss progresses at equilibrium with arthrosis, stable
Type III (disintegration)	Progressive destruction, loss of alignment, unstable

From Simmen BR, Huber H. The wrist joint in chronic polyarthritis—a new classification based on the type of destruction in relation to the natural course and the consequences for surgical therapy. Handchir Mikrochir Plast Chir 1994;26(4):183; with permission. [in German].

instability. It cannot always prevent radiological progression.[20,22,24] Compared with open synovectomy, the arthroscopic method has advantages, such as fewer postoperative complications, faster recovery time, and less restriction of joint motion.[9,10,28] Therefore, it is ideal to use the arthroscopic method when only synovectomy of the radiocarpal joint is performed without additional bony or tendon procedure.

ARTHROSCOPIC SYNOVECTOMY
The Timing and Indication of Arthroscopic Synovectomy

Surgical treatment can be considered for RA wrists refractory to medication. Although we usually expect that pain and swelling will subside within 2 to 3 months after starting antirheumatic medications, many patients have 1 or more joints resistant to medical treatment.[3] Therefore, 3 to 4 months are needed to verify the effect of antirheumatic drugs.[6,29] The generally accepted timing for synovectomy is when symptoms are not controlled, although antirheumatic drugs are used for 4 to 6 months and when radiologic change, such as erosion and joint space narrowing, is observed. If the synovitis that has been controlled starts to aggravate again, synovectomy also may be considered.

Synovectomy can provide pain relief and functional improvement, particularly in early stages of RA with joint space preservation. However, the upper extremity joints tend to maintain their functions compared with the lower extremity joints with similarly advanced stage of arthritis. In the wrist joint, decreased ROM does not have significant effect on function. Furthermore, most patients with RA have low activity levels due to chronic illnesses. Considering the advantages of minimal invasive surgery, arthroscopic synovectomy can be considered before a salvage procedure, such as arthrodesis, which has long recovery time and perioperative risk. Based on Larsen stage (see **Table 1**),[12] stage 0 with normal joint space, stage 1 with reduced joint space, stage 2 with less than 25% erosion and loss of joint surface, and stage 3 with less than 50% loss of joint surface are indications for synovectomy.[9,10,30–32]

Patients with severe joint destruction are unsuitable for arthroscopic synovectomy. Larsen stage 4 and 5 represent severe forms of arthritic joint destruction. They require arthrodesis or arthroplasty when patients have substantial disability.[5,7] When simultaneous procedures, such as extensor tendon rupture and distal ulnar arthroplasty are necessary, open synovectomy is preferred over arthroscopic procedure.[7,18]

Other Indications of Arthroscopic Synovectomy

Arthroscopic synovectomy is also indicated in wrists with undifferentiated arthritis as an initial trial of surgical intervention. Undifferentiated arthritis is usually diagnosed by exclusion based on failure to fulfill the classification criteria for definitive rheumatological conditions, such as RA, psoriatic arthritis, and ankylosing spondylitis. There is no agreement about the proper management for patients with undifferentiated arthritis. In a study of Kim and colleagues,[33] arthroscopic synovectomy was performed for mono-articular wrist synovitis not responsive to conservative treatment, including nonsteroidal anti-inflammatory drugs for at least 3 months. They demonstrated that arthroscopic synovectomy resulted in complete disappearance of symptoms in 50% of patients. Patients with recurrent symptoms were eventually diagnosed as RA, which achieved improved symptoms after antirheumatic drugs. Arthroscopic synovectomy in undifferentiated chronic mono-arthritis can provide rapid resolution of symptoms and guideline for proper management.

SURGICAL TECHNIQUE OF ARTHROSCOPIC SYNOVECTOMY

Arthroscopic synovectomy is performed under general anesthesia.[10] The forearm is suspended in a traction device with a 5.5-kg to 7.0-kg load using finger traps. A pneumatic tourniquet is applied on the upper arm. A 2.4-mm or 2.9-mm-diameter 30-degree-angled arthroscope and a motorized shaver system with a 2.0-mm or 3.5-mm-diameter synovial resector blade are used for arthroscopic synovectomy. A larger diameter arthroscope and blade are preferred, while taking care not to damage the cartilage. Joints with chronic synovitis tend to have more joint space than normal joints when pulled because joints and ligaments have laxity. In the wrist joint, a 2.0-mm-diameter shaver is used as standard. In the rheumatoid wrist, a 2.9-mm shaver is often used for synovial resection and sometimes a 3.5-mm shaver is used. A radiofrequency probe also may be used to remove synovial membrane, depending on the situation.

3-4 and 4-5 portals are used as standard portals for radiocarpal joint and midcarpal radial (MCR) and midcarpal ulnar (MCU) portals for the midcarpal joint.[34,35] To gain access to all areas of radiocarpal and midcarpal joints and to excise as much synovial tissue as possible, additional portals are used. The 1-2 portal and 6U portal are usually used as extra-portals for the radiocarpal joint. These portals are particularly useful for viewing the dorsal side of the radiocarpal joint. In the midcarpal joint, an accessory portal to the scaphoid-trapezium-trapezoid (STT) joint is frequently used. To avoid tendon and nerve injuries, the exact positions of these portals are identified by puncturing the joint with a needle and using a small hemostat to spread through the subcutaneous tissue down to the capsule.

When there is a perforation in the triangular fibrocartilage (TFC), the distal radioulnar joint (DRUJ) can be reached from the radiocarpal joint through the perforated hole. A hypertrophied synovium in the DRUJ can be easily accessed through the hole in the TFC. It is removed simply by passing the shaver through the hole. Separate portals for the DRUJ are occasionally used for the shaver while viewing the joint through the hole in the triangular fibrocartilage.

After making 3-4 portal and 4-5 portal (or 6R), the operation begins with routine arthroscopic examination. Hypertrophied synovium is often observed in the ulnar side of TFC and the TFC is often perforated. TFC perforation is a secondary lesion due to chronic inflammation. It has no clinical significance. The 6U portal is useful for removing dense synovium from the ulnar side and volar side (**Fig. 1**). Synovium of the radial side is mainly removed through the 3-4 portal. If more removal is needed, a 1-2 portal can be additionally made. Insertion of arthroscopy into the 6U portal provides better visualization of the synovium of the dorsal side, which can be removed through the 3-4 and 4-5 portal (**Fig. 2**).

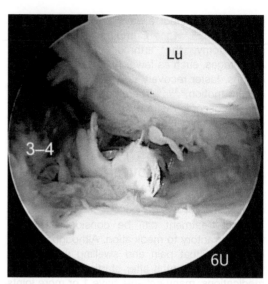

Fig. 2. The synovium of the dorsal capsule of the radiocarpal joint can be effectively visualized by arthroscopy of the 6U portal and effectively removed by shaver of 3-4 and 4-5 portals. 3-4, 3-4 portal; 6U, 6U portal; Lu, lunate.

DRUJ portal does not provide good visibility due to the narrow joint space and hypertrophied synovium. It is more effective to observe through the perforated TFC hole with the arthroscope inserted into the radiocarpal joint. The shaver inserted into the radiocarpal joint can remove synovium of the DRUJ through the TFC hole. The DRUJ portal can be made to gain direct access to the DRUJ. When marked synovitis or severe radiographic involvement of DRUJ is seen, open methods with or without arthroplastic procedures are preferable.

The MCR and MCU portals are used as standard portals for midcarpal joints. Synovium of the ulnar side can be removed from these 2 portals. As most patients with chronic synovitis have hypertrophied synovium in the STT joint space, an STT portal should be made. The synovium in the STT joint can be removed through the STT portal. The synovium in the dorsal joint capsule can be observed through the STT portal (**Figs. 3** and **4**).

Postoperatively, a compressive dressing is applied, and active motion of the wrist is permitted 2 to 3 days after the operation. All patients continue taking antirheumatic medications under the care of rheumatologists.

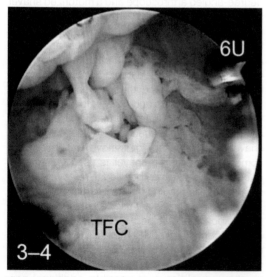

Fig. 1. Hypertrophied synovium of the ulnar side of radiocarpal joint is effectively removed by inserting a shaver into the 6U portal. 3-4, 3-4 portal; 6U, 6U portal.

RESULTS

It has been reported that arthroscopic synovectomy of rheumatoid wrists can reduce pain and improve function.[9,10,30,31,36,37] Adolfsson and Frisen[9] reported the results of arthroscopic

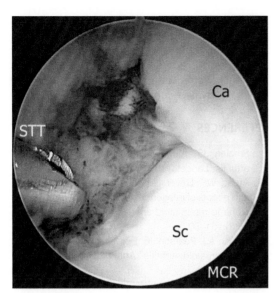

Fig. 3. The synovium of the STT joint space is removed by the shaver inserted into the STT portal while being observed by the arthroscopy of the MCR portal. Ca, capitate; MCR, MCR portal; Sc, scaphoid; STT, STT portal.

synovectomy in 24 wrists of 19 patients at a follow-up of 3.8 years. Pain was improved in 19 wrists, unchanged in 2, and worsened in 3. Average Mayo wrist score was increased from 43 to 55 points. Wei and colleagues[37] reported good to excellent results in 13 patients, fair in 3, and poor

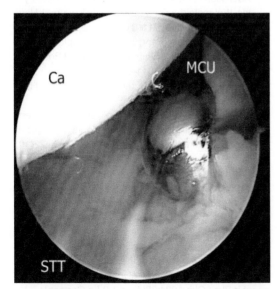

Fig. 4. The synovium overlying dorsal side of the mid-carpal joint is removed by the shaver inserted into the MCU and MCR portals while being observed by the arthroscopy of the STT portal. Ca, capitate; MCU, MCU portal; STT, STT portal.

in 1 at 12 months after office-based arthroscopic synovectomy. Although most studies have reported pain and functional improvement, improvements in ROM and grip strength are minimal.[31,32]

The results of arthroscopic synovectomy in an advanced stage of RA have been reported by Kim and colleagues[32] They reviewed 11 patients with moderately advanced arthritis (joint space narrowing of 25% to 50%) and compared with 6 patients with earlier stage of the disease. They found that patients with moderately advanced arthritis showed greater improvement in pain score and modified Mayo wrist score than the patients with earlier stage of the disease. Their study results suggested that arthroscopic synovectomy was also effective for moderate stages of RA and could be considered as a viable option before performing arthrodesis or arthroplasty. Lee and colleagues[31] have also observed that patients with rheumatoid wrists of relatively advanced radiologic stage (Larsen stage 3) have results comparable to those with rheumatoid wrists at earlier stages.

The long-term effects of arthroscopic wrist synovectomy have been reported. Lee and colleagues[31] evaluated the effects of arthroscopic synovectomy of rheumatoid wrists in a large series with a long-term follow-up. A total of 56 wrists in 49 patients underwent surgery with a mean follow-up of 7.9 years. The pain score was decreased from 6.3 to 1.7 and the mean Mayo wrist score was improved from 48 to 76. At the final follow-up, synovitis was controlled in 42 wrists (75%) but recurred in the others. The long-term effects of open wrist synovectomy also have been reported. Thirupathi and colleagues[20] evaluated 38 wrists with an average follow-up of 7.4 years and concluded that dorsal wrist synovectomy is an effective procedure with good long-term results. Brumfield and colleagues[23] performed 102 dorsal wrist synovectomies with an average follow-up of 11 years and concluded open wrist synovectomy can provide good long-term results based on pain relief and patient satisfaction. To our knowledge, no study has compared the results between open synovectomy and arthroscopic synovectomy for the rheumatoid wrist.

Although arthroscopic synovectomy shows good clinical results, it does not seem to prevent radiological progression. In the study by Kim and colleagues,[32] 9 of 19 patients showed progression of RA to a higher radiographic grade. Lee and colleagues[31] also reported similar results. At a mean follow-up of 7.9 years, 17 wrists (30%) showed no radiologic progression, 25 wrists (45%) showed a progression by 1 Larsen stage, and 14 wrists

(25%) showed a progression by 2 stages or more. Most studies on open synovectomy showed similar results on radiological progression after the surgery.[20,23,24]

It is generally accepted that arthroscopy of the wrist is a simple procedure without major complications. Lee and colleagues[31] and Adolfsson and Frisen[9] reported no complications associated with surgery. In the study of Kim and colleagues,[32] one patient showed immediate numbness of superficial radial nerve territory. However, it disappeared at 1 month after the surgery. The patients with long-standing RA might have higher risk of complications, such as wound problems after surgery, than healthy people due to nutritional deficiency and poor condition. In the study of Brumfield and colleagues,[23] 5 patients with skin necrosis and 2 patients with deep infections were reported after open dorsal synovectomies. Some investigators have reported that synovectomy can contribute to carpal instability and deformity.[38,39]

Chalmers and colleagues[40] performed a meta-analysis study for the surgical approach of synovectomy in multiple joints and found that arthroscopic and open synovectomy can provide similar pain relief at the last follow-up. Arthroscopic synovectomy of the elbow and knee might have higher rates of recurrent synovitis and radiographic progression of disease when compared with open synovectomy. For wrist joints, there was no comparison between the 2 groups (arthroscopic synovectomy and open synovectomy) due to insufficient data. However, the arthroscopic group tends to have a lower recurrence rate and radiologic progression.

SUMMARY

RA is a systemic inflammatory disorder affecting multiple joints. Wrist involvement is common. In cases of failed outcome with medical treatment, surgical procedures are necessary to relieve pain and preserve joint function. Synovectomy can be considered unless the articular cartilage is severely damaged. The generally accepted timing for synovectomy is when symptoms cannot be controlled, although antirheumatic drugs have been used for 4 to 6 months. Based on Larsen stage, synovectomy can be considered for patients with Larsen stages 1 to 3 with less than 50% loss of joint surface. Arthroscopic synovectomy has several advantages with results similar to those of conventional open surgical synovectomy. Arthroscopic synovectomy in rheumatoid wrists provides satisfactory pain relief and functional improvement. The long-term control rate of synovitis after arthroscopic synovectomy is approximately 75%. However, arthroscopic synovectomy does not seem to prevent radiological progression. Arthroscopic and open synovectomy may provide similar results. Arthroscopy is strongly recommended in that it is a safe and minimally invasive procedure.

REFERENCES

1. Smolen JS, Aletaha D, McInnes IB. Rheumatoid arthritis. Lancet 2016;388(10055):2023–38.
2. Arend WP, Dayer JM. Inhibition of the production and effects of interleukin-1 and tumor necrosis factor alpha in rheumatoid arthritis. Arthritis Rheum 1995; 38(2):151–60.
3. Silman AJ, Pearson JE. Epidemiology and genetics of rheumatoid arthritis. Arthritis Res 2002;4(Suppl 3):S265–72.
4. Alarcon GS. Epidemiology of rheumatoid arthritis. Rheum Dis Clin North Am 1995;21(3):589–604.
5. Trieb K. Treatment of the wrist in rheumatoid arthritis. J Hand Surg Am 2008;33(1):113–23.
6. Smolen JS, Landewe R, Breedveld FC, et al. EULAR recommendations for the management of rheumatoid arthritis with synthetic and biological disease-modifying antirheumatic drugs: 2013 update. Ann Rheum Dis 2014;73(3):492–509.
7. Rizzo M, Cooney WP 3rd. Current concepts and treatment for the rheumatoid wrist. Hand Clin 2011; 27(1):57–72.
8. Roth JH, Poehling GG. Arthroscopic "-ectomy" surgery of the wrist. Arthroscopy 1990;6(2):141–7.
9. Adolfsson L, Frisen M. Arthroscopic synovectomy of the rheumatoid wrist. A 3.8 year follow-up. J Hand Surg Br 1997;22(6):711–3.
10. Park MJ, Ahn JH, Kang JS. Arthroscopic synovectomy of the wrist in rheumatoid arthritis. J Bone Joint Surg Br 2003;85(7):1011–5.
11. Shapiro JS. The wrist in rheumatoid arthritis. Hand Clin 1996;12(3):477–98.
12. Rau R, Herborn G. A modified version of Larsen's scoring method to assess radiologic changes in rheumatoid arthritis. J Rheumatol 1995;22(10): 1976–82.
13. Hodgson SP, Stanley JK, Muirhead A. The Wrightington classification of rheumatoid wrist X-rays: a guide to surgical management. J Hand Surg Br 1989;14(4):451–5.
14. Simmen BR, Huber H. The wrist joint in chronic polyarthritis-a new classification based on the type of destruction in relation to the natural course and the consequences for surgical therapy. Handchir Mikrochir Plast Chir 1994;26(4):182–9 [in German].
15. Gogna R, Cheung G, Arundell M, et al. Rheumatoid hand surgery: is there a decline? A 22-year population-based study. Hand (N Y) 2015;10(2): 272–8.

16. Chim HW, Reese SK, Toomey SN, et al. Update on the surgical treatment for rheumatoid arthritis of the wrist and hand. J Hand Ther 2014;27(2):134–41 [quiz: 142].

17. Ali MKM, Khalid M. Surgical synovectomy for rheumatoid arthritis: a comprehensive literature review. Int Surg J 2016;1705–10.

18. Papp SR, Athwal GS, Pichora DR. The rheumatoid wrist. J Am Acad Orthop Surg 2006;14(2):65–77.

19. Clayton ML. Surgical treatment at the wrist in rheumatoid arthritis: a review of thirty-seven patients. J Bone Joint Surg Am 1965;47:741–50.

20. Thirupathi RG, Ferlic DC, Clayton ML. Dorsal wrist synovectomy in rheumatoid arthritis–a long-term study. J Hand Surg Am 1983;8(6):848–56.

21. Aschan W, Moberg E. A long-term study of the effect of early synovectomy in rheumatoid arthritis. Bull Hosp Jt Dis Orthop Inst 1984;44(2):106–21.

22. Allieu Y, Lussiez B, Asencio G. Long-term results of surgical synovectomies of the rheumatoid wrist. Apropos of 60 cases. Rev Chir Orthop Reparatrice Appar Mot 1989;75(3):172–8 [in French].

23. Brumfield R Jr, Kuschner SH, Gellman H, et al. Results of dorsal wrist synovectomies in the rheumatoid hand. J Hand Surg Am 1990;15(5):733–5.

24. Ochi T, Iwase R, Kimura T, et al. Effect of early synovectomy on the course of rheumatoid arthritis. J Rheumatol 1991;18(12):1794–8.

25. Ishikawa H, Hanyu T, Tajima T. Rheumatoid wrists treated with synovectomy of the extensor tendons and the wrist joint combined with a Darrach procedure. J Hand Surg Am 1992;17(6):1109–17.

26. Nakamura H, Nagashima M, Ishigami S, et al. The anti-rheumatic effect of multiple synovectomy in patients with refractory rheumatoid arthritis. Int Orthop 2000;24(5):242–5.

27. Ossyssek B, Anders S, Grifka J, et al. Surgical synovectomy decreases density of sensory nerve fibers in synovial tissue of non-inflamed controls and rheumatoid arthritis patients. J Orthop Res 2011;29(2):297–302.

28. Kim SJ, Jung KA. Arthroscopic synovectomy in rheumatoid arthritis of wrist. Clin Med Res 2007;5(4):244–50.

29. Aletaha D, Alasti F, Smolen JS. Optimisation of a treat-to-target approach in rheumatoid arthritis: strategies for the 3-month time point. Ann Rheum Dis 2016;75(8):1479–85.

30. Adolfsson L, Nylander G. Arthroscopic synovectomy of the rheumatoid wrist. J Hand Surg Br 1993;18(1):92–6.

31. Lee HI, Lee KH, Koh KH, et al. Long-term results of arthroscopic wrist synovectomy in rheumatoid arthritis. J Hand Surg Am 2014;39(7):1295–300.

32. Kim SJ, Jung KA, Kim JM, et al. Arthroscopic synovectomy in wrists with advanced rheumatoid arthritis. Clin Orthop Relat Res 2006;449:262–6.

33. Kim SM, Park MJ, Kang HJ, et al. The role of arthroscopic synovectomy in patients with undifferentiated chronic monoarthritis of the wrist. J Bone Joint Surg Br 2012;94(3):353–8.

34. Whipple TL, Marotta JJ, Powell JH 3rd. Techniques of wrist arthroscopy. Arthroscopy 1986;2(4):244–52.

35. Abrams RA, Petersen M, Botte MJ. Arthroscopic portals of the wrist: an anatomic study. J Hand Surg Am 1994;19(6):940–4.

36. Chung CY, Yen CH, Yip ML, et al. Arthroscopic synovectomy for rheumatoid wrists and elbows. J Orthop Surg (Hong Kong) 2012;20(2):219–23.

37. Wei N, Delauter SK, Beard S, et al. Office-based arthroscopic synovectomy of the wrist in rheumatoid arthritis. Arthroscopy 2001;17(8):884–7.

38. Chantelot C, Fontaine C, Flipo RM, et al. Synovectomy combined with the Sauve-Kapandji procedure for the rheumatoid wrist. J Hand Surg Br 1999;24(4):405–9.

39. Vahvanen V, Patiala H. Synovectomy of the wrist in rheumatoid arthritis and related diseases. A follow-up study of 97 consecutive cases. Arch Orthop Trauma Surg 1984;102(4):230–7.

40. Chalmers PN, Sherman SL, Raphael BS, et al. Rheumatoid synovectomy: does the surgical approach matter? Clin Orthop Relat Res 2011;469(7):2062–71.

Arthroscopic Management of Bennett Fracture

Jason Solomon, MD[a],*, Randall W. Culp, MD[b]

KEYWORDS

- Bennett • Arthroscopy • Fracture • Thumb metacarpal • Percutaneous

KEY POINTS

- Thumb carpometacarpal arthroscopy for Bennett fractures is the best method of assessing reduction while allowing for percutaneous fixation, as fluoroscopy alone may underestimate residual joint incongruity.
- If there is a severe injury to the joint, need for shaft fixation, or concomitant soft tissue repair or reconstruction, then open reduction internal fixation is preferable.
- It is important to be aware of the local anatomy surrounding the first carpometacarpal portals, as injury to the dorsal sensory nerve branches is possible.
- If using percutaneous screws for fixation, arthroscopy ensures that the tips of the screws are not too long, as they may enter the thumb/index metacarpal articulation space.

INTRODUCTION

At the British Medical Association meeting held in Cardiff in July of 1885, Edward H. Bennett, MD, a professor of surgery at the University of Dublin and president of the Royal College of Surgeons of Ireland, documented and supported his findings with pathologic specimens of the most common fracture of the base of the thumb, which later took his name.[1–5] He dedicated a large part of his career toward the study and collection of skeletal specimens, despite criticism by his peers, in the hope of improving clinical diagnosis by physicians, as well as to improve the outcomes of his patients. We now know that the mechanism of injury is typically an axial force applied to the thumb in a flexed position. This fracture produces a predictable deformity of the first metacarpal shaft in a supinated, dorsal, radial, and proximal direction while the volar ulnar fragment is held in place by the anterior oblique ligament, which is attached to the trapezium.[6–8] Forces exerted by the abductor pollicis longus, extensor pollicis longus, extensor pollicis brevis, and adductor pollicis produce this deformity. The ulnar fragment may vary in size and the metacarpal may be either subluxated or grossly dislocated (**Fig. 1**). A classification system set forth by Gedda divides this injury into 3 categories.[9] Type 1 represents a first metacarpal subluxation with an associated large volar ulnar fragment; type 2 is not associated with subluxation but includes joint impaction; and type 3 involves dislocation of the metacarpal with a small ulnar remnant attached to the anterior oblique ligament. Recognition of this injury in the emergency room or office is necessary, as missing it may lead

Disclosure Statement: Dr J. Solomon has nothing to disclose. Dr R.W. Culp is a paid speaker for Auxilium and is a consultant for Biomet, SBi, and Arthrex.

a Department of Orthopedic Surgery, Arrowhead Regional Medical Center, 400 North Pepper Avenue, Colton, CA 92324, USA; b The Philadelphia Hand Center, Thomas Jefferson University, 700 South Henderson Road, Suite 200, King of Prussia, PA 19406, USA
* Corresponding author. 1901 West Lugonia Avenue, Suite 120, Redlands, CA 92374.
E-mail address: jasonavisolomon@gmail.com

Hand Clin 33 (2017) 787–794
http://dx.doi.org/10.1016/j.hcl.2017.07.006
0749-0712/17/© 2017 Elsevier Inc. All rights reserved.

hand.theclinics.com

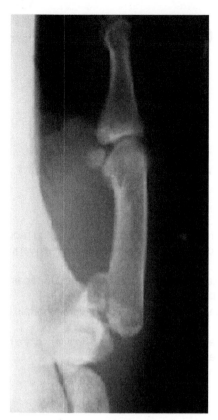

Fig. 1. Bennett fracture with dorsal, radial, proximal, and supinated deformity of the first metacarpal, and maintenance of reduction of the volar ulnar fragment to the anterior oblique ligament.

to irreversible posttraumatic arthritis and loss of function. Initial closed reduction of these injuries should be attempted, as some patients may be lost to follow-up or take a significant amount of time to present to an orthopedic physician for appropriate care.[10] A reduction maneuver should include axial traction, palmar abduction, and pronation while applying force to the metacarpal base.[11,12] Maintaining this reduction in a splint as a definitive treatment may be difficult, as prolonged pressure on the skin can lead to wounds and the fracture may displace over time as swelling subsides. Nondisplaced and stable fractures may be treated in a thumb spica cast for 4 to 6 weeks. Fractures with residual subluxation, dislocation, and a joint step off greater than 1 mm should undergo operative fixation. The exact degree of persistent joint step off that leads to long-term symptoms is unknown, but reduction of joint subluxation or dislocation should be accomplished.[13] A technique for arthroscopic evaluation of the first carpometacarpal (CMC) joint was described by Berger[14] in 1997, and since that time, has led to the ability to reduce and fix

fractures under direct visualization while causing minimal morbidity to local soft tissues. Closed reduction and percutaneous pinning under fluoroscopic guidance may lead to equivalent outcomes as open reduction internal fixation in long-term studies, but fluoroscopy may underestimate persistent joint incongruity that may be better seen with traditional radiography, arthroscopy, or open means, and may lead to long-term posttraumatic arthritis.[15] At present, no one technique of surgical management has been shown to be superior in clinical or cadaveric studies.[16,17]

INDICATIONS

Arthroscopic reduction and fixation of Bennett fractures remains a viable option of treatment for any fracture that necessitates surgery. Placement of the thumb in the arthroscopy tower with 5 to 10 pounds of traction aids in reduction and distracts the joint to allow for inspection of the articular surface with a 1.9-mm to 2.7-mm 30° angled short arthroscope (**Fig. 2**).[18] This technique obviates the need for an extensile open surgical approach and diminishes soft tissue stripping of fracture fragments and injury to the dorsal ligamentous complex, which is important for stability.[19] Evaluation with the arthroscope also helps to ensure that percutaneous screw fixation does not penetrate the joint surface and also allows for debridement of any posttraumatic loose bodies or cartilaginous flaps.[20]

CONTRAINDICATIONS

Any complex articular fracture that is not amenable to percutaneous pinning or screw fixation is not appropriate for arthroscopic treatment and may require open reduction internal fixation (**Table 1**).[21–23] Chronic injuries requiring osteotomy and reduction may also require open treatment.[24] If there is an active infection overlying the area of injury, this should be addressed appropriately with debridement and/or antibiotic treatment. Associated soft tissue injury near the first CMC joint that requires repair or reconstruction may also preclude arthroscopy.

SURGICAL TECHNIQUE
Preoperative Planning

Fractures of the base of the first metacarpal may occur by low-energy or high-energy mechanisms of injury. There may be associated fractures in the ipsilateral upper extremity, as well as soft tissue and neurovascular injuries that may preclude use of an arthroscopy tower. A reduction attempt should be performed on initial injury, but may not

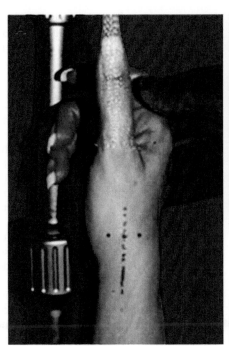
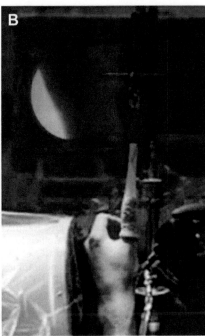

Fig. 2. (A) The thumb is placed into a finger trap and 5 to 10 pounds of traction is applied. The first dorsal compartment tendons are marked longitudinally and the 1-R and 1-U portals are marked 1 cm away on either side at the level of the first CMC joint. (B) The mini-c-arm unit is brought in perpendicular to the hand while simultaneously holding the arthroscope in the 1-R portal.

be possible if the patient presents late. Preoperative radiographic imaging should be reviewed with the patient to determine the best course of treatment to properly assess and reduce the fracture as anatomically as possible. We routinely obtain an anteroposterior, lateral, and Bett views, which requires the hand to be pronated 20 to 30° with the x-ray beam angled 15° in a distal to proximal direction at the first CMC joint. A computed tomography scan is usually not necessary for simple fracture patterns, but may be needed for more complex articular injuries.[25,26] The patient should be counseled on the risks of surgery, including deep infection, pin track infection, stiffness, dorsal sensory nerve injury/paresthesias, radial artery injury, tendon injury, and development of posttraumatic arthritis.

The local anatomy surrounding the first CMC joint also should be reviewed before surgery (Fig. 3). The 1-R, 1-U, and thenar portals have previously been described and their use may be necessary depending on the needs of instrumentation to maintain a reduction of the fracture before fixation. At the level of the first CMC joint, the 1-U portal is just ulnar to the extensor pollicis brevis tendon and the 1-R portal is just radial to the abductor pollicis longus tendon. The thenar portal (Fig. 4), described by Walsh and colleagues,[27] is placed 90° to the 1-U portal through the bulk of the thenar muscle at the level of the first CMC joint.

Table 1
Indications and contraindications of arthroscopic fixation

Indications	Contraindications
• Any Bennett fracture that also could be considered for fluoroscopic guided pinning or open reduction internal fixation with screws	• Active infection • Severe articular injury • Need for shaft fixation • Need for local soft tissue repair or reconstruction • Ipsilateral upper extremity fracture precluding use of arthroscopy tower

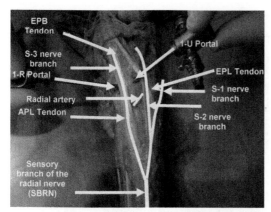

Fig. 3. Relevant neurovascular structures in relation to the 1-R and 1-U portal. APL, abductor pollicis longus; EPB, extensor pollicis brevis; EPL, extensor pollicis longus. (*From* Walsh EF, Akelman E, Fleming BC, et al. Thumb carpometacarpal arthroscopy: a topographic, anatomic study of the thenar portal. J Hand Surg Am 2005;30(2):376; with permission.)

It is a safe portal to use that is away from the radial artery, superficial radial nerve branches, and recurrent motor branch.

Preparation and Patient Positioning

The patient is positioned supine on the operating table and placed under general or regional anesthesia. Wide awake dry or wet wrist arthroscopy is also an option that allows for the patient to participate and watch the live arthroscopic procedure performed and may aid in the patient's understanding of the degree of joint injury. A

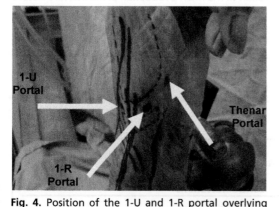

Fig. 4. Position of the 1-U and 1-R portal overlying the first CMC joint. The thenar portal is established at a 90° angle to the 1-U portal under direct visualization with an 18-gauge needle. (*From* Walsh EF, Akelman E, Fleming BC, et al. Thumb carpometacarpal arthroscopy: a topographic, anatomic study of the thenar portal. J Hand Surg Am 2005;30(2):374; with permission.)

pneumatic tourniquet is applied as high on the arm as possible and the limb is prepped in the usual sterile fashion based on the surgeon's preferences.

Surgical Approach

The surgeon may use whichever arthroscopy tower he or she is most comfortable with. We currently use the ConMed Linvatec Traction Tower system (Utica, NY). A finger trap is applied to the thumb and secured with Coban Wrap (3M Corp, St Paul, MN) and the fingers are held in the palm with Coban as well to prevent their interference with instrumentation and fluoroscopy. The 1-R portal is marked just radial to the abductor pollicis longus tendon and the 1-U portal is marked just ulnar to the extensor pollicis brevis tendon at the level of the first CMC joint. The thumb is placed into 5 to 10 pounds of traction using the arthroscopy tower, and we constantly check to maintain this level of traction during the case, as the traction routinely slips over time. An Esmarch is used to exsanguinate the limb and the tourniquet is raised to 250 mm Hg. The joint is inflated with 3 to 4 mL sterile normal saline using an 18-gauge needle to distend the joint and the placement of the needle is at times confirmed under fluoroscopy. An 11-blade is used to make an incision in the skin over the 1-R portal and a blunt instrument is used to clear structures off of the joint capsule. The capsule is then penetrated with the blunt instrument and a rush of fluid or hematoma is usually observed. A blunt trocar is then placed into the joint and a 1.9-mm short arthroscope is inserted. The 1-U portal is then established under direct visualization with an 18-gauge needle. The skin over the 1-U portal is then again incised with an 11-blade, the subcutaneous tissues spread with a blunt instrument, and the joint entered with a trocar. At this point, we typically place a 2.0-mm shaver into the 1-U portal to perform a synovectomy and debride the joint of hematoma and debris so that the joint can be visualized clearly (**Fig. 5**). A thenar portal also can be established if necessary 90° to the 1-U portal through the bulk of the thenar musculature at the level of the first CMC joint under direct visualization with an 18-gauge needle if a second instrument needs to be placed to manipulate the fracture. The fracture can be inspected with the camera through all 3 portals to gain a clear understanding of the morphology of the injury, and a 3-mm hook-probe can be placed into the joint to manipulate the volar ulnar fragment back to the metacarpal shaft (**Fig. 6**). The articular surface of the trapezium is also inspected for any injury to the cartilage and

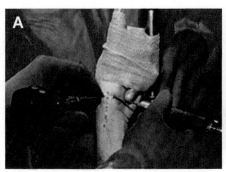
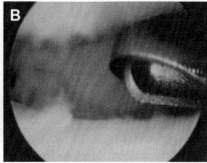

Fig. 5. (*A*) A 1.9-mm short arthroscope in the 1-R portal and 2.0-mm arthroscopic shaver in the 1-U portal. (*B*) Arthroscopic shaver in the first carpometacarpal joint viewed from the 1-R portal.

debrided. Traction provided by the tower may be insufficient to reduce the metacarpal to the volar ulnar fragment, and Kirschner wires (K-wires) introduced into the individual fragments may be used to joystick the reduction and alter malrotation. With the arthroscope in the first CMC joint, a mini C-Arm image intensifier is brought in perpendicular to the surgical field to assess the fracture and hardware placement. Depending on the size and orientation of the fracture, 0.045 K-wires, 1.0-mm to 1.5-mm percutaneous screws, or resorbable pins may be used to obtain fixation (**Fig. 7**). A pin may be placed into the fracture fragment, across the first metacarpal into the trapezium, or passed from the first metacarpal to the second metacarpal. It is important that the trapeziometacarpal or intermetacarpal pin be placed with the thumb in a relatively abducted position, as the patient may otherwise develop an adduction deformity. K wires are cut short and left out of the skin for removal in the office at a later date.

Final fluoroscopic images are obtained, and the arthroscope is removed from the joint once reduction is confirmed and all joint debris is removed. The skin is then closed with 4 to 0 nylon, a bulky dressing is applied, and the patient is placed into a forearm-based thumb spica splint. The thumb interphalangeal joint is allowed to remain free out of the splint so that the patient can begin immediate motion.

COMPLICATIONS

The incidence of deep infection and pin tract infection following arthroscopic-assisted fixation is no different from other measures of treatment (**Box 1**). Pin loosening may or may not be associated with infection. If it occurs early, it may lead to loss of reduction and need for revision surgery, although this is infrequent.[28] Patients should be counseled on the possibility of irritation of the dorsal sensory branches of the radial nerve, but

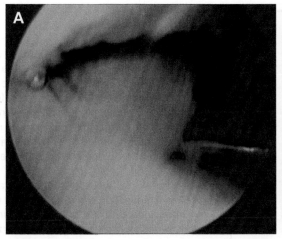
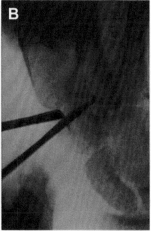

Fig. 6. (*A*) Arthroscopic view of the volar ulnar corner of the base of the first metacarpal from the 1-R portal. A 3-mm hook-probe in the 1-U portal is assisting in reduction of the fragment. (*B*) Fluoroscopic view of the reduction with the probe and arthroscope in place.

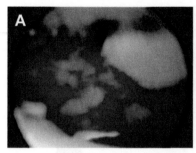
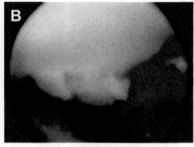
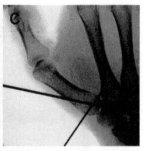

Fig. 7. (*A*) View of the volar ulnar fracture from the 1-R portal before reduction. (*B*) After reduction with 0.045 K-wire passed from the base of the metacarpal into the volar ulnar fragment. (*C*) Fluoroscopic view with 0.045 K-wire maintaining fracture reduction as well as a wire stabilizing the first metacarpal to the trapezium.

this will usually resolve with time.[29] Patients may experience stiffness following removal of hardware and may require occupational therapy. Injury to the abductor pollicis longus and extensor pollicis brevis may occur if they are not properly identified before portal creation, and repeated joint entry in direct proximity to the tendons may lead to tendon adhesions and scarring.[30,31] There is also a risk of Parsonage Turner syndrome following arthroscopy of the wrist and hand.[32] The exact etiology of this is currently unknown, but treatment is usually supportive and patients recover over time. Patients are also at risk for development of posttraumatic arthritis, even with the best efforts at restoration of articular congruity, due to the initial chondral injury.[33] Finally, iatrogenic injury to the articular cartilage is possible with the arthroscope and instrumentation. Small joint tools should be used when possible and traction between 5 and 10 pounds should be maintained to keep the joint distracted during the case. Instruments should be inserted into the joint at precise angles predetermined by the path of an 18-gauge needle.

Tsujii and colleagues[29] evaluated the incidence of complications associated with the use of the 1-R, 1-U, and thenar portals. Two of 21 patients undergoing first CMC arthroscopy developed paresthesias of the dorsal sensory branches of the radial nerve, but there were no paresthesias associated with the 1-U or thenar portals. The paresthesias resolved by 2 months with no intervention. Three patients complained of scar tenderness of the thenar portal, but this was not associated with the 1-U or 1-R portals. They pointed out that use of the thenar portal allows the surgeon to place instruments at angles that may be difficult to obtain with standard portals, and limits the amount of stretching of surrounding structures that occurs when trying to manipulate objects that are out of reach. There was also a decrease in the number of 1-R portal penetrations with instrumentation when using a thenar portal, which may have limited injury to the radial sensory branches.

Box 1
Potential complications

- Pin tract infection
- Pin loosening
- Deep infection
- Dorsal sensory nerve injury
- Tendon injury
- Iatrogenic articular cartilage injury
- Malunion
- Nonunion
- Stiffness
- Posttraumatic arthritis
- Complex regional pain syndrome
- Parsonage Turner syndrome

REHABILITATION

Patients are seen in the office 7 to 10 days after surgery and sutures are removed if the wound is deemed appropriate. A thermoplastic forearm-based thumb spica splint is fabricated for the patient with the thumb interphalangeal joint left free; however, a plaster splint or cast may be necessary if the patient is unable to cooperate with restrictions. Percutaneous pins are usually removed at 4 weeks, and gentle motion of the thumb is allowed at 4 to 6 weeks if the clinical and radiographic examination warrants it. Full motion of the index, long, ring, and small fingers are encouraged immediately after surgery. Return to play for athletes following this injury is dependent on age, sport, position, handedness, and level of play. Injuries to the nonthrowing hand and athletes in nontackling positions at the college and professional levels may return to sport in a protective brace in approximately 3 weeks. Injuries to the throwing hand and players in tackling positions at the college and professional levels return to play at approximately 6 weeks. Children may be treated more conservatively and delay to return to sport may be extended to 10 weeks.[34,35]

OUTCOMES

Pomares and colleagues[20] assessed the outcome of arthroscopically assisted screw fixation of Bennett fractures versus open reduction internal fixation. They reported fewer complications (1 of 11 vs 6 of 11), shorter immobilization time (3.9 weeks vs 7.1 weeks), and diminished tourniquet time (42 minutes vs 56 minutes) in the arthroscopic group compared with the open fixation group. There was also a higher return to work in the percutaneous group (91%) versus the open group (70%). Another recent study by Zemirline and colleagues[36] suggested that at short-term follow-up, arthroscopic-assisted percutaneous screw fixation of Bennett fracture led to satisfactory reduction of the joint in all cases, key pinch was 73% and grip strength 85% of the contralateral side. It was noted, however, that 4 patients had subsequent displacement of the surgical reduction at final follow-up of 4.5 months.[36]

A limited number of series with small sample sizes are available for this technique so far, and only short-term follow-up data are available, yet the potential benefit of directly visualizing reduction and fixation with minimal soft tissue stripping remains an attractive option, as obtaining the best possible reduction may correlate with development of arthritis in the long term.[37] Excellent outcomes can be achieved with fluoroscopically guided percutaneous pinning as well as open reduction and internal fixation, but each technique carries its own complications.[38,39] Viewing the fracture line can be difficult with an open procedure, as forceful manipulation of the fracture fragments may be necessary, whereas use of the arthroscope obviates the need for this. Outcomes of arthroscopic-assisted fixation in our experience are encouraging and it continues to be our treatment of choice for Bennett fracture when appropriate patients are identified.

SUMMARY

Bennett fracture is the most common fracture of the thumb. Choosing the appropriate approach to fracture fixation requires a thorough knowledge of the anatomy surrounding the first CMC joint, which is necessary to prevent injury to local sensory nerves and tendons. Although no study has shown superior outcomes compared with open reduction internal fixation and fluoroscopically guided closed reduction and percutaneous pinning, arthroscopic-assisted fixation allows for debridement of the CMC joint, direct visualization of the articular surface during reduction, and has minimal morbidity and associated complications.

REFERENCES

1. Zhang X, Shao X, Zhang Z, et al. Treatment of a Bennett fracture using tension band wiring. J Hand Surg Am 2012;37:427–33.
2. Byrne AM, Kearns SR, Morris S, et al. "S" Quattro external fixation for complex intra-articular thumb fractures. J Orthop Surg (Hong Kong) 2008;16:170–4.
3. Pavic R, Malovic M. Operative treatment of Bennett's fracture. Coll Antropol 2013;37:169–74.
4. Culp RW, Johnson JW. Arthroscopically assisted percutaneous fixation of Bennett fractures. J Hand Surg Am 2010;35:137–40.
5. Bennett EH. On fracture of the metacarpal bone of the thumb. Br Med J 1886;2(1331):12–3.
6. Ellis H. Edward Hallarran Bennett: Bennett's fracture of the base of the thumb. J Perioper Pract 2013;23:59–60.
7. Bettinger PC, Linscheid RL, Berger RA, et al. An anatomic study of the stabilizing ligaments of the trapezium and trapeziometacarpal joint. J Hand Surg 1999;24:786–98.
8. Bettinger PC, Berger RA. Functional ligamentous anatomy of the trapezium and trapeziometacarpal joint. Hand Clin 2001;17:151–68.
9. Gedda KO. Studies on Bennett's fracture; anatomy, roentgenology, and therapy. Acta Chir Scand Suppl 1954;193:1–114.
10. Griffiths JC. Fractures at the base of the first metacarpal bone. J Bone Joint Surg Br 1964;46:712–9.
11. Burkhalter WE. Closed treatment of hand fractures. J Hand Surg Am 1989;14:390–3.
12. Burkhalter WE, Reyes FA. Closed treatment of fractures of the hand. Bull Hosp Jt Dis Orthop Inst 1984;44:145–62.
13. Livesley PJ. The conservative management of Bennett's fracture-dislocation: a 26-year follow-up. J Hand Surg Br 1990;15:291–4.
14. Berger RA. A technique for arthroscopic evaluation of the first carpometacarpal joint. J Hand Surg 1997;22:1077–80.
15. Capo J, Kinchelow T, Orillaza N, et al. Accuracy of fluoroscopy in closed reduction and percutaneous fixation of simulated Bennett's fracture. J Hand Surg Am 2009;34(4):637–41.

16. Rivlin M, Fei W, Mudgal C. Bennett fracture. J Hand Surg Am 2015;40(8):1667–8.

17. Deml C, Smekal V, Kastenberger T, et al. Pressure distribution in carpometacarpal joint, due to step-off in operatively treated Bennett's fractures. Injury 2014;45(10):1574–8.

18. Menon J. Arthroscopic management of trapeziometacarpal arthritis of the thumb. Arthroscopy 1996;12: 581–7.

19. Ladd AL, Crisco JJ, Hagert E, et al. The 2014 ABJS Nicolas Andry Award: the puzzle of the thumb: mobility, stability, and demands in opposition. Clin Orthop Relat Res 2014;472(12):3605–22.

20. Pomares G, Strugarek-Lecoanet C, Dap F, et al. Bennett fracture: arthroscopically assisted percutaneous screw fixation versus open surgery: functional and radiographic outcomes. Orthop Traumatol Surg Res 2016;102(3):357–61.

21. Buchler U, Fischer T. Use of a minicondylar plate for metacarpal and phalangeal periarticular injuries. Clin Orthop Relat Res 1987;214:53–8.

22. Buchler U, McCollam SM, Oppikofer C. Comminuted fractures of the basilar joint of the thumb: combined treatment by external fixation, limited internal fixation, and bone grafting. J Hand Surg Am 1991;16:556–60.

23. Chen SH, Wei FC, Chen HC, et al. Miniature plates and screws in acute complex hand injury. J Trauma 1994;37:237–42.

24. Brüske J, Bednarski M, Niedźwiedź Z, et al. The results of operative treatment of fractures of the thumb metacarpal base. Acta Orthop Belg 2001; 67:368–73.

25. Foster RJ, Hastings H. Treatment of Bennett, Rolando, and vertical intraarticular trapezial fractures. Clin Orthop Relat Res 1987;214:121–9.

26. Carlsen B, Moran S. Thumb trauma: Bennett fractures, Rolando fractures, and ulnar collateral ligament injuries. J Hand Surg Am 2009;34(5):945–52.

27. Walsh E, Akelman E, Fleming B, et al. Thumb carpometacarpal arthroscopy: a topographic, anatomic study of the thenar portal. J Hand Surg Am 2005; 30:373–9.

28. Botte MJ, Davis JL, Rose BA, et al. Complications of smooth pin fixation of fractures and dislocations in the hand and wrist. Clin Orthop Relat Res 1992; 276:194–201.

29. Tsujii M, Lida R, Satonaka H, et al. Usefulness and complications associated with thenar and standard portals during arthroscopic surgery of thumb carpometacarpal joint. Orthop Traumatol Surg Res 2015; 101(6):741–4.

30. Creighton JJ, Steichen JB. Complications in phalangeal and metacarpal fracture management: results of extensor tenolysis. Hand Clin 1994;10:111–6.

31. Green DP. Complications of phalangeal and metacarpal fractures. Hand Clin 1986;2:307–28.

32. Buckley T, Culp RW. Brachial plexopathy following wrist arthroscopy. J Hand Surg Am 2016;41(2): 320–2.

33. Van Heest AE, Kallemeir P. Thumb carpal metacarpal arthritis. J Am Acad Orthop Surg 2008;16: 140–51.

34. Evans P, Pervaiz K. Sport-specific commentary on Bennett and metacarpal fractures in football. Hand Clin 2012;28:393–4.

35. Singletary S, Freeland AE, Jarrett CA. Metacarpal fractures in athletes: treatment, rehabilitation, and safe early return to play. J Hand Ther 2003;16: 171–9.

36. Zemirline A, Lebailly F, Taleb C, et al. Arthroscopic assisted percutaneous screw fixation of Bennett's fracture. Hand Surg 2014;19(2):281–6.

37. Timmenga EJ, Blokhuis TJ, Maas M, et al. Long-term evaluation of Bennett's fracture: a comparison between open and closed reduction. J Hand Surg Br 1994;19:373–7.

38. Leclere FM, Jenzer A, Husler R, et al. 7-year follow-up after open reduction and internal screw fixation in Bennett fractures. Arch Orthop Trauma Surg 2012; 132:1045–51.

39. Lutz M, Sailer R, Zimmermann R, et al. Closed reduction transarticular Kirschner wire fixation versus open reduction internal fixation in the treatment of Bennett's fracture dislocation. J Hand Surg Br 2003;28:142–7.

Arthroscopic Management of Thumb Carpometacarpal Joint Arthritis

CrossMark

Clara Wing-yee Wong, MBChB, MRCS, FRCSEd (Orth), FHKAM (Orth Surg), FHKCOS[a],[*],
Pak-cheong Ho, MBBS, FRCS (Edinburg), FHKCOS, FHKAM (Orth Surg)[b]

KEYWORDS

- Thumb basal joint arthritis • Arthroscopy • Thumb carpometacarpal joint
- Suture button suspensionplasty

KEY POINTS

- Thumb carpometacarpal joint (CMCJ1) is born to have good freedom of motion. This excellent mobility at the CMCJ1 and the thumb biomechanics predispose to the occurrence of CMCJ1 arthritis.
- Current evidence suggests that trapeziectomy and ligament reconstruction/tendon interposition are not superior to simple trapeziectomy, whereas simple trapeziectomy has the problem of subsidence and debilitating weakness. Complications from prosthetic replacement are not uncommonly reported.
- Arthroscopic technique, which includes debridement, synovectomy, thermal shrinkage, partial trapeziectomy, CMCJ1 excision, and K-wire stabilization, is minimally invasive, simple, and effective. It preserves vascularity, promotes healing and stability, and shows rewarding results.
- The operative decision on choosing arthroscopic procedures should be based on the patient's demand for strength, mobility, and expectation of pain reduction.
- The use of suture button suspensionplasty in addition to arthroscopic procedures obviates the surgical trauma from extensive approaches to prevent subsidence and maintain stability. It helps to maintain the metacarpal height and the space after arthroscopic partial trapeziectomy as forming a "new joint" while providing some mobility in this "new joint"; to provide stability after K-wire removal in arthroscopic CMCJ1 excision; and to create a painless fibrous union at the CMCJ1. Preliminary results showed good pain relief and strength improvement.

 Video content accompanies this article at www.hand.theclinics.com.

INTRODUCTION/NATURE OF THE PROBLEM
Thumb Carpometacarpal Joint Is Born to Have Good Freedom of Motion

With only 2 phalanges on the thumbs, they should have less mobility and dexterity than other fingers, which have 3 phalanges. However, the thumb accounts for approximately 50% of the overall hand function and is regarded as the most important digit of the hand.[1] "The hand without a thumb is at worst nothing but an animated fish-slice and at best a pair of forceps whose points don't meet

Disclosure Statement: The authors have no disclosures to report.
[a] Division of Hand and Microsurgery, Department of Orthopaedic and Traumatology, Prince of Wales Hospital, Chinese University of Hong Kong, 16/F, The Club Lusitano, 16 Ice House Street, Central, Hong Kong SAR;
[b] Division of Hand and Microsurgery, Department of Orthopaedic and Traumatology, Prince of Wales Hospital, Chinese University of Hong Kong, 5F, Lui Che Woo Clinical Sciences Building, 30-32 Ngan Shing Street, Shatin, NT, Hong Kong SAR
* Corresponding author.
E-mail address: clarawong@ort.cuhk.edu.hk

hand.theclinics.com

properly," as said by John Napier.[2] Good stability, strength, and for sure, mobility and dexterity are essentials for the thumb to carry out its prominent functions. Nature creates a biconcave saddle geometry at the thumb carpometacarpal joint (CMCJ1) to compensate for the mobility of thumb. The radius of curvature of the metacarpal base is 34% greater than that of the trapezium. These differing radii of curvature of this saddle construct give a wider range of motion.[3,4] The saddle-shaped joint surfaces allow for motions of radial abduction/adduction and palmar abduction/adduction. Capsular laxity gives an additional motion, rotation, of the metacarpal on the trapezium. The osseous construct and soft tissue characteristics enable circumduction motion at the CMCJ1, which distinguishes the thumb from the other 4 fingers.[4] Studies show that CMCJ1 mobility was significantly correlated with hand grip force and dexterity, and therefore, important for mechanical thumb function.[5]

Good Mobility at the Thumb Carpometacarpal Joint Predisposes Attenuation of Capsuloligamentous Structures, Joint Incongruity, Instability, and Thumb Carpometacarpal Joint Osteoarthritis

However, good mobility at the CMCJ1 predisposes it to have subluxation, joint incongruity, and instability. Three-dimensional computed tomography, stereophotogrammetric, or casting investigations on contact surface areas of the CMCJ1 in normal individuals and cadavers showed that about 50% of the articular area of the thumb metacarpal base was in contact with trapezium in opposition, and 25% in palmar abduction and radial abduction.[3,6–8] With the strong extrinsic and intrinsic tendons across the thumb to produce strong pinching and grasping action, 1 kg of applied force at the thumb tip can produce joint compression forces, averaging 13 kg at the CMCJ1 and 120 kg at the CMCJ1 when grasping.[9] This limited joint contact with localized stress peaks on the dorsoradial and volar-ulnar regions of CMCJ1 could lead to cartilage erosion, progressing to osteoarthritis (OA) of the CMCJ1.[10–12] The subluxation, joint incongruity, and instability could stretch out and attenuate the capsuloligamentous structures, further worsening the joint stability, overload, and grind of the CMCJ1, producing further cartilage wear and tear, and causing pain, loss of grip and pinch strength, web space, and disability.[13–19]

Prevalence of Radiographic and Symptomatic Thumb Carpometacarpal Joint Osteoarthiritis

The age-standardized prevalence of radiographic hand OA was 44.2% in women and 33.7% in men, whereas that of CMCJ1 OA was 32.9% in women and 30.3% in men.[20] CMCJ1 OA is the second most common site of degenerative disease in the hand after arthritis of the distal interphalangeal joints (DIPJ),[21] but is associated with more pain and functional disability than DIPJ OA.[19] The correlation between symptomatic OA and radiographic OA has been shown to be inconsistent.[13,22] The prevalence of radiographic CMCJ1 OA in people older than 55 years of age (mean age 66.6) was 35.8%,[13] whereas symptomatic CMCJ1 OA in the elderly (older than 70 years old) was only 1.9% to 5.3%.[22–24] The study also found that only 28% of women having radiographic features of CMC1 OA had symptoms.[25]

Why Is Thumb Carpometacarpal Joint Osteoarthritis Painful?

Many people with radiographic CMCJ1 OA have minimal symptoms. However, for those with symptoms, the pain can be very disabling.[13,23–25] Subchondral bone, periosteum, periarticular ligaments, joint capsule, and synovium are all richly innervated and are the source of nociception in CMCJ1 OA.

The pain can be aroused from the following:
  i. The degenerative synovitis causing inflammatory pain,
  ii. from the high subchondral pressure at the limited contact areas, and
  iii. The capsule and periarticular ligaments with stretching pain from joint instability on loading, and with irritation from the adjacent prominent osteophytes.

The pain severity depends on the following:
  i. The degree of synovitis,
  ii. The amount of subchondral pressure, and
  iii. The degree of joint mobility.

The amount of subchondral pressure also depends on the following:
  i. How much the joint is subluxed,
  ii. How good the remaining cartilage is to help unload the pressure,
  iii. How much the load the patient usually applies on the joint,
  iv. How much the patient demands of the thumb, and
  v. How unstable the joint is, which creates an additional grinding pressure on the joint.

If the patient has a very advanced radiographic CMCJ1 OA, with narrowed joint space, significant subluxation, and large osteophytes but does not put demand on the thumb while the joint becomes ankylosed with minimal CMCJ1 mobility, he or she may not complain of pain or anticipate any functional impairment (**Fig. 1**).

Operation Decision

Therefore, the surgical decision not only depends solely on the radiograph findings but also should be judged by how much the patient demands of their thumb, how unstable the joint is, how much strength the patient needs, how much mobility is needed to handle their work and life, and their expectation of how much pain can be relieved after the surgery.

Options of Surgical Intervention for Established Thumb Carpometacarpal Joint Osteoarthritis

Trapeziectomy, total or partial, should be an effective procedure to alleviate pain because there will be no further CMCJ1 synovitis, and no pain arising from the joint pressure or from the irritation to the capsule and ligaments. However, subsidence of the thumb metacarpal could result in thumb metacarpal/scaphoid impingement, thumb metacarpal/second metacarpal impingement, or impingement onto the remnant trapezium in partial trapeziectomy, and create a new source of pain.[26] Loss of support at the thumb metacarpal base, and loss of thumb axial length and thus the lever arm for pinching, could also result in loss of hand strength despite an improvement in overall hand function with a decrease in pain.[27–29]

In an effort to prevent proximal metacarpal migration, an additional suspension with or without interposition was popularized, including hematoma distraction, tendon interposition, different kinds of suspensionplasty, and the combination with tendon interposition. However, multiple prospective randomized controlled trials comparing each of different surgical procedures showed no significant difference between simple trapeziectomy and the different types of suspensionplasty/tendon interposition in terms of pain relief, strength, and hand function, and there is also no evidence to suggest that any of the above surgical procedures was superior to another.[30–37] However, the fear of subsidence and debilitating weakness drives the surgeons away from simple trapeziectomy despite the current evidence.[38–40]

Trapeziectomy with or without suspensionplasty/tendon interposition would never provide enough strength for high-demand patients. CMCJ1 fusion should be a reasonable procedure if strength is crucial. This trapezium-preserving procedure allows easier and better salvage options when it fails than a failed trapezoidal reaction procedure. However, there are still complications like inability to lay the hand flat, pantrapezial arthritis, and fusion site nonunion.[41]

Prosthetic arthroplasty should theoretically preserve joint mechanics, avoid metacarpal subsidence, and improve stability. However, it has a higher failure rate and does not excel ligament reconstruction and tendon interposition currently in pain, strength, disability, and patient satisfaction.[42]

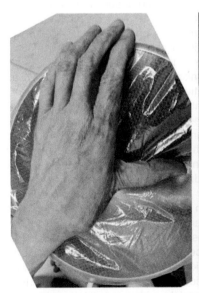
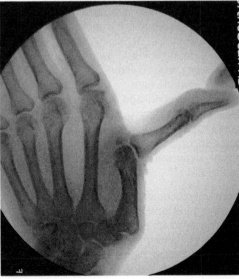

Fig. 1. A 75-year-old woman who presented with bilateral knee pain. She was noticed to have a deformed left thumb with radiographic features of CMCJ1 OA. However, she had no complaint on the thumb. She did not have pain at the CMCJ1.

Problems of subluxation, dislocation, persistent pain, loosening, and patient dissatisfaction were not uncommonly reported.[43–47]

Is There Any Procedure That Is Simpler, Less Invasive, and More Effective to Relieve Patients' Pain and Meet Their Demands?

With the refinement of arthroscopic instrumentation and advancement of small joint arthroscopic techniques, the role of arthroscopic surgeries on wrist and hand diseases is emerging. Menon[48] first published the use of arthroscopic techniques in treating CMCJ1 OA in 1996. He did 25 cases of arthroscopic partial trapeziectomy and interposition arthroplasty with autogenous tendon graft, Gore-Tex, or fascia late allograft. A promising place in treating CMCJ1 OA by arthroscopy was mentioned by Culp and Osterman[49] in 1997. Culp and Rekant[50] did 24 cases of arthroscopic debridement, shrinkage, partial/complete trapizectomy with 88% good to excellent outcomes. They concluded that arthroscopic debridement and synovectomy offered an exciting alternative in Eaton I and II arthritis. Badia[51] described an arthroscopic staging system to determine treatment of CMCJ1 OA in 2006. Currently described arthroscopic techniques have shown efficacy and success in treatment of CMCJ1 OA. The options in arthroscopic management on CMCJ1 OA are as follows:

1. Arthroscopic staging of the disease,[51]
2. Arthroscopic debridement, synovectomy, capsuloligamentous shrinkage,[52,53]
3. Arthroscopic debridement, synovectomy, capsuloligamentous shrinkage, hemitrapeziectomy,[54–56]
4. Arthroscopic debridement, synovectomy, interposition,[57]
5. Arthroscopic debridement, synovectomy, hemitrapeziectomy, interposition,[57–62]
6. Arthroscopic debridement, synovectomy, capsuloligamentous shrinkage, hemitrapeziectomy/total trapeziectomy, suture button suspensionplasty,[63,64]
7. Arthroscopic debridement, synovectomy, hemitrapeziectomy, ligament reconstruction,[65] and
8. Arthroscopic fusion.[66]

Good to excellent outcomes were obtained from all of the above arthroscopic procedures, except that complication rates with synthetic materials in interposition series[67] and interposition without partial trapeziectomy were higher,[57] and Cobb and Edwards, respectively, suggested that interposition was not necessary following arthroscopic resection arthroplasty for thumb basal joint arthritis.[55,68]

The next section discusses how this minimally invasive surgery helps patients.

ARTHROSCOPIC DEBRIDEMENT, SYNOVECTOMY, WITH MINIMAL BONE WORK
Patient Series

From April 2002 to August 2013, the authors performed arthroscopic debridement and synovectomy on 76 CMCJ1 in 65 patients with CMCJ1 OA. There were 51 women and 14 men. The average age was 56 (range 28–76). Thirty-nine thumbs were involved on the left side and 37 on right side. The average duration of symptoms was 2 years, and all failed conservative treatment for more than 6 months. There were one case of Eaton and Littler[11] stage I disease, 38 cases of stage II disease, 36 cases of stage III, and one case of stage IV. According to Badia arthroscopic staging,[51] 4 cases were stage I, in which the articular cartilage was intact while the anterior oblique ligament was attenuated; 23 cases were stage II, in which there was frank eburnation of the articular cartilage; and 49 cases were stage III disease with widespread full-thickness cartilage loss and frayed volar ligaments with instability. The average operation duration was 68 minutes.

Surgical Techniques

The authors now routinely perform this arthroscopic procedure under portal site local anesthesia (PSLA). For this study series, 72 thumbs were operated under PSLA, 2 thumbs were operated under intravenous local anesthesia, and 1 thumb was operated under forearm intravenous regional anesthesia. Local anesthetic procedure allows for the patient to watch the arthroscopic monitor and understand the degree of joint degeneration and the nature of the procedure. The patient is placed in the supine position with the operated arm placed on a hand table (**Fig. 2**). Standard wrist arthroscopy tower and equipment with a 1.9-mm arthroscope are used. A tourniquet is not necessary. The shoulder should not be abducted 80° or more, because too much shoulder abduction in addition to forearm supination can cause patient discomfort. Moreover, if subsequent imaging or manipulation for other procedures with the hand put back on the hand table is necessary, too much shoulder abduction will make proper imaging views and hand positioning difficult. The arm is secured on the traction tower baseplate with a positioning strap (see **Fig. 2**). Padding is placed between the arm and the baseplate and between the arm and the strap. The

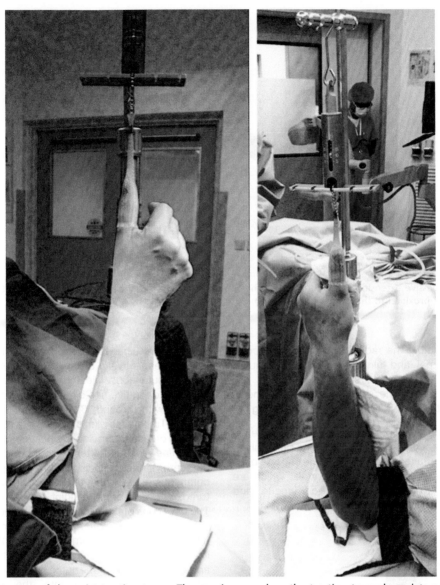

Fig. 2. The setup of the wrist traction tower. The arm is secured on the traction tower baseplate with a positioning strap. Padding is placed between the arm and the baseplate and between the arm and the strap. The elbow is flexed 90°. The thumb is suspended with a single nylon finger trap, and a vertical traction force of about 8 lbs is applied. The forearm is supinated by wrapping the other 4 fingers onto the tower stand so that the dorsum of the thumb base is directly facing the surgeon. Padding is placed between the forearm and the tower, and between the fingers and the stand, to promote patient comfort and avoid direct contact with metal.

elbow is flexed 90°. The thumb is suspended with a single nylon finger trap and vertical traction force of about 8 lbs is applied. The forearm is supinated by wrapping the other 4 fingers onto the tower stand (see **Fig. 2**) so that the dorsum of the thumb base is directly facing the surgeon. Padding is placed between forearm and the tower, and between the fingers and the stand, to promote patient's comfort and to avoid direct contact with metal (see **Fig. 2**). Continuous irrigation is achieved with a 3-L bag of normal saline

suspended 1.5 m above the patient and instilled under gravity.

Fluoroscopic identification of the CMCJ1 is not necessary. It can be identified by the following 2 methods:

i. By releasing the thumb from traction, passively extending and adducting the thumb, the radial base of the metacarpal becomes prominent and the CMCJ1 is palpable just proximal to the prominence (**Fig. 3**).

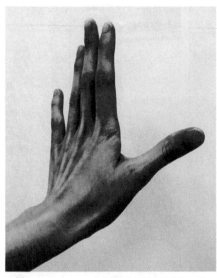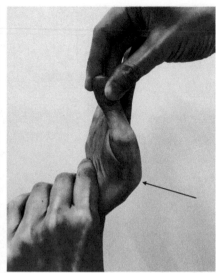

Fig. 3. By passive extension and adduction of the thumb, the metacarpal base becomes prominent. CMCJ1 is located just proximal to this prominence (*arrow*).

ii. By palpating the radial border of the second metacarpal and ulnar border of the thumb metacarpal from its shaft to the base, the confluence of the second and thumb metacarpal base is the CMCJ1 ulnar aspect (**Fig. 4**).

Xylocaine (2%) in 1:200,000 adrenaline is injected through a 25-G needle to the portal sites, to the subcutaneous layer, and to the capsule only. The authors use 1-R and 1-U portals, which are just radial to the abductor pollicis longus, and

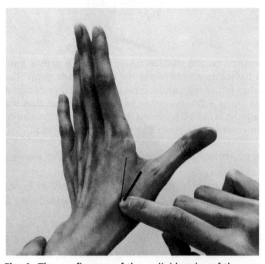

Fig. 4. The confluence of the radial border of the second metacarpal shaft (*thinner line*) and the ulnar border of the thumb metacarpal (*thick line*) is the level of the CMCJ1.

about 2 mm ulnar to the extensor pollicis brevis tendon, respectively, at the level of the CMCJ1. The subcutaneous injected adrenaline helps to minimize operative site bleeding. The joint is distended with around 3 mL of normal saline (**Fig. 5**). Transverse skin incisions are made along the skin crease to provide the best cosmetic healing. A fine mosquito artery is used to dissect underneath the skin incision and to spread the cutaneous nerve. Then, the joint capsule is punctured, and an egress of joint fluid is observed. The directions of the portals should be pointing toward the thenar region. A 1.9-mm arthroscope is used. The correct placement of the arthroscope into the CMCJ1 can be confirmed with the saddle appearance of the trapezium. If by accident the arthroscope is inserted into the scaphoid-trapezium-trapezoid joint (STTJ), the inferior articular surface will appear convex and dome shaped, which is the scaphoid, whereas there are 2 articular facets in the distal articular surface. The 1-R and 1-U portals are interchangeable for viewing and working. Outflow can be made with an 18-G needle at the thenar portal, which is 90° perpendicular to the 1-U portal, through the thenar muscle bulk. The second or third portals can be established under direct arthroscopic visualization. Synovectomy is performed with a 2-mm shaver, to remove any inflamed synovium and frayed capsule (**Fig. 6**). Loose bodies floating or adhered to the capsule are removed. Radiofrequency ablation is used to ablate the capsule. In the authors' series, 25 out of 76 cases had loose bodies removal. Thermal shrinkage is performed

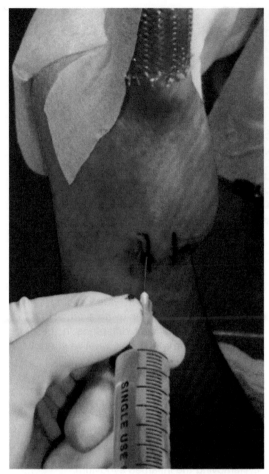

Fig. 5. The 1-R and 1-U portal sites are marked, and injection of normal saline through the 1-U portal is shown.

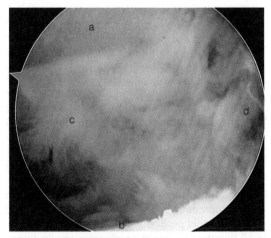

Fig. 6. Arthroscopic view of CMCJ1. (*a*) Proximal articular surface of thumb metacarpal; complete loss of articular cartilage. (*b*) Distal articular surface of trapezium. (*c*) Frayed joint capsule. (*d*) Inflamed synovium.

on the intact ligaments. The authors did 30 cases of thermal shrinkage in their series. Minimal bone work is performed. Only prominent osteophytes are blurred in order to create a smooth opposing articular surface (**Fig. 7**). Xylocaine with adrenaline can be injected through the joint to the opposite volar joint capsule if the patient feels some pain. The operation is concluded by releasing the thumb, asking the patient to actively flex, extend, abduct, and adduct the thumb to confirm tendon integrity. Suture is not necessary. Steristrips are applied to the portal sites. Bulky dressing is applied for soft tissue swelling. No cast or immobilization is necessary. Patients can start free range of motion immediately after the operation as tolerated (Video 1). For those who had thermal shrinkage on the CMCJ1 ligaments, cast or splint immobilization is given for 4 to 6 weeks.

Results

The 76 cases in 65 patients were followed up for an average of 59 months (4–144).

Subjective exertion pain
Sixty-nine patients (91%) experienced pain relief after the operation from an average of 8.6/10 on the visual analogue scale (VAS) to 2.4/10. The pain relief occurred on average 3 months after the operation. Patients were asked to quantify the degree of pain relief. Pain relief for more than 90% occurred in 20 thumbs and lasted until the day of the final follow-up, which was graded as "excellent pain relief." Pain relief for more than 70% occurred in 14 thumbs and lasted until the final follow-up, which was graded as "good pain relief." Twenty-four thumbs had pain relief improved for less than 70%, but the pain was not a nuisance to the patients, which was graded as "fair pain relief." However, 7 cases had similar pain as their preoperative condition after the operation, which was graded as "poor pain relief." There was pain improvement in 11 thumbs, but was short lasting, which was also graded as "poor pain relief." These 18 thumbs were reoperated on an average of 14 months after the arthroscopic debridement because the patients found the initial surgery did not help their symptoms. There was no complication encountered, and the scar was inconspicuous (**Fig. 8**).

Thumb mobility
The Kapandji score was similar as the preoperative status (8 ± 1.6).

Palmar abduction range
The palmar abduction range was averaged 3.75° ($P = .038$) more than the preoperative range.

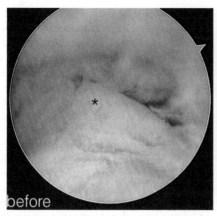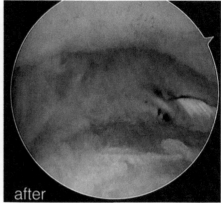

Fig. 7. Arthroscopic view of CMCJ1 (*asterisk*). Prominent osteophyte before burring. Minimal bone work was performed. Only prominent osteophytes were removed.

Strength

For pinch power and grip power, there was no significant difference from the preoperative strength.

Satisfaction and complications

For the patient's subjective satisfaction, the mean score was 77/100 with 0 the worst and 100 the best.

There were no complications from this procedure. The surgical scar was inconspicuous (see **Fig. 7**).

Seven patients requested the same operation on their opposite thumb, and 3 patients requested the same operation on the same thumb 2 to 5 years after the initial one, because the pain relief was not lasting. All had excellent pain relief after the second operation.

Correlation of pain symptoms

Statistical analysis showed that the degree of pain relief was not statistically correlated with the patient's age, sex, duration of symptoms, metacarpophalangeal joint hyperextendibility, radiologic staging, size of the impinging osteophytes, arthroscopic cartilage status (Badia classification), presence of loose bodies and their removal, and presence of postoperative radiologic progression. However, statistically better outcomes were correlated with the osteophytes burring (see **Fig. 6**), thermal shrinkage, or casting/splintage given after the operation.

Analysis of the trends for 2 years more

After this study series, the authors further followed up these 65 patients for another 2 years. Lasting excellent or good pain relief could be maintained on those 34 thumbs (44.7% of the patients). The authors found that there was further improvement in pain score, with VAS averaged 1.63 one year after the above study period, and VAS 0.88

two years after the above study period. The improvement in pain score was statistically significant. In these 2 years, there was a decrease in the range of palmar abduction by an average of 4.72°. There was no significant difference in the pinch and grip power from the preoperative strength.

Discussion

Sustaining excellent to good pain relief occurred in 44.7% of the patients in an average follow-up of 7 years.

This procedure may help to alleviate pain by

i. Removing the inflamed synovium,
ii. Denerving by means of debridement of the frayed joint capsule and radiofrequency ablation,
iii. Promoting CMCJ1 stability by thermal shrinkage, postoperative immobilization, and postoperative fibrosis,
iv. Relieving the subchondral pressure by burring the impinging prominent osteophytes growing from the side of the joint, because statistical findings showed that better outcomes occurred in cases with prominent osteophytes burring, thermal shrinkage, and a period of immobilization.

The analysis at the 2-year follow-up showed further mild improvement of pain despite mild deterioration of palmar abduction range. Less motion at the CMCJ1 should induce less mechanical loading and therefore less pain at the CMCJ1.

The authors could not achieve better strength after this procedure. Moreover, they did encounter poor outcomes (no pain relief, or short-term pain relief) from this procedure. They had poor results in 18 thumbs (23.7%) in which other surgical procedures were subsequently performed.

This procedure is not an ideal operation to provide improvement in all the 3 parameters of pain,

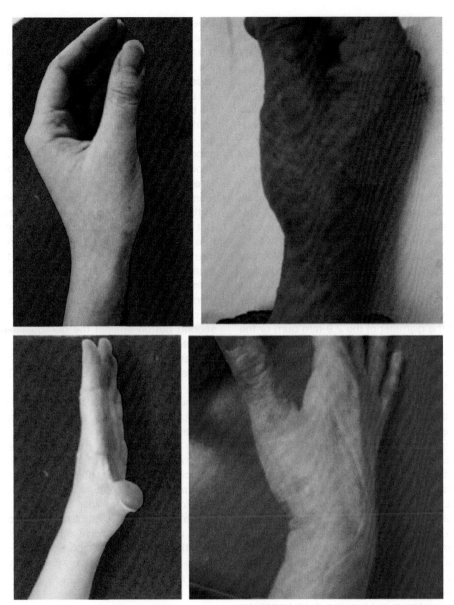

Fig. 8. Four patients had arthroscopic CMCJ1 arthroscopic debridement, synovectomy, and thermal shrinkage performed. The scars were inconspicuous.

strength, and mobility. Pain relief is also not a guarantee. Excellent pain relief occurred in only 26.3% of the patients. However, this is a minimally invasive procedure that is safe and technically easy, gives better visualization of the joint, helps for better clinical judgment, and can be performed under local anesthesia with fast rehabilitation and minimal complications. The authors saw 91% of the patients had pain relief after the operation, 44.7% had excellent to good long-lasting pain relief, slight improvement in abduction range, and high patient satisfaction, preservation of the trapezium, and therefore, no subsidence problem, and preservation of grip and pinch strength. It can be

a definitive procedure, especially for patients who do not demand better thumb strength, want to preserve the motion, or would like to try a minimally invasive, simpler procedure. It retains the possibility of later joint reconstruction, should that become necessary. It could be a procedure to buy time, especially if the cartilage is still viable.

ARTHROSCOPIC PARTIAL TRAPEZIECTOMY + SUTURE BUTTON SUSPENSIONPLASTY

If better strength is needed while preserving CMCJ1 mobility, especially in widespread cartilage loss in the distal articular surface of the trapezium (Badia stage III), arthroscopic partial trapeziectomy and suture button suspensionplasty may be good options.

Surgical Technique

Arthroscopy is performed similarly as the arthroscopic debridement as mentioned above. It can be performed with the patient wide awake with lignocaine mixed with adrenaline, or under plexus anesthesia, or general anesthesia. A tourniquet is used and placed at the upper arm if it is performed under plexus or general anesthesia. After debridement, synovectomy, and radiofrequency ablation, the distal trapezium is burred with a 2.9-mm arthroscopic burr (Smith & Nephew DYONICS) through the various portals, including 1-U/1-R/thenar portals. About 3 to 4 mm of distal trapezium is removed. The depth of the bone being removed can be measured by the burr. About 1.5 times the diameter of the 2.9-mm burr, or the diameter of the burr sheath (for the Smith & Nephew DYONICS 2.9-mm burr, the burr sheath is 3.9 mm in diameter), is the appropriate amount of bone to be removed. An even thickness of distal trapezium removal should be achieved. After the distal trapezium is removed, the amount of the space created should be enough that the thumb metacarpal would not grind onto the remaining trapezium. The thumb should be released from the traction tower and check with the fluoroscope. The dorsoradial subluxation and adduction deformity of the thumb metacarpal should be passively reduced. Fluoroscopy is helpful to assess whether the bone removal is enough and even, and whether the osteophytes, especially at the volar-ulnar aspect of the trapezium, are adequately removed without causing impingement. The thumb should be suspended in the traction tower and burr the distal trapezium until adequate.

To insert the suture button, release the thumb and put it on the hand table. Extend the 1-R portal radially along volar-radial skin crease. Dissect with a mosquito artery to the volar-radial aspect of the thumb metacarpal base. Use a fine periosteal elevator to elevate the radial border of the thenar muscle and the periosteum from the bone so that the suture button does not compress onto the periosteum and produce pain. The authors prefer to reduce the thumb metacarpal dorsoradial subluxation and adduction deformity, restore its normal height, pin it to the trapezium at 40° of palmar abduction, 15° of radial abduction, and the thumb pulp facing the finger pulp of the middle finger. The 1.1-mm

tapered Suture Passing K-wire (Arthrex) is inserted through the incision, 2 to 3 mm distal to the thumb metacarpal base articular surface, at the volar-radial border of the thumb metacarpal base, aiming toward the proximal one-third of the second metacarpal, exiting at the ulnar border of the second metacarpal. The trajectory is confirmed under fluoroscopy. Another longitudinal incision is made over the exit site. Dissect subcutaneously to avoid and retract any cutaneous nerve. A fine periosteal elevator is used to elevate the interosseous muscle and periosteum from the bone. The Suture Passing K-wire (Arthrex) is advanced and pulled through the exit wound while the attached suture and the suture button are advanced with the K-wire. The suture button sits on the volar-radial cortex of the thumb metacarpal base and is covered by the thenar muscle, while another suture button is placed over the sutures onto the second metacarpal. The sutures are then tightened to sit the second button against the dorsoulnar cortex of the second metacarpal. One provisional knot is tied and held with a mosquito artery. The pin across the CMCJ1 is then removed. The alignment, mobility, and resistance to subsidence are then checked under fluoroscopy. Tensioning is adjusted accordingly, and the remaining knots are tied.

The radial border of the thenar muscle fascia and the radial border of the interosseous fascia are closed to their origins, respectively, for coverage of the 2 suture buttons. The wounds are closed with fine nylon sutures. A short arm thumb spica slab is applied for 5 to 7 days. Then, a thumb spica splint is offered for 4 weeks, and the patient is encouraged to do active range-of-motion exercises without the splint 6 times per day.

Case Example

A 51-year-old car repairman had left thumb base pain for 3 years and failed nonoperative treatments for 1 year. A radiograph showed Eaton and Littler stage III disease (**Fig. 9**). Badia arthroscopy classification was stage III disease. Arthroscopic debridement, synovectomy, partial trapeziectomy, and suture button suspensionplasty were performed. **Fig. 9**C and Video 2 show the condition at 4 weeks after the operation. At 6 months after the operation, the resting pain improved from preoperative VAS 3/10 to 0/10, while the exertion pain improved from 8/10 to 0/10. The pinch power improved from 2 kg to 11 kg. The grip power improved from 12 kg to 29 kg. A radiograph showed the CMCJ1 space was maintained and mobile (Video 3).

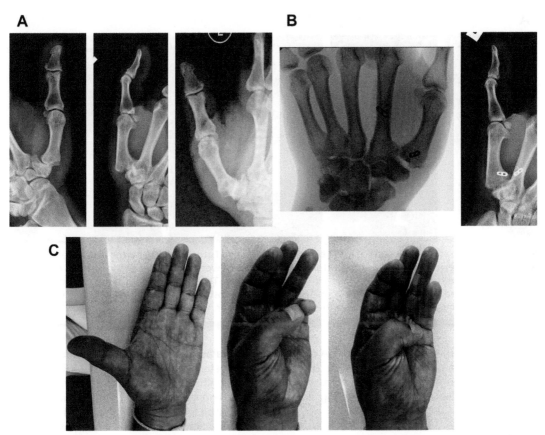

Fig. 9. A 51-year-old car repairman had left CMCJ1 OA with arthroscopic partial trapeziectomy and suture button suspensionplasty performed. (*A*) Preoperative radiograph shows Eaton and Littler stage III disease. (*B*) Postoperative radiographs. (*C*) The patient was able to move the thumb well 4 weeks after the operation.

Results and Discussion

The authors have performed only 9 cases of this procedure from May 2015 to March 2017. There were 7 women and 2 men. The average age was 59.5 (range 51–75). Six cases were on the left side. All were Badia stage III disease. The average follow-up duration was 9.3 months (range 2–24).

Preoperatively, the resting pain score VAS was averaged 2.78 (range 0–7), exertion pain score VAS averaged 6.67 (range 3–8), grip power 14.67 kg (range 10–22), and pinch power 4.56 kg (range 2–7). Postoperatively, the resting pain score VAS was averaged 0.56 (0–5), exertion pain VAS 2.11 (0–7), grip power 18.89 kg,[11–29] pinch power 6.58 kg (3.5–9.25).

The average improvement in resting pain after the operation was VAS 2.22 (0–4), exertion pain VAS 4.56 (0–8), grip power 4.22 kg (0–17), and pinch power 2.02 kg (−1.5–9).

All patients had rest pain improved. No complication was encountered.

The authors had 1 case of unsatisfactory results, and 2 cases of fair results.

Unsatisfactory results
A 75 year-old man had improvement of rest pain from VAS 7 to 5, but only mild improvement in exertion pain from VAS 8 to 7 (**Fig. 10**A). There was no improvement in grip power (remained the same at 11 kg) and deterioration in pinch power (from 5 kg to 3.5 kg) at the final follow-up 8 months after the operation, although he did not feel any deterioration in the strength. A radiograph showed that the CMCJ1 was still subluxed, and the osteophytes at the ulnar side were not removed adequately (see **Fig. 10**B).

Fair results
A 64-year-old woman had improvement in rest pain from VAS 3 to 0, exertion pain from VAS 8 to 3 four months after the operation (**Fig. 11**A). However, her pinch and grip power did not change. Her performance was also affected by the preexisting pain at the metacarpophalangeal

A   **B**

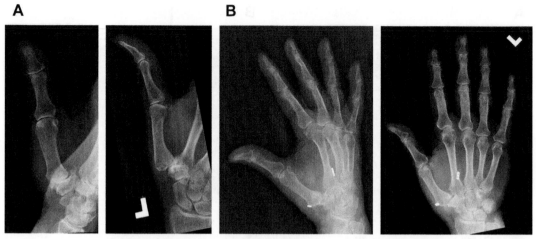

Fig. 10. (*A*) Preoperative radiograph of a 75-year-old man who had Eaton and Littler stage III disease. (*B*) Arthroscopic partial trapeziectomy and suture button suspensionplasty were performed. Postoperative radiographs show that the thumb metacarpal base was still radially subluxed. The osteophytes at the ulnar side were not adequately removed, which impeded the reduction. The residual osteophytes at the radial side may also cause irritation pain to the capsuloligamentous structures. The suspension was not adequate.

joint, which also showed features of OA. A radiograph showed inadequate removal of the osteophytes at the ulnar side of the trapezium, which may account for the limited power (see **Fig. 11**B).

Fair results

A 59-year-old woman had thumb metacarpal corrective osteotomy for CMCJ1 arthritis 14 years ago. The pain reappeared 3 years ago (**Fig. 12**. Three months after the arthroscopic partial trapeziectomy and suture button suspensionplasty, there was only mild improvement in pain score, but rest pain improved from VAS 1 to 0, and exertion pain was the same at VAS 5. Her grip power

deteriorated from 22 kg to 15 kg, whereas pinch power deteriorated from 6.5 kg to 4.5 kg, although the strength improved slowly with time. According to the improvement trend, the authors expect there will be further improvement in her symptoms with time. However, for the other patients, they enjoyed better outcomes than the preoperative status at around 2 months after the operation. Possibly, there was insufficient distal trapezium resection especially at the ulnar side. Moreover, the suspension suture was tensioned too much, and the suture button was not placed proximal enough at the thumb metacarpal base, which resulted in thumb metacarpal adduction, and

A   **B**

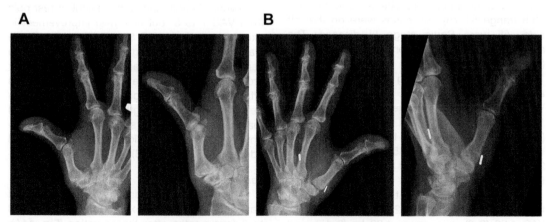

Fig. 11. (*A*) A 64-year-old woman who had left thumb Eaton and Littler stage IV disease. She also had pain at the metacarpophalangeal joint. (*B*) Postoperative radiographs show that the osteophyte at the ulnar side of the trapezium was not removed adequately, the distal trapezium was not removed adequately, and the space at the CMCJ1 was very limited.

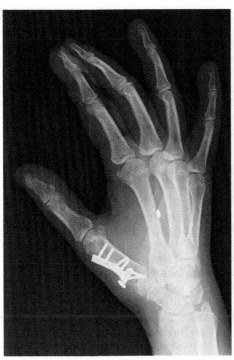
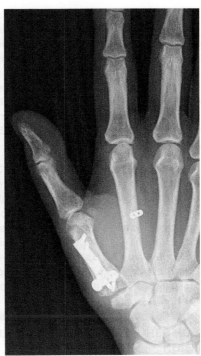

Fig. 12. A 59-year-old woman had previous corrective osteotomy of thumb metacarpal 14 years ago. She then had arthroscopic partial trapeziectomy and suture button suspensionplasty. The rest pain improved, but the pinch and grip power was worse than the preoperative status at 3 months after the operation. A radiograph showed that the ulnar side of the thumb metacarpal base was in contact with the trapezium. The suture button was not placed proximal enough at the thumb metacarpal base, which might result in thumb metacarpal adduction and therefore created pressure at the ulnar side of CMCJ1.

therefore, created pressure between the thumb metacarpal base and the ulnar aspect of the remaining trapezium.

Although the experience is limited, the authors find that consistent excellent to good results can be obtained if the following points are followed:

i. Adequate removal of the distal trapezium, including the osteophytes, especially at the ulnar-volar side, so that a space is created between the trapezium and thumb metacarpal in all ranges of CMCJ1 motion under mild suspension. Then, a pseudo "new joint" is created (**Fig. 13**).

ii. Adduction deformity of the thumb metacarpal and the CMCJ1 subluxation is adequately reduced, so that no localized pressure will be created in this newly created "pseudo-joint," and no excessive tension will be created at the capsule-ligamentous structures at the dorsoradial side of the CMCJ1.

iii. A suture button is placed at the most basal side of the thumb metacarpal, in order to effectively maintain the abduction of the thumb metacarpal. If the button is placed too distally, the

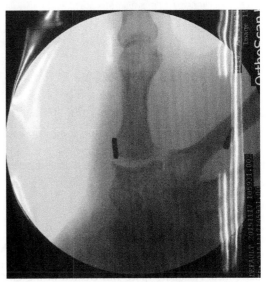

Fig. 13. Radiograph shows an adequate space was created in the CMCJ1 after arthroscopic partial trapeziectomy and suture button suspensionplasty. A pseudo "new joint" was created.

suture will pull the thumb metacarpal into adduction and the CMCJ1 into dorsal/radial subluxation. The CMCJ1 motion will also be hindered by the suspension suture, which is too far away from the CMCJ1 center of motion (**Fig. 14**). Thumb function and strength may be affected because the degree of the first web space and the thumb abduction range determines hand grip forces and mechanical thumb function.[5]

If the above factors were achieved, and those 3 cases of unsatisfactory/fair/poor cases were excluded, all patients enjoyed improvement in all 4 parameters of rest pain, exertion pain, pinch power, and grip power, with the improvement of rest pain for VAS 2.2 (range 0–4, 0 improvement as the patient had preoperative VAS 0 and postoperative VAS 0), exertion pain for VAS 5.86 (range 5–8), grip power for 7.5 kg (range 1–17), and pinch power for 3.5 kg (range 1–9).

ARTHROSCOPIC THUMB CARPOMETACARPAL JOINT EXCISION + SUTURE BUTTON SUSPENSIONPLASTY + K-WIRE FIXATION

Although pain improvement was consistently good and there was improvement in strength in arthroscopic partial trapeziectomy and suture button suspensionplasty, the extent of strength improvement was found to be variable and unpredictable so far in the few cases the authors have seen. The improvement in grip power ranged from 1 kg to 17 kg, and pinch power ranged from 1 kg to 9 kg. Arthroscopic CMCJ1 excision together with suture button suspensionplasty and K-wire may be a better option to achieve a fibrous union at the CMCJ1. Sturdy CMCJ1 should theoretically provide a stronger thumb. It may be indicated for those who demand better strength.

Surgical Technique

The surgical technique is similar to the arthroscopic partial trapeziectomy and suture button suspensionplasty, but just the subchondral bone and osteophytes are removed in the trapezium. About 2 mm of distal trapezium and 1 to 2 mm of proximal thumb metacarpal base are burred in order to create opposing bleeding bone surfaces. CMCJ1 subluxation and adduction deformity are corrected and held with 2 K-wires. Suture buttons are then applied as mentioned above.

K-wires are then removed 3 weeks after the operation.

Case Example

A 70 year-old man had right thumb base arthritis for 3 years with arthroscopic CMCJ1 excision

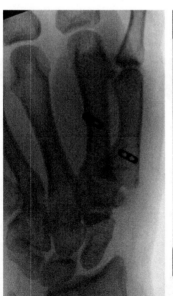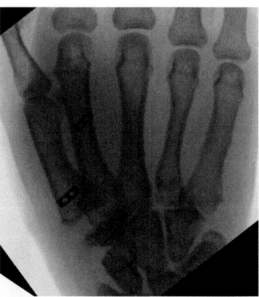

Fig. 14. A 54-year-old woman who had arthroscopic partial trapeziectomy and suture button suspensionplasty performed. Adequate space was created in the CMCJ1. Adequate osteophytes were removed. The rest pain improved from VAS 3 to 0, exertion pain from VAS 8 to 3. However, the improvement in strength was not remarkable. At 9 months after the operation, the grip power was improved from 14 kg to 15 kg, and pinch power from 5 kg to 7 kg. The suture button at the thumb metacarpal was placed too distally. Motion and the first web space at the "new" CMCJ1 were hindered by the suspension suture.

A   **B**

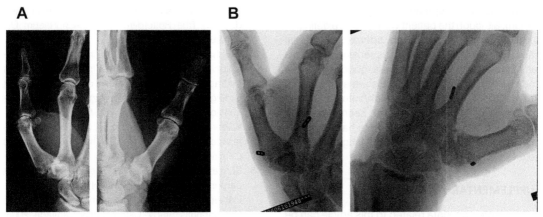

Fig. 15. (*A*) Preoperative radiographs of a 70-year-old man who had arthroscopic CMCJ excision and suture button suspensionplasty and K-wire fixation performed for right CMCJ1 OA. (*B*) Postoperative radiographs.

and suture button suspensionplasty and K-wire fixation performed (**Fig. 15**). Four months after the operation, grip power improved from 28 kg to 36 kg, pinch power from 3 kg to 8 kg, rest pain VAS 5 to 0, and exertion pain VAS 8 to 2. A radiograph showed that there was fibrous union at the CMCJ1 with minimal mobility at passive motion (Video 4).

Results and Discussion

The authors have performed only 4 cases of this procedure from August 2015 to February 2017. There were 2 women and 2 men. The average age was 60 (range 49–70). Three cases were on the right side. All were Badia stage III disease and had no STTJ arthritis. The average follow-up duration was 9 months (range 2–21).

Preoperatively, the rest pain score VAS averaged 4.7 (range 3–6), exertion pain score VAS averaged 8.3 (range 8–9), grip power 20 kg (range 10–28), and pinch power 3.3 kg (range 3–4). Postoperatively, the rest pain score VAS averaged 0, exertion pain VAS 1.0 (0–3), grip power 30.7 kg,[26–36] and pinch power 7.8 kg (6–9.5).

The average improvement in rest pain after the operation was VAS 4.7 (3–6), exertion pain VAS 7.3,[5–9] grip power 10.7 kg,[8–16] and pinch power 4.5 kg (3–5.5).

All patients had improvement in all 4 parameters of rest pain, exertion pain, grip power, and pinch power.

K-wires are temporary to secure initial CMCJ1 stability, whereas the subsequent stability is provided by the suture button. Long-term CMCJ1 stability is provided by the fibrosis around and between the trapezium and the thumb metacarpal.

Painful CMCJ1 is removed. The pain arising from this joint should theoretically be tackled as

evidenced from these 4 cases. The fibrous connection between the thumb metacarpal base and distal trapezium provides thumb metacarpal stability while some mobility at this fibrous union site may slow down the problem in formal arthrodesis, pantrapezial arthritis.[41] A complication of formal open CMCJ1 arthrodesis is well known to be nonunion.[41] However, long-term follow-up has shown that many nonunions are asymptomatic. Some surgeons deliberately created a narrow pseudoarthrosis of the CMCJ1 as alternative treatment of CMCJ1 arthritis, with satisfactory short-term results.[69] Painless pseudoarthrosis also reflects in the authors' 4 cases in which good pain relief was achieved.

SUMMARY

So far, there is no single ideal surgery to treat all stages of CMCJ1 arthritis and all kinds of patients. Trapeziectomy and ligament reconstruction/interposition or prosthetic replacement has not been superior to trapeziectomy alone. However, subsidence and weakness are inevitable in trapeziectomy alone. Advancement in arthroscopy may give a better alternative. It is a minimally invasive technique, can be performed under local anesthesia, helps to assess cartilage condition and determine treatment, achieves synovectomy, radiofrequency ablation, denervation, thermal shrinkage, and helps to remove impinging osteophytes. Arthroscopic synovectomy/debridement/thermal shrinkage/minimal osteophytes burring gave sustained excellent to good pain relief in 44.7% of the patients but minimal improvement in strength. It can be a minimally invasive, simple, time-buying procedure and helps patients through the painful period until the CMCJ1 becomes secondarily stabilized, and the patients have adapted and become accustomed to the use of their thumbs in daily life.

When there is widespread cartilage loss in the trapezium, although the patient wants a more definitive surgery with a stronger thumb, arthroscopic partial trapeziectomy/suture button suspensionplasty is a reasonable technique to provide good pain relief and strength if the surgical details are emphasized. Arthroscopic CMCJ1 excision/suture button suspensionplasty/K-wire fixation seems a more guaranteed technique if the patients have high demand on strength. A larger and longer study is necessary.

SUPPLEMENTARY DATA

Supplementary data related to this article can be found online at http://dx.doi.org/10.1016/j.hcl.2017.07.007.

REFERENCES

1. Moran SL, Berger RA. Biomechanics and hand trauma: what you need. Hand Clin 2003;19:17–31.
2. Napier J. Revised edition. Hands, vol. 55. Princeton (NJ): Princeton University Press; 1993.
3. Goto A, Leng S, Sugamoto K, et al. In vivo pilot study evaluating the thumb carpometacarpal joint during circumduction. Clin Orthop Relat Res 2014;472: 1106–13.
4. Katarincic JA. Thumb kinematics and their relevance to function. Hand Clin 2001;17:169–74.
5. Herck I, Steenwerckx A, De Smet L, et al. Is there a correction between mobility of the thumb and mechanical hand function. Acta Orthop Belg 1996; 62(1):30–3.
6. Ateshian GA, Ark JW, Rosenwasser MP, et al. Contact areas in the thumb carpometacarpal joint. J Orthop Res 1995;13:450–8.
7. Momose T, Nakatsuchi Y, Saitoh S. Contact area of the trapeziometacarpal joint. J Hand Surg Am 1992;24(3):491–5.
8. Halilaj E, Moore DC, Got CJ, et al. Articular shape of the carpometacarpal joint differs with age but not sex. ORS 2014 Annual Meeting. Poster 0209. New Orleans (LA), 15-18 March, 2014.
9. Cooney WP, Chao EY. Biomechanical analysis of static forces in the thumb during hand function. J Bone Joint Surg Am 1977;59(1):27.
10. Aune S. Osteoarthritis in the first carpometacarpal joint. Acta Chir Scand 1955;109:449–56.
11. Eaton RG, Littler JW. Ligament reconstruction for the painful thumb carpometacarpal joint. J Bone Joint Surg Am 1973;55:1655–6.
12. Eaton RG, Glickel SZ. Trapeziometacarpal osteoarthritis: staging as a rationale for treatment. Hand Clin 1987;3:455–71.
13. Dahaghin S, Bierma-Zeinstra SMA, Gina AZ, et al. Prevalence and pattern of radiographic hand

osteoarthritis and association with pain and disability (the Rotterdam study). Ann Rheum Dis 2005;64:682–7.
14. Marshall M, van der Windt D, Nicholls E, et al. Radiographic thumb osteoarthritis: frequency, patterns and associations with pain and clinical assessment findings in a community-dwelling population. Rheumatology (Oxford) 2011;50:735–9.
15. Wilder FV, Barrett JP, Farina EJ. Joint-specific prevalence of osteoarthritis of the hand. Osteoarthritis Cartilage 2006;14:953–7.
16. Sonne-Holm S, Jacobsen S. Osteoarthritis of the first carpometacarpal joint: a study of radiology and clinical epidemiology. Results from the Copenhagen Osteoarthritis Study. Osteoarthritis Cartilage 2006; 14:496–500.
17. Dominick KL, Jordan JM, Renner JB, et al. Relationship of radiographic and clinical variables to pinch and grip strength among individuals with osteoarthritis. Arthritis Rheum 2005;52:1424–30.
18. Spacek E, Poiraudeau S, Fayad F, et al. Disability induced by hand osteoarthritis: are patients with more symptoms at digits 2–5 interphalangeal joints different from those with more symptoms at the base of the thumb? Osteoarthritis Cartilage 2004;12:366–73.
19. Bijsterbosch J, Visser W, Kroon HM, et al. Thumb base involvement in symptomatic hand osteoarthritis is associated with more pain and functional disability. Ann Rheum Dis 2010;69:585–7.
20. Haugen ID, England M, Aliabadi P, et al. Prevalence, incidence and progression of hand osteoarthritis in the general population: the Framingham Osteoarthritis Study. Ann Rheum Dis 2011;70:1581–6.
21. Batra S, Kanvinde R. Osteoarthritis of the thumb trapeziometacarpal joint. Orthopaedic Trauma 2007; 21:135–44.
22. Niu J, Zhang Y, LaValley M, et al. Symmetry and clustering of symptomatic hand osteoarthritis in elderly men and women: the Framingham Study. Rheumatology (Oxford) 2003;42:343–8.
23. Dillon CF, Hirsch R, Rasch EK, et al. Symptomatic hand osteoarthritis in the United States: prevalence and functional impairment estimates from the third, U.S. National Health and Nutrition Examination Survey, 1991–1994. Am J Phys Med Rehabil 2007;86: 12–21.
24. Wolf JM, Turkiewicz A, Atroshi I, et al. Prevalence of doctor-diagnosed thumb carpometacarpal joint osteoarthritis: an analysis of swedish health care: thumb arthritis consultations in Sweden. Arthritis Care Res 2014;66(6):961–5.
25. Armstrong AL, Hunter JB, Davis TR. The prevalence of degenerative arthritis of the base of the thumb in post-menopausal women. J Hand Surg Br 1994;19: 340–1.
26. Lins RE, Gelberman RH, McKeown L, et al. Basal joint arthritis: trapeziectomy with ligament

reconstruction and tendon interposition arthroplasty. J Hand Surg 1996;21A:202–9.

27. Kvarnes L, Reikeras O. Osteoarthritis of the carpometacarpal joint of the thumb: an analysis of operative procedures. J Hand Surg Br 1985;10:117–20.

28. Murley AHG. Excision of the trapezium in osteoarthritis of the first carpometacarpal joint. J Bone Joint Surg Br 1960;42:502–9.

29. Burton RI, Pelligrini VD. Surgical management of basal joint arthritis of the thumb. Part II. Ligament reconstruction with tendon interposition arthroplasty. J Hand Surg Am 1986;11:324–32.

30. De Smet L, Sioen W, Spaepen D, et al. Treatment of basal joint arthritis of the thumb: trapeziectomy with or without tendon interposition/ligament reconstruction. Hand Surg 2004;9:5–9.

31. Kriegs-Au G, Petje G, Fojtl E, et al. Ligament reconstruction with or without tendon interposition to treat primary thumb carpometacarpal osteoarthritis: a prospective randomized study. J Bone Joint Surg Am 2004;86:209–18.

32. Davis TR, Brady O, Dias JJ. Excision of the trapezium for osteoarthritis of the trapeziometacarpal joint: a study of the benefit of ligament reconstruction or tendon interposition. J Hand Surg Am 2004; 29:1069–77.

33. Gangopadhyay S, McKenna H, Burke FD, et al. Five- to 18-year follow-up for treatment of trapeziometacarpal osteoarthritis: a prospective comparison of excision, tendon interposition, and ligament reconstruction and tendon interposition. J Hand Surg Am 2012;37:411–7.

34. Davis TR, Brady O, Barton NJ, et al. Trapeziectomy alone, with tendon interposition or with ligament reconstruction? J Hand Surg Br 1997;22:689–94.

35. Davis TR, Pace A. Trapeziectomy for trapeziometacarpal joint osteoarthritis: is ligament reconstruction and temporary stabilisation of the pseudarthrosis with a Kirschner wire important? J Hand Surg Eur Vol 2009;34:312–21.

36. Salem H, Davis TR. Six year outcome excision of the trapezium for trapeziometacarpal joint osteoarthritis: Is it improved by ligament reconstruction and temporary Kirschner wire insertion? J Hand Surg Eur Vol 2012;37:211–9.

37. Wajon A, Carr E, Edmunds I, et al. Surgery for thumb (trapeziometacarpal joint) osteoarthritis. Cochrane Database Syst Rev 2009;(7):CD004631.

38. Aliu O, Davis MM, DeMonner S, et al. The influence of evidence base in surgical treatment of thumb basal joint arthritis. Plast Reconstr Surg 2013; 131(4):816–28.

39. Brunton LM, Wilgis EF. A survey to determine current practice patterns in the surgical treatment of advanced thumb carpometacarpal osteoarthrosis. Hand (N Y) 2010;5:415–22.

40. Wolf JM, Delaronde S. Current trends in nonoperative and operative treatment of trapeziometacarpal osteoarthritis: a survey of US hand surgeons. J Hand Surg Am 2012;37:77–82.

41. Kenniston JA, Bozentka DJ. Treatment of advanced carpometacarpal joint disease: arthrodesis. Hand Clin 2008;24:285–94, vi.

42. Vandenberghe L, Degreef I, Didden K, et al. Long term outcome of trapeziectomy with ligament reconstruction/tendon interposition versus thumb basal joint prosthesis. J Hand Surg Eur Vol 2013; 38:839–43.

43. Athwal GS, Chenkin J, King GJ, et al. Early failures with a spheric interposition arthroplasty of the thumb basal joint. J Hand Surg Am 2004;29:1080–4.

44. Nicholas RM, Calderwood JW. De la Caffinière arthroplasty for basal thumb joint osteoarthritis. J Bone Joint Surg Br 1992;74:309–12.

45. Parker WL, Rizzo M, Moran SL, et al. Preliminary results of nonconstrained pyrolytic carbon arthroplasty for metacarpophalangeal joint arthritis. J Hand Surg Am 2007;32:1496–505.

46. Martinez de Aragon JS, Moran SL, Rizzo M, et al. Early outcomes of pyrolytic carbon hemiarthroplasty for the treatment of trapezial-metacarpal arthritis. J Hand Surg Am 2009;34:205–12.

47. Colegate-Stone TJ, Garg S, Subramanian A, et al. Outcome analysis of trapezectomy with and without pyrocarbon interposition to treat primary arthrosis of the trapeziometacarpal joint. Hand Surg 2011;16: 49–54.

48. Menon J. Arthroscopic management of trapeziometacarpal joint arthritis of the thumb. Arthroscopy 1996;12:581–7.

49. Culp R, Osterman A. Arthroscopic evaluation and treatment of thumb carpometacarpal joints. Atlas Hand Clin 1997;2(2):23–8.

50. Culp RW, Rekant MS. The role of arthroscopy in evaluating and treating trapeziometacarpal disease. Hand Clin 2001;17:315–9.

51. Badia A. Trapeziometacarpal arthroscopy: a classification and treatment algorithm. Hand Clin 2006;22: 153–63.

52. Furia JP. Arthroscopic debridement and synovectomy for treating basal joint arthritis. Arthroscopy 2010;26(1):34–40.

53. Chu PJ, Lee HM, Chung LJ, et al. Electrothermal treatment of thumb basal joint instability. Arthroscopy 2009;25:290–5.

54. Hofmeister EP, Leak RS, Culp RW, et al. Arthroscopic hemitrapeziectomy for first carpometacarpal arthritis: results at 7-year follow-up. Hand (N Y) 2009;4:24–8.

55. Edwards SG, Ramsey PN. Prospective outcomes of stage III thumb carpometacarpal arthritis treated with arthroscopic hemitrapeziectomy and thermal

capsular modification without interposition. J Hand Surg Am 2010;35:566–71.

56. Jones NF, Maser BM. Treatment of arthritis of the trapeziometacarpal joint with trapeziectomy and hematoma arthroplasty. Hand Clin 2001;17:237–43.

57. Diaconu M, Mathoulin C, Facca S, et al. Arthroscopic interposition arthroplasty of the trapeziometacarpal joint. Chir Main 2011;30:282–7.

58. Earp BE, Leung AC, Blazar PE, et al. Arthroscopic hemitrapeziectomy with tendon interposition for arthritis at the first carpometacarpal joint. Tech Hand Up Extrem Surg 2008;12:38–42.

59. Adams JE, Merten SM, Steinmann SP. Arthroscopic interposition arthroplasty of the first carpometacarpal joint. J Hand Surg Eur 2008;32:268–74.

60. Pegoli L, Parolo C, Ogawa T, et al. Arthroscopic evaluation and treatment by tendon interpositional arthroplasty of first carpometacarpal joint arthritis. Hand Surg 2007;12:35–9.

61. Park MJ, Lee AT, Yao J. Treatment of thumb carpometacarpal arthritis with arthroscopic hemitrapeziectomy and interposition arthroplasty. Orthopaedics 2012; 35(12):e1759–64.

62. Chuang MY, Huang CH, Lu YC, et al. Arthroscopic partial trapeziectomy and tendon interposition for thumb carpometacarpal arthritis. J Ortho Surg Res 2015;10:184.

63. Cox CA, Zlotolow DA, Yao J. Suture button suspensionplasty after arthroscopic hemitrapeziectomy for treatment of thumb carpometacarpal arthritis. Arthroscopy 2010;26(10):1395–403.

64. Yao J. Suture-button suspensionplasty for the treatment of thumb carpometacarpal joint arthritis. Hand Clin 2012;28:579–85.

65. Desmoineaux P, Delaroche C, Beaufils P. Partial arthroscopic trapeziectomy with ligament reconstruction to treat primary thumb basal joint osteoarthritis. Orthop Traumatol Surg Res 2012;98:834–9.

66. Zhang X, Wang T, Wan S. Minimally invasive thumb carpometacarpal joint arthrodesis with headless screws and arthrodesis assistance. J Hand Surg Am 2015;40(1):152–8.

67. Adams JE. Does arthroscopic debridement with or without interposition material address carpometacarpal arthritis? Clin Orthop Relat Res 2014;472: 1166–72.

68. Cobb TK, Walden AL, Cao Y. Long-term outcome of arthroscopic resection arthroplasty with or without interposition for thumb basal joint arthritis. J Hand Surg Am 2015;40:1844–51.

69. Rubino M, Civani A, Pagani D, et al. Trapeziometacarpal narrow pseudarthrosis: a new surgical technique to treat thumb carpometacarpal joint arthritis. J Hand Surg Eur 2013;38:844–50.

Arthroscopic Management of Scaphoid-Trapezium-Trapezoid Joint Arthritis

Loris Pegoli, MD*, Alessandro Pozzi, MD

KEYWORDS

- STT arthritis • Arthroscopy • Scaphoid-trapezium-trapezoid joint • Wrist • Arthritis

KEY POINTS

- Scaphoid-trapezium-trapezoid (STT) joint arthritis is a condition that can lead to hand impairment and chronic pain if untreated.
- Several solutions have been proposed, although the arthroscopic management of this condition showed advantages compared with other techniques.
- The arthroscopic management of STT joint arthritis reduces the symptoms without impairing the function of the hand for a long time.

INTRODUCTION

It is now widely accepted that the thumb constitutes the most important part of the human hand and it defines the whole function of the organ its belongs to. The scaphoid-trapezium-trapezoid (STT) joint is crucial to the proper functioning of the thumb and therefore of the hand. STT joint arthritis, although it is reported to be less common than the carpometacarpal (CMC) joint arthritis, still represents 16% of arthritis in the hand.[1] The classic clinical presentation of this condition consists of pain on the radial side of the wrist and at the base of the thumb, swelling, and tenderness over the STT joint. Limitation of the thumb range of motion due to pain can occur, especially during thumb abduction and opposition. Grip strength reduction is often present too. STT joint arthritis may be associated as well with flexor carpi radialis tenosynovitis or a palmar ganglion cyst.

Both conservative and surgical treatments have been proposed for the treatment of STT joint arthritis. The role of arthroscopic surgery in this field has constantly grown over the past decade, from being considered a mere curiosity or an adjunctive gesture to a traditional procedure to a valuable option for the management of this condition. The evident advantages to an arthroscopic approach are the reduced invasiveness, the possibility of sparing precious intracarpal ligaments, and finally the capacity to better visualize the articular surfaces.

The aim of this article is to review the arthroscopic management of the STT joint arthritis in its entirety.

SCAPHOID-TRAPEZIUM-TRAPEZOID ARTHROSCOPY FOR ARTHRITIS
Anatomy and Pathogenesis of Scaphoid-Trapezium-Trapezoid Arthritis

The STT joint consists of a complex structure that is mainly stabilized by 3 ligaments: the scaphotrapezial ligament, the scaphocapitate ligament, and the capitate-trapezium ligament.[2] In cases of partial or total failure of 1 or more of these structures,

Disclosure Statement: The authors have nothing to disclose.
Hand and Reconstructive Microsurgery Department, Humanitas Pio X Clinic, Via Francesco Nava, 31, Milano 20159, Italy
* Corresponding author.
E-mail address: info@drpegoli.com

STT arthritis develops. Continuous mechanical overload could also lead to STT arthritis. The radial artery and the sensory branches of the radial nerve pass closely to the joint and they should be spared during any surgical procedure in the area.

As happens in other circumstances (such as in the CMC joint), compressive forces and repetitive loading of the thumb produce mechanical stress and inflammatory factors released leading to ligament partial or total rupture, followed by instability, cartilage degeneration, and subchondral bone sclerosis. The most common location of degenerative changes in the scaphoid is considered the ulnar area of articular facet of the distal scaphoid.

Alteration of the fine anatomy at this level may produce joint inflammation, volar rotation of the scaphoid, and rupture of the joint capsule. All 3 events may cause synovitis of the flexor carpi radialis tendon that, as discussed previously, is often associated with STT arthritis together with volar ganglion cysts.[3]

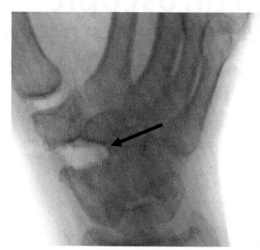

Fig. 1. Intraoperative radiograph of a right hand after an arthroscopic resection arthroplasty for STT arthritis. The arrow points toward the radial aspect of the capitate that remained intact, showing that a selective débridement has been performed.

Classification and Traditional Treatment Options

The most widely used classification for STT arthritis is the radiographic classification proposed by Crosby and colleagues,[4] who divided this pathology into 3 different stages[5]: in the first stage there are signs of arthritis without reduction of the articular space; in the second, the articular line is still visible but reduced, whereas in the last stage the articular line is not entirely visible anymore and bone scleroses, erosion, and irregularity are present. The classification also includes a stage zero where no sign of arthritis can be recognized on radiographs.

Traditionally the conservative treatments aim to reduce pain and to improve grip strength. These therapies consist of splinting, nonsteroidal anti-inflammatory drugs, and physical therapy. Usually conservative treatments have been advocated for patients who suffer from symptomatic STT arthritis in Crosby stage I or II. Conservative treatments for advanced stages can be proposed in those cases of patients declining any kind of surgical procedure or when the latter is not advisable due to the general health condition of the patient.

In cases of failure of conservative treatments or of isolated advanced symptomatic STT arthritis, surgical treatment has been previously proposed. Surgical options include silicone implants,[6] STT arthrodesis,[7,8] and resection arthroplasties,[9,10] with or without tendon or capsular interposition,[11,12] and prostheses or spacer was also suggested.[13–15] Resection arthroplasty of the STT joint (**Fig. 1**) with or without a prosthetic spacer

has been previously described by our group, by means of both open and arthroscopic surgery,[5,16] to prevent the dorsal intercalated segmental instability (DISI) deformity that might follow after resection of the distal scaphoid.

Indications and Contraindications for Scaphoid-Trapezium-Trapezoid Arthroscopy

Indications for STT arthroscopy are all the conditions where a patient is suffering from symptomatic isolated STT arthritis and there was a previously failed attempt to treat the condition conservatively for a minimum period of 2 months. The arthroscopic approach can be proposed independently of the Crosby radiographic degenerative stage.

In cases of both CMC joint arthritis and STT arthritis, the indication has to be weighed case by case. In cases of STT joint arthritis accompanied by early arthritis of the CMC joint, the indication of arthroscopy is still good and no contraindication should be present. STT arthroscopy can also be combined with CMC joint arthroscopy for the treatment of both conditions.

STT arthroscopy is, therefore, not indicated in all cases of combined severe STT and CMC joint arthritis where other more aggressive procedures may be indicated, such as trapeziectomy.

In cases of isolated STT arthritis combined with a wide scapholunate angle or in the presence of DISI, may be indicated after having completed the resection arthroplasty, to insert a pyrocarbon spacer to give more stability to the scaphoid.

Surgical Procedure

Trough an arthroscopic approach a surgeon is able to perform a diagnostic arthroscopy of the STT joint, a joint débridement, a resection arthroplasty, and finally an arthroplasty associated with an implant interposition (inserted through a small access connecting 2 arthroscopic portals).

Patients are usually treated under brachial plexus anesthesia and tourniquet control. With the thumb suspended in 2-kg to 3-kg traction in Chinese finger traps, a 2-portal approach to the STT joint is created. Both portals are located dorsally at the level of the midcarpal row—1 ulnar to the tendons of the first compartment and the other radial to the tendons of the third compartment, as described by Carro and colleagues.[17] A 1.9-mm arthroscope is strongly recommended in this case to minimize the risk of iatrogenic damage to the articular cartilage, to avoid an excessive disruption of the joint capsule and to obtain greater mobility within this small articular space.

After the scope is inserted and the portals are created, the first step is to perform a diagnostic arthroscopy of the STT joint, searching for area of chondral lesion, synovitis, and ligament rupture.

The next step of the procedure is to carefully débride any synovitis using a 2.5-mm full radius shaver to gain a better view of the joint and to evaluate the cartilage damage. In cases of severe dorso-ulnar arthritis or in presence of narrow joints, it is sometimes hard with the dorsal portal to evaluate correctly the presence of osteophytes in the ulnar side of the joint, especially in the dorsal portion. In these cases, performing a volar approach is strongly suggested.[17] This portal allows a great view of the dorso-ulnar portion of the STT joint and eventual osteophytes can be safely removed without damaging the dorsal capsule.

A resection of at least 3-mm to 4-mm of the distal pole of the scaphoid can then be performed using a 2.5-mm bur and occasionally a 3.5-mm bur. Great care must be taken to preserve as much as possible of the main ligament system of the joints, such as the scaphotrapezial and scaphocapitate ligaments, because these two are the most important to avoid a DISI deformity.[2]

In cases of an increased scapholunate angle, to prevent an increase, or again in the presence of DISI deformity, some investigators suggest that it may be necessary to insert a pyrocarbon spacer. In these cases, creating a slight slope from the radial side to the ulnar side of the bone to minimize the chance of dislocation of the implant is strongly suggested (**Fig. 2**).

In the case a DISI deformity is present or the scapholunate angle is wide, the 2 arthroscopic portal incisions can then be joined by a small transverse incision and the appropriate size prosthesis can be chosen with the help of a template and then placed into the STT space. Intraoperative testing to assess the proper positioning and stability of the spacer can be performed without traction.

Postoperative Protocol

The postoperative rehabilitation protocol is described as follows: the same day as or the day after the surgical procedure, a static thermoplastic removable splint, which includes the wrist and the metacarpophalangeal joint of the thumb, can be applied (**Fig. 3**). The splint has to be worn continuously for 3 weeks during which time the patient is instructed to perform active exercises to control

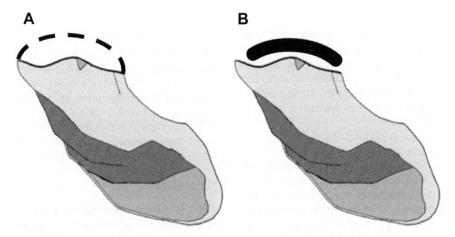

A   **B**

Fig. 2. Drawing of the scaphoid from an anterior perspective. (A) The dotted line should represent the original anatomic profile of the distal pole of the scaphoid that has been gently removed during the arthroscopic arthroplasty of the STT joint. The area on the distal and ulnar aspect of the distal pole of the scaphoid has been removed (B) to allocate the pyrocarbon spacer and give it more stability.

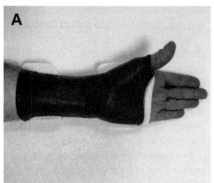
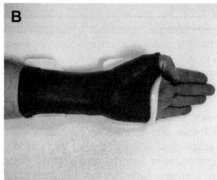

Fig. 3. (*A*) The pictures show the postoperative cast that should be applied after an arthroscopic arthroplasty of the STT joint. (*B*) Note the interphalangeal joint of the thumb has been left free to allow tendon gliding and to promote a safe early recovery of the hand function.

edema. This exercise includes long finger flexion–extension exercise and flexion–extension of the interphalangeal joint of the thumb. At 3 weeks after the surgery, a removable splint, which is similar to that described previously, is applied and gentle active and passive mobilization of the base of the thumb and wrist is allowed. Strengthening exercises are started at 4 weeks postoperative. On average, the removable splint can be used for an additional 3 weeks.

RESULTS

Conservative treatment rarely is successful for the treatment of STT arthritis due to the difficulty in isolating this joint with a splint, and painkillers cannot be considered a solution in the long term. Arthritis of the STT joint is an often asymptomatic condition that can lead, in its advanced stages, to an important impairment of hand function and, therefore, should be treated as soon as it is diagnosed.

For the treatment of STT arthritis in stage I, the arthroscopic approach is considered the best option, because it allows removal of all the inflammatory tissue that is present inside the articular space as well providing a possibility of removing osteophytes without damaging the intracarpal ligaments. It is also possible to perform a ligament shrinkage if necessary.

The possible solutions for STT arthritis at stages II and III, the main alternative to a resection arthroplasty is the STT arthrodesis that is related to a high rate of nonunion, and great care must be taken in the proper positioning of the bones (especially the scaphoid); it often needs a secondary surgical procedure for fixation removal.[18] After such a procedure, the radioscaphoid joint could also develop secondary arthritis.

Due to the fact that it does not lead to secondary arthritis, the resection of the scaphoid distal pole, which allows prompt pain relief and a fast return to normal activities, can on the contrary be considered the best solution at present for STT arthritis. Usually, the STT joint resection arthroplasty is performed with a traditional open approach.[19] The traditional procedure is simple and reliable but does not give the same view as the arthroscopic one, cannot be considered minimally invasive, and is more disruptive on the intracarpal ligaments. These are the reasons that suggest that the arthroscopic approach for STT arthritis should be considered the best option.

From recent studies, the long-term results of the traditional arthroplasty approach and those of the arthroscopic approach are similar, but data suggest that the short-term results are better for the arthroscopic approach. It also seems that arthroscopy allows performing a better resection of the distal pole of the scaphoid, especially on the anterior portion that cannot be well visualized during a traditional open arthroplasty procedure.

The choice between simple resection arthroplasty and association with an implant interposition is debated. There is no clinical evidence at the moment that the implant is always necessary but it seems that in those cases of signs of scapholunate instability prior to surgery (such as widening of the S-L angle or the presence of DISI), the implant is required to improve the stability of the scaphoid, reduce the DISI, and slow down the radiocarpal joint degeneration.

SUMMARY

There is enough evidence to support that patients affected by STT arthritis who have been operated with joint arthroplasty showed better results in terms of pain reduction, strength recovery, and wrist motion compared with their performances before the surgery.

The arthroscopic approach has better results in the short term compared with the traditional approach, mainly due to lower invasiveness. Another advantage is that in this way, there is more selectivity in the scaphoid distal pole resection and the ligaments that provide stability to this particular joint are spared in the process.

The arthroscopic approach is not used as widely as it should be in this field, mainly because the indications are rare compared with other hand districts, such as the CMC joint or the radiocarpal joint, and the STT joint arthroscopy is often considered an advanced technique; therefore, many surgeons do not receive enough training in this field.

Moreover, as often happens in such a small and specific field, data are outdated or the studies that have been published do not include series large enough to obtain statistical relevance. Finally, it is strongly suggested to approach STT arthritis arthroscopically for all the reasons discussed previously.

ACKNOWLEDGMENTS

The authors would like to thank Judy Chang for editing this article.

REFERENCES

1. Scordino LE, Bernstein J, Nakashian M, et al. Radiographic prevalence of scaphotrapeziotrapezoid osteoarthrosis. J Hand Surg Am 2014;39(9): 1677–82.

2. Moritomo H, Viegas SF, Nakamura K, et al. The scaphotrapezio-trapezoidal joint. Part 1: an anatomic and radiographic study. J Hand Surg Am 2000;25(5): 899–910, 19.

3. Parellada AJ, Morrison WB, Reiter SB, et al. Flexor carpi radialis tendinopathy: spectrum of imaging findings and association with triscaphe arthritis. Skeletal Radiol 2006;35(8):572–8.

4. Crosby B, Linscheid R, Dobyns H, et al. Traiment de l'arthrose isole de l'arthrose scapotrapezotrapezoi-dienne. J Hand Surg 1978;3:223–34 [in French].

5. Pegoli L, Pozzi A, Pivato G, et al. Arthroscopic resection of distal pole of the scaphoid for scaphotrapeziotrapezoid joint arthritis: comparison between simple resection and implant interposition. J Wrist Surg 2016;5(3):227–32.

6. Kessler I, Baruch A, Hecht O, et al. Osteoarthritis of the base of the thumb. Acta Orthop Scand 1976;47: 361–9.

7. Watson HK. Scaphotrapeziotrapezoid arthrodesis for arthritis. J Hand Surg Am 1988;13:66–77.

8. Wollstein R, Watson HK. Scaphotrapeziotrapezoid arthrodesis for arthritis [review]. Hand Clin 2005; 21(4):539–43, vi.

9. Meier R, Prommersberger KJ, Krimmer H. Scaphotrapezio-trapezoid arthrodesis (triscaphe arthrodesis). Handchir Mikrochir Plast Chir 2003;35(5): 323–7 [in German].

10. Linscheid RL, Lirette R, Dobin JH. L'artrose degenerative scaphotrapezienne. In: Saffar P, editor. La rizoarthrose (monographies du GEM). Paris: Expansion Scientifique Francaise; 1990. p. 185–94 [in French].

11. Garcia-Elias M, Lluch A, Ferreres A. Treatment of scaphotrapeziotrapezoid arthrosisby distal scaphoid resection and capsular interposition arthroplasty. In: Dunitz M, editor. Current practice in hand surgery. 1997;vol. 29. p. 181–5.

12. Da Rin F, Mathoulin C. Traitement arthroscopique de l'arthrose scapotrapezotrapezoidienne (STT). [Arthroscopic treatment of osteoarthritis of scapho-trapezotrapezoid joint]. Chir Main 2006;25(Suppl 1):S254–8 [in French].

13. Wolf JM. Treatment of scaphotrapezio-trapezoid arthritis. Hand Clin 2008;24(3):301–6.

14. Pequignot JP, D'asnieres de Veigy L, Allieu Y. Arthroplasty for scaphotrapeziotrapezoidal arthrosis using a pyrolytic carbon implant. Preliminary results. Chir Main 2005;24(3–4):148–52 [in French].

15. Low AK, Edmunds IA. Isolated scaphotrapeziotrapezoid osteoarthritis: preliminary results of treatment using a pyrocarbon implant. Hand Surg 2007;12(2): 73–7.

16. Pegoli L, Zorli IP, Pivato G, et al. Scaphotrapeziotrapezoid joint arthritis: a pilot study of treatment with the scaphoid trapezium pyrocarbon implant. J Hand Surg Br 2006;31(5):569–73.

17. Carro LP, Golano P, Fariñas O, et al. The radial portal for scaphotrapeziotrapezoid arthroscopy. Arthroscopy 2003;19(5):547–53.

18. Watson HK, Wollenstein R, Joseph E, et al. Scaphotrapeziotrapezoid arthrodesis: a follow-up study. J Hand Surg 2003;28A:397–404.

19. Garcia-Elias M. Excisional arthroplasty for scaphotrapeziotrapezoidal osteoarthritis. J Hand Surg Am 2011;36(3):516–20.

Progress and Role of Finger Joint Arthroscopy

Isato Sekiya, MD, PhD[a],*, Masaaki Kobayashi, MD, PhD[b], Hideki Okamoto, MD, PhD[b], Takanobu Otsuka, MD, PhD[b]

KEYWORDS

- Finger joint arthroscopy • Metacarpophalangeal joint • Proximal interphalangeal joint
- Distal interphalangeal joint

KEY POINTS

- Arthroscopy of finger joints provides more precise information regarding the status of the intra-articular structures than alternative imaging modalities.
- Because the metacarpophalangeal joint is suitable for arthroscopic surgery, many attempts to treat various conditions, such as arthritis, intra-articular fractures, and ligament injuries, have been reported.
- There are technical limitations in arthroscopy and arthroscopic surgery in the proximal interphalangeal and distal interphalangeal joints, because the joint cavity is very small.
- The arthroscope and instruments should be manipulated gently to avoid iatrogenic cartilage damage and slippage out of the joint.

INTRODUCTION

Arthroscopy is useful for the evaluation and treatment of intra-articular disorders and causes minimal surgical trauma. It is the gold standard for the assessment of articular cartilage, synovium, and ligaments of large joints. Upper extremity arthroscopy has been used mostly in the shoulder, elbow, wrist joints, and carpometacarpal joint of the thumb.

Arthroscopy for finger joints was first described by Chen[1] in 1979, and the standard technique for this method was established. However, few attempts at metacarpophalangeal (MCP), proximal interphalangeal (PIP) and distal interphalangeal (DIP) joint arthroscopy have been made since that time, because it requires a specially designed small arthroscope and instruments. Arthroscopy is not essential for the diagnosis of most finger joint disorders, and its therapeutic use in finger joint has not yet been established.

This article discusses the role and surgical techniques of finger joint arthroscopy.

INSTRUMENTS

Specially designed small arthroscopes and instruments are necessary for arthroscopic surgery in finger joints because the joint cavity is very small.

Small Joint Arthroscope

A review of the literature reveals reports using various sizes and types of arthroscopes. Arthroscopes 1.9 mm in diameter are most commonly used,[2–17] although others with diameters of 1.7,[18,19] 2.0,[20] 2.2,[21] 2.3,[22] and 2.5 mm[23] have also been reported. There were 2 reports using a

Conflicts of Interest: The authors declare no conflicts of interest in association with this article.
[a] Department of Orthopaedic Surgery, Kainan Hospital, The Aichi Prefectural Federation of Agricultural Cooperative for Health and Welfare, 396, Minamihonden, Maegasu-cho, Yatomi, Aichi 498-8502, Japan; [b] Department of Orthopaedic Surgery, Graduate School of Medical Sciences, Nagoya City University, 1 Kawasumi, Mizuho-cho, Mizuho-ku, Nagoya 467-8601, Japan
* Corresponding author.
E-mail address: i_sekiya@yahoo.co.jp

1.0-mm needle arthroscope for biopsy and staging procedures.[4,24] The authors use a 1.5-mm arthroscope at our facility (**Fig. 1**).[25,26]

Shaver System

The 2.0-mm shaver cutter[2,5,7,9,12–14,17–19,27] has been used most often, although others with diameters of 1.9,[20] 2.5,[22,23] 2.9,[3] and 3.0 mm[18] have also been used. The authors use a shaver system with a 2.5-mm full-radius cutter for synovectomy at our facility (see **Fig. 1**).[25,26]

Grasping Forceps

Although synovial biopsy samples are obtained with a grasping forceps,[2,4,6,15,24] there were no reports describing the details of grasping forceps. The authors have been using miniforceps for biopsies and the removal of foreign bodies at our facility (see **Fig. 1**).[25,26]

Radiofrequency Probes

For the treatment of shoulder instability, thermal shrinkage is commonly used. Although the authors have no experience with using radiofrequency probes in finger joints, there have been several reports using radiofrequency probes for synovectomy and thermal shrinkage of the MCP joint capsule.[8–10,12–14,17]

Traction Apparatus

In the early reports, no articles mentioned any finger traction apparatus, and the hand and arm were placed on the operating table horizontally.[1,18,20] Traction with a Chinese finger trap was first described by Declercq and colleagues[2] in 1994. The hand was hung up in a finger trap, with the weight of the hand and arm alone providing sufficient traction. Ryu and Fagan[19]

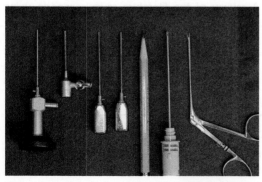

Fig. 1. Instruments for small joint arthroscopy and arthroscopic surgery. From left to right: arthroscope, arthroscope sheath, semiblunt and blunt trocars, shaver cutter, and grasping forceps.

also reported that a wrist tower and finger trap were used to suspend the hand vertically, with the weight of the arm serving as traction. A finger trap made of plastic is preferred to one of metal for maximizing the patient's comfort.

Traction tension applied per digit was first mentioned in 1999.[3,22,23] Recently, there have been many reports of the affected digit being suspended with a finger trap using a traction device with 2.3 to 5.5 kg (5–12 lb) of tension: 2.3 kg (5 lb),[7,23] 2.3 to 3.6 kg (5–8 lb),[27] 2.3 to 4.5 kg (5–10 lb),[11] 2.5 to 4.5 kg (5.5–10 lb),[13] 3.6 kg (8 lb),[3] 3.6 to 5.5 kg (8–12 lb),[22] 4.5 kg (10 lb),[10] and 5.0 kg (11 lb).[17]

When finger traps provide poor traction, Slade and Gutow[22] advocate the placement of a transfixing Kirschner wire through the phalanx to secure the finger trap to the finger. For this technique, after the finger trap is applied, a single 0.9-mm (0.035-inch) Kirschner wire is drilled through the phalanx under radiographic guidance.

Fluid Management System

Berner[10] described a fluid management system in which an arthroscopic fluid pump is used to facilitate fluid management, provided a low-pressure setting is used. However, he has not found this necessary, because the volume of the joint is small, and a pressure bag system using a 1-L bag of saline solution at 100 mm Hg has proved adequate. The authors have no experience in using a fluid management system, and continuous injection by an assistant is sufficient to obtain good visualization when needed.

GENERAL TECHNIQUE
Anesthesia

Although regional or general anesthesia has been reported often in such procedures, there seems to be no strong reason to perform anesthesia instead of a digital block. Although a tourniquet applied either to the upper arm or on the digit should be used in most cases, all procedures can be performed on an outpatient basis under axillary block, wrist block, digital block, or local anesthesia.

Portals

For MCP, PIP, and DIP joints, the portals from both the radial and ulnar side to the central extensor tendon were established by Chen.[1] Two dorsal portals were developed for each joint (**Fig. 2**). The dorsal joint line is located by palpation for all joints, and by inspection of 2 depressions

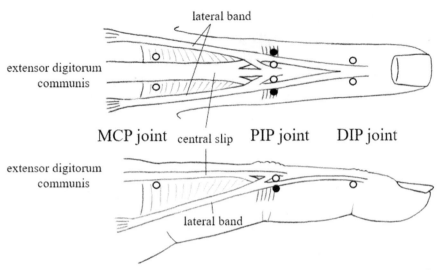

Fig. 2. Arthroscopic approaches in the MCP, PIP, and DIP joints. Dorsal portal (○) proposed by Chen[1], and dorsal-lateral portal (●) proposed by the authors.[25] (*Courtesy of* I. Sekiya, MD, PhD, Yatomi, Aichi, Japan.)

alongside the central extensor tendon under manual traction for the MCP joints.

For arthroscopy of PIP joints, Chen[1] advocated the portals between the central slip and the lateral bands. The same portals were used by Johnson.[21] However, the authors established new portals of PIP joints on the dorsal-lateral aspect.[25,26] These new portals were applied from both the radial and ulnar positions to the lateral bands of the extensor mechanism, which is more lateral than previous portals described by Chen[1] and allows for the observation of the entire joint cavity.

Standard Surgical Procedure

The patient is positioned supine with the shoulder abducted, the arm positioned horizontally, with or without suspension of the affected finger using a traction device and a finger trap at the surgeon's preference.

A 25-gauge needle was first introduced into the dorsal joint cavity, and 2 mL or less of normal saline solution were then injected to expand the joint. Two small, longitudinal skin incisions, 2 to 3 mm in length, were made with a no. 11 blade. Care should be taken not to injure the terminal branches of the nerve during the procedure. Subcutaneous tissue was dissected with a blunt trocar or a mosquito clamp after skin incision. An arthroscopic sheath with a semiblunt trocar was used to open the joint capsule and was inserted into the dorsal joint cavity using gentle pressure, avoiding damage to the articular surfaces. Inflow with normal saline solution through the arthroscopic sheath or a 20-gauge or 22-gauge needle introduced through the dorsal extensor tendon was established, and

the arthroscope was then placed into the joint (**Figs. 3** and **4**). If an outflow tract is necessary, a large-bore needle may be introduced, or a shaver may be used to evacuate excess fluid.

A comprehensive inspection of the intra-articular structures in the joint is performed. Magnified observation of the articular cartilage, synovial membrane, and collateral ligaments is possible (**Figs. 5** and **6**). However, immediately after arthroscope insertion, the articular cartilage could not be visualized in patients with an inflamed hypertrophic synovium, because severely hypertrophic synovial tissue blocked the view of the arthroscope. To obtain good visualization, an assistant continuously injected saline solution into the cavity while the operator held the arthroscope to maintain adequate distention of the joint cavity. It may also be necessary to debride excess synovial tissue in order to visualize the articular cartilage

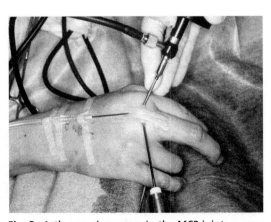

Fig. 3. Arthroscopic surgery in the MCP joint.

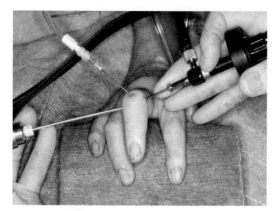

Fig. 4. Arthroscopic surgery in the PIP joint.

and the ligaments using the shaver cutter introduced via another portal. The portals for the arthroscope and instruments were interchanged to allow inspection of the entire joint.

For MCP joints, the joint space was able to be expanded with finger traction, thereby allowing insertion of the arthroscope and instruments into the palmar joint cavity. However, because the joint space of the PIP joints was not wide enough to insert the arthroscope into the palmar cavity, the palmar portion of the articular cartilage and the volar synovium could not be inspected.

The arthroscope and instruments should be moved gently to avoid injury and slippage out of the joint because the joint cavity is very small, making it difficult to handle the arthroscope and instruments. Wei and colleagues[3] described a pencil-grip position using the tip of the arthroscopist's middle finger as a guide/fulcrum to overcome this problem.

After arthroscopy, each portal is closed with 1 suture or sterile strip.

Authors' Preferred Methods

A traction apparatus is not necessary for arthroscopy and arthroscopic synovectomy in PIP and MCP joints. For PIP joint arthroscopy, because the interval between the head of the proximal phalanx and the base of the middle phalanx is narrow and cannot be expanded, the volar joint space cannot be accessed, even with strong traction force. With MCP joint arthroscopy, the joint space can be expanded, making it possible to insert the arthroscope and instruments into the palmar joint cavity with finger traction. However, synovectomy of the palmar capsule was difficult to perform, because handling the instruments in the palmar cavity can damage the articular surfaces. Limited operative arthroscopy and arthroscopic synovectomy in the dorsal joint cavity can be performed easily without traction. Gentle manual traction is applied on the finger by the assistant when inspection of the articular surfaces is required. Thomsen and colleagues[5] also used the same technique for PIP joint arthroscopy, which allowed for free movement of the PIP joint.

In addition to this, the authors recommend arthroscopy with the finger positioned horizontally, as performed by Wilkes.[18] The patient was placed in a supine position with the shoulder abducted, the arm positioned horizontally, and the forearm pronated on the operating table. Whether the finger should be positioned horizontally or vertically is a matter of habit, and arthroscopy of the finger joint should be performed using a well-practiced method. Hidalgo-Diaz and colleagues[16] compared the advantages and disadvantages of horizontal versus vertical traction. Because the setup time and the tourniquet time were shorter and ergonomics better, they concluded that MCP joint arthroscopy may be best performed with horizontal traction.

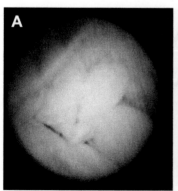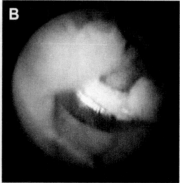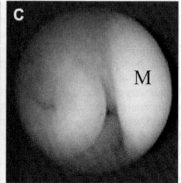

Fig. 5. Arthroscopic images of the MCP joint. (*A*) Synovial villus proliferation in the dorsal capsule. (*B*) Arthroscopic synovectomy using a shaver cutter. (*C*) Metacarpal head (M) and synovial villus.

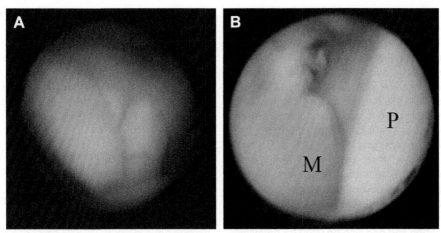

Fig. 6. Arthroscopic images of the PIP joint. (*A*) Synovial villus proliferation in the dorsal capsule. (*B*) The head of the proximal phalanx (P) and middle phalanx (M).

INDICATIONS AND DETAILS FOR EACH CLINICAL CONDITION
Metacarpophalangeal Joint Arthroscopy

The MCP joint is suitable for arthroscopy and arthroscopic surgery, and many attempts have been reported. Because the joint space can be expanded, allowing insertion of the arthroscope and instruments into the palmar joint cavity, most of the synovium in the dorsal and volar joint capsule and radial and ulnar recesses and the entire articular surfaces of both the metacarpal and the proximal phalanx are visualized. However, there remains a blind and inaccessible area: the palmar joint cavity between the volar plate and the volar aspect of the metacarpal head.

Inflammatory arthritis
Arthroscopy is useful for the evaluation, staging, and treatment of inflammatory arthritis. Synovectomy of the dorsal capsule under visual control can be performed with a shaver system or a radiofrequency probe using the 2-portal technique (see **Figs. 3** and **5**). If a biopsy of the synovial tissue is required, it can be readily obtained from the dorsal joint capsule under visual guidance through standard portals with grasping forceps. The biopsy sample size is sufficient for a histologic examination.

Pyogenic arthritis
In cases of septic arthritis, irrigation and debridement of septic MCP joint are easily accomplished with the arthroscope and a shaver.[27] Cultures can be obtained by sampling the initial aspirate. A large volume of normal saline can be passed through the joint by running the shaver in the joint space while connecting the inflow to a wide-open source of fluid.

Degenerative arthritis
Shin and Osterman[12] described arthroscopic debridement and synovectomy of the MCP joint. In patients who have mild osteoarthritis or synovitis of the MCP joint, arthroscopic synovectomy using the 2-portal technique permits a diagnostic and therapeutic approach. An arthroscopic evaluation helps to determine the location and extent of cartilage lesions and also provides an opportunity to determine whether treatment should be performed by debridement of loose cartilage or thermal capsulorrhaphy or other means.

Intra-articular fractures
Fractures involving the articular surfaces and supporting subchondral bone of the MCP joint can be assessed and treated with an arthroscopically assisted approach.

Arthroscopic reduction and internal fixation for avulsion fracture at the MCP joint were reported by Badia.[7] A 2.0-mm full-radius shaver is initially used to remove any hematoma or minute fragments. Aggressive synovectomy is then performed to more clearly delineate the avulsed fracture fragment. The probe is inserted through the portal, and the fragment is hooked with gentle traction leading to reduction. The shaver can be inserted into the fracture site for debridement and assists in achieving adequate reduction without step-off. A 0.9-mm (0.035-inch) Kirschner wire is manually introduced into the joint just proximal to the bony fragment that has been reduced. The arthroscopic view confirms the tip of the wire in the proper position. Once in place and manually held, the Kirschner wire is drilled through the phalanx under fluoroscopic guidance. Both fluoroscopy and arthroscopy are used to determine the quality of fragment reduction as well as to confirm proper wire placement and stability. The wire is cut just underneath the skin, and a bulky splint is applied. Final fluoroscopic pictures are taken and the tourniquet is released.

Arthroscopically assisted reduction of metacarpal head fracture was reported by Choi and colleagues.[13] MCP joint arthroscopy can be used for direct visualization to achieve anatomic reduction of the intra-articular fracture fragment. The fracture was temporarily fixed with a 0.9-mm Kirschner wire and then fixed with 2 absorbable pins in a retrograde manner. After surgery, the patient was placed in a bulky dressing for 1 to 2 days and then allowed free mobilization as tolerated.

Kirschner wires may be used as joysticks to assist reduction and can also be used for definitive fixation.[10] Depending on the fracture pattern and surgeon's preference, it may be possible to use a small conventional screw or a headless screw.

Removal of loose bodies
Removal of loose body using a grasping forceps and shaver under visual guidance was easily accomplished through standard portals in the MCP joints.

Collateral ligament injury
Treatment of an ulnar collateral ligament tear also has been managed arthroscopically. In the thumb, reduction of Stener lesions has been reported by Ryu and Fagan.[19] A small probe, inserted through the radial portal, was introduced along the metacarpal head, passed through the proximal edge of the aponeurosis around the anticipated origin site of the ulnar collateral ligament, and pulled toward the joint. This maneuver, which may be repeated if necessary, brings the distal end of the ulnar collateral ligament inside the joint. After the ligament's end was placed at its point of proximal phalangeal base insertion, a Kirschner wire was inserted to immobilize the MCP joint in a 20° to 30° flexed position. Good results from immobilization with a cast for 4 weeks without insertion of a Kirschner wire were also reported by Choi and colleagues.[13]

Chronic pain and instability
Persistent pain despite ample conservative treatment in the MCP joint injury is an indication for arthroscopy.[9] An arthroscopic evaluation determines the location and extent of injury and gives an opportunity to provide treatment, by simple debridement and/or thermal capsulorrhaphy. Occult pain often associated with chronic swelling may be another indication.[9] This pain may be from an unrecognized injury, early presentation of osteoarthrosis, or an idiopathic synovitis. Arthroscopy is performed after conservative treatment fails, providing precise information about the intra-articular structures. Arthroscopic debridement is easily performed with a shaver system using the 2-portal technique. The use of a radiofrequency probe to induce thermal shrinkage of the joint capsule, especially the volar plate structure, can relieve the symptoms in patients with capsular laxity and joint instability.[13,17]

Stiff fingers
MCP joint stiffness in fingers may be disabling. Choi and colleagues[13] selectively performed an arthroscopic release of a stiff MCP joint in 2 cases caused by prolonged immobilization in an extended position with a subsequent loss of flexion. Intra-articular fibrosis was removed arthroscopically, and limited extensor tenolysis was performed through the dorsal portals.

Proximal Interphalangeal Joint Arthroscopy

Arthroscopy of the PIP joint has not been widely accepted as a useful technique because of the restricted number of indications caused by the technical limitations. Because the joint space of PIP joints was not wide enough to insert the arthroscope into the palmar cavity, the palmar portion of articular cartilage and the volar synovium could not be inspected. The indications for PIP joint arthroscopy are essentially the same as those for the MCP joint.

Inflammatory arthritis
Arthroscopy is useful for the evaluation, staging, and treatment of inflammatory arthritis, even in PIP joints. Synovectomy of the dorsal capsule under visual control can be performed with a shaver system using the 2-portal technique (see **Figs. 4** and **6**).[25,26] A synovial biopsy from the dorsal joint capsule using grasping forceps can be performed under visual guidance through standard portals, and the biopsy sample size is sufficient for a histologic examination.

Pyogenic arthritis
In cases of septic arthritis, irrigation and debridement of the septic PIP joint are easily accomplished with an arthroscope and a shaver.[27] Cultures can be obtained by sampling the initial aspirate. A large volume of normal saline can be passed through the joint by running the shaver in the joint space while connecting the inflow to a wide-open source of fluid.

Removal of foreign bodies
Removal of foreign bodies under visual guidance can be performed with grasping forceps and a shaver using the 2-portal technique. There is 1

report of a 1.5-mm metal splinter being removed using a 2.0-mm shaver.[5]

Distal Interphalangeal Joint Arthroscopy

Only 2 attempts at DIP joint arthroscopy have been reported.

Arthritis

Chen[1] performed arthroscopy for gouty arthritis of the DIP joint. He reported that, after repeated irrigation with normal saline solution, necrotic villi with whitish crystals on the tips and crystal masses in the joint space became visible.

Arthrodesis

Arthrodesis of the DIP joint of the fingers or interphalangeal joint of the thumb is indicated for pain, deformity, or instability. Common causes include posttraumatic joint deformity, degenerative osteoarthritis, and chronic tendon injury. Cobb[11] presented an arthroscopic technique for arthrodesis using a headless screw. The digit is suspended with finger trap traction and secured with a 0.9-mm (0.035-inch) Kirschner wire through the distal phalanx. Between 2.3 and 4.5 kg (5–10 lb) of traction is applied. After the collateral ligaments are released through longitudinal incisions (5–6 mm in length) placed over the medial and lateral sides of the joint, an elevator is placed into the joint, which is opened enough to create a working space. An arthroscope and a shaver are then inserted into the joint, and the joint is cleared of debris, allowing visualization. Next, a hooded bur is brought into the joint, and 1 to 2 mm of bone is removed from the proximal and distal sides of the joints. The amount of bone resection is assessed visually through the scope and with the aid of fluoroscopy. After resection of the joint, the traction devices are removed. A longitudinal guidewire is then placed in the central axis under fluoroscopic control. A cannulated drill is used to drill across the DIP joint, followed by the placement of a headless screw (a mini-Acutrak screw).

POSSIBLE COMPLICATIONS
Articular Cartilage Damage

Iatrogenic injury to the articular surfaces occurs easily without gentle handling of the arthroscope and instruments. The arthroscopic sheath with a semiblunt trocar should be used to open the joint capsule, and insertion into the dorsal joint cavity should be performed using gentle pressure, avoiding damage to the articular surfaces. Intra-articular manipulation may injure the cartilage, because the joint cavity is very small. Shaver blades should not be turned toward the cartilage, and sharp

instruments should not be used in the narrow joint space. The arthroscope and instruments should be moved gently to avoid cartilage damage. A pencil-grip position using the tip of the arthroscopist's middle finger as a guide/fulcrum, as described by Wei and colleagues,[3] overcomes this problem.

Tendon Injuries

Because of the proximity to the portals, the extensor tendon is at risk of damage. To avoid damage to the extensor tendon, care should be taken while inserting instruments through the portals and performing synovectomy with a shaver or a radiofrequency probe.

Choi and colleagues[13] reported a case of flexor pollicis longus rupture 3 weeks after thermal shrinkage of the volar plate. The flexor tendon is prone to damage by indirect thermal injury when using the radiofrequency probes, because it is located adjacent to the volar recess. They mentioned that several precautions are needed when using a radiofrequency probe:

1. Intermittent transmission of radiofrequency signal should be used, instead of a continuous long duration of transmission.
2. Continuous flow of irrigation fluid should be used.

These precautions avoid overheating the surrounding structures, especially the flexor tendon and the neurovascular bundles, which are in close proximity to the volar capsule.

Neurovascular Bundle Injuries

The terminal branches of the nerve may be damaged, causing either sensory dysfunction or painful neuroma. Therefore, incisions should be restricted to the skin alone.[5] Subcutaneous tissue is dissected with a blunt trocar or a mosquito clamp to expose the joint capsule.

The digital neurovascular bundles are close to the volar recesses. Therefore, they are prone to indirect thermal injury by the radiofrequency probes.[13] Close attention must be paid when using the radiofrequency probes in the volar joint space. The use of portal-site local anesthesia without a tourniquet helps preserve intact sensation of the finger during the surgery, providing useful feedback from the patient on any impaling injury to the neurovascular bundle.

ROLE OF FINGER JOINT ARTHROSCOPY

Because the MCP joint is suitable for arthroscopy and arthroscopic surgery, many attempts at finger joint arthroscopy have been reported. However, there are technical limitations in arthroscopy and arthroscopic surgery in the PIP and DIP joints.

Arthritis

Compared with alternative imaging modalities, arthroscopy provides more precise information regarding the status of the articular cartilage, which may aid in planning future procedures.

Rheumatoid arthritis

Rheumatoid arthritis is characterized by an inflamed, hypertrophic synovium that causes destruction of cartilage and ligaments. Obtaining tissue samples from affected joints might improve understanding of the disease. Because small finger joints are mostly involved in the early stages of rheumatoid arthritis, blind biopsies using needle equipment have been performed in finger joints. However, arthroscopically guided biopsies of the dominantly affected finger joint are useful because this technique is minimally invasive, provides tissue samples from areas of special interest with the highest inflammation, and decreases the risk of sampling errors.[4]

Recent rapid developments in immunology, molecular biology, and biotechnology have led to a dramatic increase in the number of new targeted therapies for rheumatoid arthritis, and serial synovial biopsy samples are increasingly being used for the evaluation of novel therapies. Kraan and colleagues[6] compared synovial biopsy samples from knee joints with those from paired wrist or MCP joints and concluded that the inflammation in one inflamed joint is generally representative of that in other inflamed joints, and, therefore, it is possible to use serial samples from the same joint, selecting either large or small joints, for the evaluation of antirheumatic therapies. Vordenbaumen and colleagues[15] also discussed this issue and concluded that some histologic findings in arthroscopically guided biopsies of the dominantly affected MCP joint reflect global disease activity measures and their changes in patients with rheumatoid arthritis. Furthermore, repeated MCP synovial biopsies may distinguish true responders from individuals with residual disease activity, who are otherwise not readily recognized by clinical means.

Synovectomy for the treatment of rheumatoid arthritis has been widely performed, and a large number of studies have evaluated this technique. Progressive joint synovitis that stretches the capsule, ligamentous structures, and the extensor mechanism in the MCP and PIP joints results in typical rheumatoid finger deformity. Therefore, excision of hypertrophic synovium has been thought to be effective in the relief of symptoms and in the prevention or delay of aggravation of irreversible damage to the joint. Recently, remarkable advances in the medical treatment of rheumatoid arthritis have been achieved, and the disease can be controlled with medication in most patients. However, inflammatory synovium remains resistant to medication in some patients; thus, synovectomy remains an important treatment option in these cases.

The use of open synovectomy remains controversial, because studies have yielded contradictory results. Thompson and colleagues[28] reported the 2-year follow-up results of a controlled trial of synovectomy of MCP joints in patients with rheumatoid arthritis and observed significant and sustained improvement with respect to clinical symptoms and function. In contrast, the results of controlled trials of MCP joint synovectomy in the United Kingdom[29] were discouraging, with no marked differences noted between synovectomized and control MCP joints at 1-year, 2-year, and 3-year follow-up, as determined both clinically and roentgenologically. Furthermore, a multicenter study in the United States[30,31] reported no evidence of benefit in MCP or PIP joints at 3-year follow-up or over a period of 5 years after surgery. Despite these results, minimally invasive excision of hypertrophic synovium of the small joints in the hand should result in a better outcome than synovectomy performed using open surgical methods.

In 1987, Wilkes[18] first described arthroscopic synovectomy of MCP joints in rheumatoid arthritis, with successful results. In 1999, Wei and colleagues[3] reported this technique in detail and concluded that it could be performed safely and effectively. The authors[25] also described rheumatoid synovectomy in MCP and PIP joints under arthroscopic visualization in 2002, and this was the first description of arthroscopic synovectomy of PIP joints in rheumatoid patients. Our assessment[26] at a mean follow-up of 84 months revealed that approximately 20% of joints showed slight swelling; however, the swelling was not as severe as that before synovectomy. Although only limited operative arthroscopy is possible with this technique, swelling of each joint disappeared after the procedure and did not return for a long period in the other 80% of joints. Furthermore, no joints required reoperation (**Fig. 7**). Thomsen and colleagues[5] also reported the use of this technique in a single PIP joint during the same period.

Synovectomy is performed in the patients with rheumatoid arthritis who have not responded to standard medical treatment. The most favorable indications for arthroscopic synovectomy are

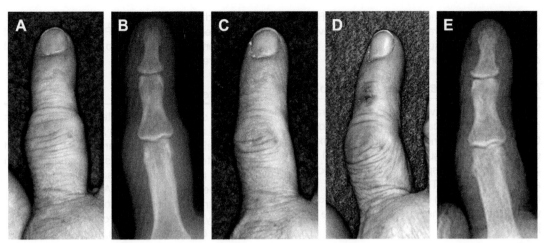

Fig. 7. A 50-year-old woman with rheumatoid arthritis. Arthroscopic synovectomy of the PIP joint in the right index finger was performed. (*A, B*) Before the operation. (*C*) Ten months after the operation. (*D, E*) Ten years after the operation. Swelling of the PIP joint disappeared after the procedure and did not return for 10 years. Destruction of the articular surfaces was prevented.

sustained joint swelling without finger deformity and radiographic changes of grade 2 or less according to the system of Larsen and colleagues.[32]

If progressive finger deformity and dysfunction are present, arthroscopic treatment neither corrects the deformity nor improves the function. A variety of surgical procedures are recommended to correct such deformity. Synovectomy is useful, with short-term improvement in symptoms. However, long-term benefits have not yet been established.[10]

Degenerative arthritis

Although the role of finger joint arthroscopy is not established in patients with osteoarthritis, no other diagnostic or imaging modalities provide accurate, detailed information about the location and extent of cartilage lesions. An arthroscopic evaluation helps to determine the location and extent of cartilage lesions and also helps physicians decide treatment.

In the earliest stages of osteoarthritis, arthroscopic debridement may be the best option if symptoms recur despite adequate conservative treatment.[9] However, there are no established guidelines outlining a treatment algorithm for degenerative arthritis.[10,14]

Pyogenic arthritis

Incision, drainage, and the administration of antibiotics are important treatments for pyogenic arthritis. Irrigation with a large volume of normal saline and debridement of septic MCP and PIP joints are easily accomplished using the arthroscope and a shaver system with minimal surgical trauma.[27]

Intra-articular Fractures

Among several internal fixation techniques suggested for intra-articular fractures at the MCP joint, arthroscopy-assisted reduction and percutaneous fixation of the avulsed fragment have various advantages compared with open reduction.[7] Using this technique, there is no need to violate the joint capsule to achieve reduction, so the rehabilitation period can be shortened. Total surgical and tourniquet times are shorter than with open reduction, and less scarring is involved, improving the cosmetic appearance without sacrificing the function or stability as the main goals of the surgical procedure. In addition, a thorough assessment of the entire joint surface prevents any residual articular step-off.

Collateral Ligament Injury

Most ligament injuries of the MCP joints are treated well with closed means. However, as in the Stener lesion, the distally avulsed collateral ligament is displaced and trapped under the free proximal edge of the extensor hood, so nonoperative treatment yields unpredictable results.[19] Although injury to the ulnar collateral ligament of the thumb is the most common injury associated with Stener lesions, cases of such injury in the fingers have been reported.[27]

Stener lesions can be diagnosed with ultrasonography or an MRI scan, but these methods are less sensitive than direct visualization using an arthroscope. The role of arthroscopy includes identifying the presence of a Stener lesion and reduction of the lesion in any of the digits by minimally invasive means, if necessary. Repositioning of the collateral ligament was achieved under arthroscopic visualization, and good clinical outcomes were reported.[13,19]

Removal of Loose Bodies or Foreign Bodies

The minimally invasive approach is preferable to open arthrotomy because it permits a rapid return to activity by obviating an incision in the extensor expansion and capsulotomy.[10] There is 1 report of a 1.5-mm metal splinter being removed using a 2.0-mm shaver.[5] The removal of loose bodies or foreign bodies can be achieved arthroscopically without difficulty if they are situated in the dorsal joint space.

Chondral Lesions

MCP joint arthroscopy is useful for intra-articular cartilage defects. Ostendorf and colleagues[33] showed that MCP joint arthroscopy was more sensitive in the detection of intra-articular cartilage abnormalities than plain radiograph or MRI.

Pain improvement can be further achieved with debridement of the cartilage defects, although pain control is not guaranteed. Good results were reported with chondroplasty for chondral defects in the thumb MCP joint of a professional golfer.[20] Persistent pain and a mechanical block caused by an unstable cartilage flap can be treated by the removal of the cartilage flap and smoothing the joint surface under arthroscopic visualization, achieving a good functional outcome. However, the prognosis depends on the severity of the cartilage damage.[13]

Arthrodesis

There is 1 report of arthroscopy-assisted fusion of DIP joints,[11] but this is a technically challenging procedure and should be reserved only for experienced arthroscopists. The advantages of this technique include smaller scars, avoidance of incisions/scars on the dorsum of the digit, no disruption of the dorsal venous system or extensor tendon, and possible faster healing. Care must be taken not to damage the scope, because the working space is limited.

Chronic Pain and Instability

Persistent pain associated with chronic swelling and/or instability in the MCP joint is often managed by conservative treatment. However, if conservative treatment fails, an arthroscopic evaluation and debridement and/or thermal capsulorrhaphy are promising backup options. There have been several reports[9,13,17] on this method, and Wall

and Goldfarb[17] concluded that arthroscopic debridement of painful MCP joints is a useful assessment tool that also provides clinical improvement.

Stiff Fingers

Choi and colleagues[13] reported the arthroscopic release of a stiff MCP joint in 2 cases. Intra-articular fibrosis was removed arthroscopically, and limited extensor tenolysis was performed through the dorsal portals, achieving satisfactory improvement in the range of motion. Arthroscopic release may be an option in MCP joint stiffness mainly caused by intra-articular fibrosis, because there are many causes of stiffness, both intra-articular and extraarticular. Compared with open methods, minimal surgical trauma of the joint capsule and extraarticular tissue may shorten the postoperative rehabilitation period. Less scarring is associated with a better cosmetic appearance.

REFERENCES

1. Chen Y-C. Arthroscopy of the wrist and finger joints. Orthop Clin North Am 1979;10(3):723–33.
2. Declercq G, Schmitgen G, Verstreken J. Arthroscopic treatment of metacarpophalangeal arthropathy in haemochromatosis. J Hand Surg Br 1994;19(2):212–4.
3. Wei N, Delauter SK, Erlichman MS, et al. Arthroscopic synovectomy of the metacarpophalangeal joint in refractory rheumatoid arthritis: a technique. Arthroscopy 1999;15(3):265–8.
4. Ostendorf B, Dann P, Wedekind F, et al. Miniarthroscopy of metacarpophalangeal joints in rheumatoid arthritis. Rating of diagnostic value in synovitis staging and efficiency of synovial biopsy. J Rheumatol 1999;26(9):1901–8.
5. Thomsen NOB, Nielsen NS, Jorgensen U, et al. Arthroscopy of the proximal interphalangeal joints of the finger. J Hand Surg Br 2002;27(3):253–5.
6. Kraan MC, Reece RJ, Smeets TJM, et al. Comparison of synovial tissues from the knee joints and the small joints of rheumatoid arthritis patients. Arthritis Rheum 2002;46(8):2034–8.
7. Badia A. Arthroscopic reduction and internal fixation of bony gamekeeper's thumb. Orthopedics 2006; 29(8):675–8.
8. Erdos J, Gannon C, Baratz ME. Arthroscopy of the metacarpophalangeal joint. Oper Tech Orthop 2007;17(2):133–9.
9. Badia A. Arthroscopy of the trapeziometacarpal and metacarpophalangeal joints. J Hand Surg Am 2007; 32(5):707–24.
10. Berner SH. Metacarpophalangeal arthroscopy: technique and applications. Tech Hand Up Extrem Surg 2008;12(4):208–15.

11. Cobb TK. Arthroscopic distal interphalangeal joint arthrodesis. Tech Hand Up Extrem Surg 2008; 12(4):266–9.

12. Shin EK, Osterman AL. Treatment of thumb metacarpophalangeal and interphalangeal joint arthritis. Hand Clin 2008;24:239–50.

13. Choi AKY, Chow ECS, Ho PC, et al. Metacarpophalangeal joint arthroscopy: indications revisited. Hand Clin 2011;27:369–82.

14. Cobb TK, Berner SH, Badia A. New frontiers in hand arthroscopy. Hand Clin 2011;27:383–94.

15. Vordenbaumen S, Sewerin P, Logters T, et al. Inflammation and vascularisation markers of arthroscopically-guided finger joint synovial biopsies reflect global disease activity in rheumatoid arthritis. Clin Exp Rheumatol 2014;32(1):117–20.

16. Hidalgo-Diaz JJ, Ichihara S, Taleb C, et al. Metacarpophalangeal joint arthroscopy in the fingers other than the thumb: retrospective comparison of horizontal versus vertical traction. Chir Main 2015; 34(3):105–8.

17. Wall LB, Goldfarb CA. Metacarpophalangeal joint arthroscopy: outcomes for the painful, radiographically normal joint. J Hand Surg Eur 2016;39(8): 887–8.

18. Wilkes LL. Arthroscopic synovectomy in the rheumatoid metacarpophalangeal joint. J Med Assoc Ga 1987;76(9):638–9.

19. Ryu J, Fagan R. Arthroscopic treatment of acute complete thumb metacarpophalangeal ulnar collateral ligament tears. J Hand Surg Am 1995;20(6): 1037–42.

20. Vaupel GL, Andrews JR. Diagnostic and operative arthroscopy of the thumb metacarpophalangeal joint: a case report. Am J Sports Med 1985;13(2): 139–41.

21. Johnson LL. Finger joints, arthroscopic surgery-principles and practice. 3rd edition. St Louis (MO): Mosby; 1986. p. 1486–90.

22. Slade JF III, Gutow AP. Arthroscopy of the metacarpophalangeal joint. Hand Clin 1999;15(3):501–27.

23. Rozmaryn LM, Wei N. Metacarpophalangeal arthroscopy. Arthroscopy 1999;15(3):333–7.

24. Gaspar L, Szekanecz Z, Dezso B, et al. Technique of synovial biopsy of metacarpophalangeal joints using the needle arthroscope. Knee Surg Sports Traumatol Arthrosc 2003;11(1):50–2.

25. Sekiya I, Kobayashi M, Taneda N, et al. Arthroscopy of the proximal interphalangeal and metacarpophalangeal joints in rheumatoid hands. Arthroscopy 2002;18(3):292–7.

26. Sekiya I, Kobayashi M, Okamoto H, et al. Arthroscopic synovectomy of the metacarpophalangeal and proximal interphalangeal joints. Tech Hand Up Extrem Surg 2008;12(4):221–5.

27. Berger RA. Small-joint arthroscopy in the hand and wrist. In: Geissler WB, editor. Wrist arthroscopy. New York: Springer; 2005. p. 155–66.

28. Thompson M, Douglas G, Davison EP. Synovectomy of the metacarpophalangeal joints in rheumatoid arthritis. Proc R Soc Med 1973;66:197–9.

29. Arthritis and Rheumatism Council and British Orthopaedic Association. Controlled trial of synovectomy of knee and metacarpophalangeal joints in rheumatoid arthritis. Ann Rheum Dis 1976;35:437–42.

30. Arthritis Foundation Committee on Evaluation of Synovectomy. Multicenter evaluation of synovectomy in the treatment of rheumatoid arthritis. Report of results at the end of three years. Arthritis Rheum 1977;20:765–71.

31. McEwen C. Multicenter evaluation of synovectomy in the treatment of rheumatoid arthritis. Report of results at the end of five years. J Rheumatol 1988; 15:765–9.

32. Larsen A, Dale K, Eek M. Radiographic evaluation of rheumatoid arthritis and related conditions by standard reference films. Acta Radiol Diagn (Stockh) 1977;18:481–91.

33. Ostendorf B, Peters R, Dann P, et al. Magnetic resonance imaging and miniarthroscopy of metacarpophalangeal joints: sensitive detection of morphologic changes in rheumatoid arthritis. Arthritis Rheum 2001;44(11):2492–502.

Complications of Wrist and Hand Arthroscopy

Zahab S. Ahsan, MD[a], Jeffrey Yao, MD[b],*

KEYWORDS

- Wrist arthroscopy • Complications • Neurovascular structures • Tendon injury
- Surgeon experience

KEY POINTS

- A detailed review of the wrist arthroscopy literature yields a complication rate of 4.8%.
- A number of safety precautions have been identified to mitigate the incidence of iatrogenic injury with wrist arthroscopy.
- The rate of complications decreases when a surgeon performs more than 25 cases/year and also decreases significantly after more than 5 years of operative experience.

INTRODUCTION

Arthroscopy of the wrist continues to evolve and advance as a valuable clinical technique in hand surgery that facilitates effective diagnosis and therapy. First introduced in 1979[1] and further detailed in the literature in 1988,[2,3] wrist arthroscopy provides a wide range of current indications and continues to adapt and yield minimally invasive alternatives to open surgical procedures. With increasing adaptation of wrist arthroscopy and an escalating volume of cases performed worldwide, further insights have been gained regarding the complications of wrist arthroscopy over the past 5 years. Specifically, a systematic review of the incidence of complications,[4] systematic review of cadaveric studies reporting structures at risk,[5] and a large multicenter trial[6] have been introduced into the literature for wrist arthroscopy.

Largely regarded as a safe procedure, incidence of complications in the literature ranges from 1.2% to 7.9%.[4,7–14] The most recent study is a multicenter retrospective review of 10,107 cases by Leclercq and colleagues[6] with a finding of 5.98%

complications, with 5.07% listed as serious and 0.91% as minor. Serious complications were defined as laceration of tendon, nerve, artery, large cartilage lesion, loose body requiring arthrotomy, hematoma formation, compartment syndrome, pyogenic arthritis, wrist stiffness, chronic regional pain syndrome, and newly defined "failure to achieve the procedure."[6] Minor complications include transient neuropraxia, small cartilage lesion, loose body not requiring arthrotomy, synovial fistula, local swelling, superficial sepsis, portal site pathology (ganglia, adhesion, pain), and miscellaneous self-limiting problems.

Possible complications may be related to traction and positioning of the arm, portal placement, procedure-specific injuries, and general complications involved in wrist arthroscopy.[8,15] Complications that are universal to wrist arthroscopy include infection, articular surface damage, and equipment failure.[15] The establishment of portals and introduction of instruments requires a thorough knowledge of the regional anatomy and appropriate tactile sensitivity of the surgeon. Poor positioning of portals and forceful insertion of instruments may damage articular cartilage,

---

Disclosure Statement: The authors have no disclosures to report.
[a] Department of Orthopaedics and Sports Medicine, University of Washington, 325 9th Avenue, Box 359798, Seattle, WA 98104, USA; [b] Department of Orthopaedic Surgery, Robert A. Chase Hand and Upper Limb Center, Stanford University Medical Center, 770 Welch Road, Suite 400, Palo Alto, CA 94304, USA
* Corresponding author. 450 Broadway Street, Suite C-442, Redwood City, CA 94063.
E-mail address: jyao@stanford.edu

Hand Clin 33 (2017) 831–838
http://dx.doi.org/10.1016/j.hcl.2017.07.008

ligaments, tendons, cutaneous nerves, and vascular structures.[16]

An evolving figure, the true incidence of complications is likely dependent on the definition of complications as well as the willingness of surgeons to report their complications. Regardless, a thorough knowledge and understanding of the possible consequences of our interventions as surgeons can help to mitigate complications and optimize patient outcomes. The objective of this article is to summarize the current literature to guide clinicians implementing wrist arthroscopy into their respective practices.

A comprehensive review of the literature was performed, identifying 12 multiple patient trials that address complications of wrist arthroscopy (**Table 1**). There were 4 case reports that described unique incidence of wrist arthroscopy complications (**Table 2**).

Cadaveric Studies

Prior to overviewing the clinically reported wrist arthroscopy complications in the literature, a review of the relevant anatomy is warranted. This primarily pertains to the dorsal structures, as most arthroscopic procedures are performed via a dorsal approach (**Fig. 1**). The 6 extensor compartments delineate the margins for instrumentation into the wrist joint. The spaces intervening the compartments (1–2, 3–4, 4–5), as well as the ulnar and radial aspects of the sixth compartment comprise the primary portals. Structures of importance include the deep branch of the radial artery (RA), superficial branch of the radial nerve (SBRN), dorsal sensory branch of the ulnar nerve (DSBUN), and the distal posterior interosseous nerve (PIN).[11,15,17] The deep branch of the RA enters the anatomic snuffbox under the tendons of the first dorsal compartment and crosses the base of the thumb metacarpal to enter the palm.[8,18] The SBRN travels deep to the brachioradialis and changes course at the intersection of the first and second extensor compartments with arborization to supply sensation to the thumb, index, and long fingers.[8,15] The DSBUN arises from the ulnar nerve deep to the flexor carpi ulnaris tendon, runs subcutaneously and wraps around the distal ulna within 1 cm of the ulnar head. Near the level of the ulnar styloid, 5 variable branches of the DSBUN are typically noted, giving rise to higher risk of injury, particularly when using the 6U portal.[18–20] The DSBUN consistently travels intimately around the extensor carpi ulnaris (ECU) and can be found on either side of the tendon, in close proximity to the 6 radial (6R) and 6 ulnar

---

Table 1
Multiple patient studies presenting wrist arthroscopy complications

Author, Year	Study Design	Level of Evidence	Number of Complications	Number of Patients in Study	Percentage
Lourie et al,[20] 1994	Prospective cohort	II	3	15	20.0
Warhold and Ruth,[15] 1995	Case series	IV	4	205	2.0
de Smet,[16] 1996	Case series	IV	2	129	1.6
Doi et al,[42] 1999	Randomized controlled study	I	7	34	20.5
Hofmeister et al,[10] 2001	Prospective cohort	II	1	89	1.1
Beredjiklian et al,[7] 2004	Case series	IV	11	211	5.2
Pell and Uhl,[27] 2004	Case series	IV	4	47	8.5
Darlis et al,[30] 2005	Case series	IV	2	16	12.5
Rocchi et al,[31] 2008	Prospective randomized study	I	2	20	10.0
Gallego and Mathoulin,[32] 2010	Case series	IV	6	114	5.3
Chen et al,[33] 2010	Case series	IV	1	15	6.6
Leclercq et al,[6] 2016	Multicenter case series	IV	605	10,107	6.0
Total			648	11,002	5.9

Table 2
Summary of case reports of wrist arthroscopy complications

Author, Year	Study Design	Level of Evidence	Description of Injury
del Piñal et al,[34] 1999	Case report	V	Avulsion of distal PIN at 3–4 portal
Tsu-Hsin Chen et al,[38] 2006	Case report	V	Strangulation of DSBUN with suture after TFCC repair (inside-out technique)
Shirley et al,[37] 2008	Case report	V	Extensor tendon sheath fistula formation
Nguyen et al,[41] 2011	Case report	V	Transection of ulnar nerve trunk at 6U portal

Abbreviations: DSBUN, dorsal sensory branch of the ulnar nerve; PIN, posterior interosseous nerve; TFCC, triangular fibrocartilaginous complex; 6U, 6 ulnar.

(6U) portals. The distal PIN travels along the floor of the fourth compartment and supplies sensation to the joint capsule. It is less mobile than the surrounding sensory nerves.[8,15]

In an effort to establish the anatomic basis for complications of wrist arthroscopy, Shyamalan and colleagues[5] conducted an anatomic study of 10 cadaveric wrists and simultaneously performed

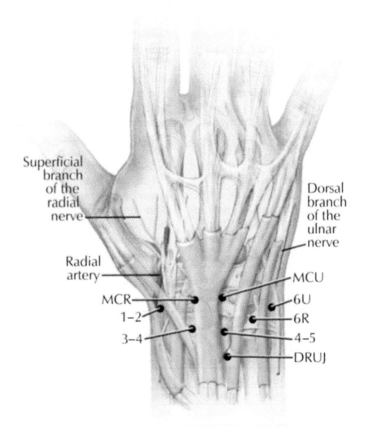

Fig. 1. Portal anatomy of the dorsal aspect of the wrist. DRUJ, distal radioulnar joint; MCR, midcarpal radial; MCU, midcarpal ulnar; R, radial; U, ulnar. (*From* El-Gazzar Y, Baker CL. Complications of elbow and wrist arthroscopy. Sports Med Arthrosc 2013;21(2):80–8; with permission.)

a systematic review of cadaveric studies pertaining to wrist arthroscopy and the proximity of neighboring anatomic structures. The specimens underwent 60 to 180 minutes of arthroscopic surgery by experienced surgeons involving a diagnostic arthroscopy followed by repair of the triangular fibrocartilaginous complex (TFCC). During these procedures the 1–2, 3–4, 4–5, 6R, 6U, ulnar midcarpal, and radial midcarpal portals were created with aid of a 22-gauge needle. Additional portals including distal radioulnar joint (DRUJ), volar radial, and volar ulnar portals have been described,[21,22] although were not the focus of this study. Subsequent dissection of the cadaveric wrists was performed to identify the proximity of the DSBUN, SBRN, PIN, and extensor tendons to the portals. Digital calipers were used to measure the distances from the portals and damage to any nerves or tendons was recorded. The average distances of each sensory nerve from the portals was documented and is outlined in **Table 3**.

All 7 portals were within close proximity of the 3 nerves (DSBUN, SBRN, and PIN). During dissection of the wrist following completion of the arthroscopy, one nerve injury was identified during a capsulodesis stitch placement; all 3 nerves were noted to run under a skin portal in at least 1 specimen. Six extensor tendon injuries were noted including the extensor digitorum communis (EDC) to the index finger, EDC to the middle finger, ECU, and extensor digiti minimi.

Seven publications were included in the systematic review of cadaveric studies addressing susceptibility to injury during wrist arthroscopy. Three of these were performed on fresh frozen cadavers[22–24] and 4 on preserved cadavers.[19,21,25,26]

Among these studies, the DSBUN was a risk from the 6U, 6R, and ulnar midcarpal portals in the study by Shyamalan and colleagues.[5] The 6R had a mean distance of 8 mm and the 6U portal was documented as a zero-distance due to several adjacent data points. Tryfonidis and colleagues[19] reported the DSBUN at risk only from

the 6U portal, not the 6R or ulnar midcarpal portal. The DSBUN was documented as a mean of 2.4 cm (range 1.8–2.8 mm) from the ulnar styloid along a straight line in the trajectory of the fourth webspace. It was concluded that portal placement in the proximal fifth of this line was "safe."[26] The SBRN was at risk from the 1 to 2 portal with mean distance of 1.6 mm (range 0–8 mm) and the radial midcarpal portal was a close second with mean distance of 24 mm.[5] The reviewed studies supported this finding along with risk from the 3 to 4 portal.[19,23] The PIN was at risk in the study by Shyamalan and colleagues[5] at the 3 to 4 portal and had the shortest mean distance of 4.4 mm (range 0–10) and at the 4 to 5 portal with a distance of 12.6 mm (range 2–25).[5] This is a new finding, undocumented in the reviewed cadaveric literature.[14,19,21–23,25]

Clinical Studies

Lourie and colleagues[20] reported a series of 15 patients who underwent DRUJ arthroscopy. Three of these patients presented with transection of the transverse radioulnar branch of the DSBUN. Persistent dysesthesia with a positive Tinel sign, consistent with neuroma formation was noted for each of these instances. The patients were treated with secondary operative excision of the neuroma and this relieved all symptoms but left a small region of hypesthesia of the skin. The transverse radioulnar branch of the DSBUN is particularly vulnerable to injury in the region of the 6R portal because of its variable arborization. Injury to this nerve has potential to cause persistent pain due to neuroma formation.

A study by Warhold and Ruth in 1995[15] provided a review of complications from a series of 205 wrist arthroscopies. Four complications were described, amounting to a 2% incidence. These complications consisted of 1 suture abscess, which resolved on removal of the suture; 1 inclusion cyst, which required surgical removal 6 months after the initial arthroscopy; and 2 cases

Table 3
Anatomic distance of DSBUN, SBRN, PIN from arthroscopic portals (mm)

Nerve	1–2	3–4	4–5	6 Radial	6 Ulnar	Ulnar Midcarpal	Radial Midcarpal
DSBUN	51–82	30–60	13–32	2–14	0–8	9–56	27–54
SBRN	0–8	15–33	23–52	44–76	51–84	30–64	13–42
PIN	18–35	0–10	2–25	10–36	18–40	10–16	0–20

Abbreviations: DSBUN, dorsal sensory branch of the ulnar nerve; PIN, posterior interosseous nerve; SBRN, superficial branch of the radial nerve.

From Shyamalan G, Jordan RW, Kimani PK, et al. Assessment of the structures at risk during wrist arthroscopy: a cadaveric study and systematic review. J Hand Surg Eur Vol 2016;41(8):854; with permission.

of mild reflex sympathetic dystrophy (RSD). The RSD resolved spontaneously in 1 patient; however, it remained as persistent wrist pain in the second patient. De Smet and colleagues[9] presented a retrospective review of 129 patients with wrist arthroscopy with 2 identified complications (1.6%). These were 1 case of tendon rupture over a Kirschner wire and 1 superficial infection at a portal site. Hofmeister and colleagues[10] presented a series of 89 wrist arthroscopies in 2001 with a single reported complication. This complication was a partial laceration of the EDC tendon to the small finger. An extension lag was noted immediately in the postoperative period but no treatment was necessary. Beredjiklian and colleagues[7] reviewed 211 patients with wrist arthroscopy, identifying 11 complications (5.2%). These complications were further categorized into major and minor complications based on whether the complications resolved with observation or conservative treatment. There were 2 cases of major complications: 1 patient developed permanent wrist stiffness (25° extension and 30° flexion) after 12 months of therapy. The other involved ganglion cyst development that required surgical excision 12 months postoperatively. Minor complications in the remaining 9 patients consisted of transient sensory neuropraxia of DSBUN, transient stiffness of the wrist and finger joints, superficial portal infection, first-degree burn, and ECU tendinitis.

Pell and Uhl[27] reviewed 47 patients who underwent thermal ablation procedures during wrist arthroscopy and reported 3 tendon ruptures and 1 case of a full-thickness skin burn as a result of use of the electrothermal frequency probe. Extensor tendon function was maintained immediately after arthroscopy and rupture was noted 1 to 3 months postoperatively. The minimal soft tissue between the dorsal wrist capsule and the surrounding structures places them at additional risk with use of the thermal ablation. Shellock and Shields[28] suggest that monopolar radiofrequency may not properly regulate the delivery of energy-induced heat, and bipolar devices are recommended due to a linear relationship between surface temperature and time. Ultimately, the extent of thermal injury is dependent on the surgeon's regulation.[29] A 2005 study by Darlis and colleagues[30] evaluated the treatment of partial scapholunate ligament injuries with arthroscopic debridement and thermal shrinkage. Two of 16 patients undergoing treatment experienced postoperative complications during the follow-up period: one instance of carpal tunnel syndrome (CTS) managed with splinting and another patient developed de Quervain tenosynovitis requiring a corticosteroid injection to alleviate symptoms. A direct correlation with the thermal capsulorrhaphy and CTS or de Quervain was not apparent, although the investigators advocated for judicious use of radiofrequency probe application for thermal shrinkage.

Rocchi and colleagues[31] present a prospective randomized study comparing the treatment of articular ganglia via arthroscopic resection and open excision. Among 20 patients in the arthroscopic resection group, there were 2 complications: 1 case of neuropraxia of the SBRN to the dorsal aspect of the thumb and 1 injury to a branch of the radial artery. The neuropraxia recovered spontaneously in 3 months and the arterial injury was converted to an open operation to obtain hemostasis. Gallego and Mathoulin[32] evaluated 114 patients for arthroscopic resection of dorsal wrist ganglia. Six arthroscopy-related complications were noted: 2 hematomas required surgical drainage, 1 case of tenosynovitis of the extensor pollicis longus tendon, 1 case of tenosynovitis of the EDC tendon, and 2 patients with transient neuropraxia of the SBRN and DSBUN. Fourteen patients experienced recurrence of the ganglion cyst, which were not classified as isolated wrist arthroscopy complication, although merits acknowledgment. Chen and colleagues[33] present a case series of 15 patients who underwent arthroscopic ganglionectomy with a mean follow-up of 15.3 months. There was a single arthroscopy-related complication, transient paresthesias along the radial side, which resolved in 1 month. Recurrence of the ganglion cyst was appreciated in an additional case, although not considered a complication of the arthroscopic procedure.

The largest study of wrist arthroscopy complications to date was presented by Leclercq and colleagues[6] in conjunction with the European Wrist Arthroscopy Society (EWAS) in April 2016. A large multicenter retrospective review identified 36 series comprising 10,107 wrist arthroscopy procedures; 605 complications (5.85%) were noted, of which 5.07% were considered major and 0.91% minor. The review was performed by the administration of a questionnaire to members of the EWAS, with contribution from 36 of 180 members. Scrutiny of the data for each surgeon's experience with wrist arthroscopy and its relation to complications demonstrated that average complication rate is 6 times greater in small series (<50 cases: 22.6% complications) than in large series (>600 cases: 3.7% complications). Higher incidence of complications was correlated with less than 25 wrist arthroscopy procedures performed annually or less than 5 years of practice of wrist arthroscopy. This finding supports the existence of a learning curve, as with all acquired technical skills in surgery. The most common complication (118 cases, 1.17%) was "failure to achieve the procedure," defined as need to proceed with open surgery to achieve surgical goals. More than 50% of these cases involved ganglion excision. Nerve lesions were the second most common (0.8% incidence), with 59 nerve lacerations (0.59%) occurring at the site of the wrist portals. Most of these were sensory nerve injuries, although 2 involved the median nerve proper during volar ganglia excision. Fifteen of these lesions required revision surgery. Cartilage lesions were further categorized as minimal (unlikely to create future problems) and large (more than 5 mm^2). Minimal cartilage lesions occurred in most series (33 of 36) with 51 total large lesions identified throughout the total cohort (0.5%). The presence of a "tight wrist," making navigating within the joints difficult, irrespective of procedure, was most likely to generate a cartilage lesion.

Chronic regional pain syndrome, wrist stiffness, loose bodies, hematoma formation, and tendon lacerations were noted in declining incidence. Finger traction and arm countertraction were also identified as sources of complication, responsible for neuropraxia at the finger or arm level. Also, there were 3 reported cases of burns due to the hot traction tower.[6,8] This emphasizes the importance of diligence throughout each part of the procedure, including preparation, draping, and patient positioning.

In 1999, del Piñal and colleagues[34] presented a case report of distal PIN avulsion following wrist arthroscopy. Instrumentation into the wrist joint was performed via the 3–4, 6R, and radial midcarpal portals. A scapholunate injury was visualized and an open repair was deemed necessary.[35] On an open approach with a longitudinal incision centered at the Lister tubercle, the distal PIN was found to be avulsed at the level of the 3–4 portal. This is the only reported case of this injury in the literature. The lack of other reports may be attributed to the rarity of the injury or that most arthroscopies do not require an open procedure that may reveal distal PIN injury that may otherwise remain occult. This study presents the possibility of distal PIN injury during wrist arthroscopy that may lead to chronic dorsal wrist pain. On the contrary, it is possible that complete avulsion of the distal PIN provides symptomatic relief via partial sensory denervation for patients experiencing prior chronic dorsal wrist pain.[36]

Shirley and colleagues[37] presented a case report of extensor tendon sheath fistula formation in a 45-year-old man who underwent diagnostic arthroscopy after sustaining a scapholunate ligament (SL) disruption. When the patient returned for SL ligament reconstruction, a tender fluctuant swelling (6 × 3 × 1 cm) was noted on the dorsum of the hand. The collection of fluid was identified around the extensor pollicis longus tendon within the tendon sheath. A patent opening from the tendon sheath into the radiocarpal joint was noted at the location of the previous 3–4 portal. This was treated with fluid evacuation and surgical diathermy to preserve the tendon sheath. A case report of DSBUN injury during repair of a Palmer Class 1B TFCC lesion has been presented in the literature by Tsu-Hsin Chen and colleagues.[38] The mechanism of injury involved strangulation of the nerve during arthroscopic TFCC repair by a pull-out suture placed in the joint capsule. Three percutaneous sutures were used with an arthroscope-assisted inside-out technique, the most distal of which entrapped the nerve. Postoperatively, the patient experienced severe pricking pain in the distribution of the DSBUN and local tenderness over the TFCC scar, worsening with forearm pronation/supination and percussion. Treatment entailed the segmental excision of the nerve 2 cm proximal and distal to the suture site. In a cadaveric study of arthroscopic TFCC repair, it has been demonstrated by McAdams and Hentz[39] that the inside-out sutures may be as close as 0.4 mm to the main trunk of the DSBUN, suggesting that if the nerve is not located and protected before passing of the sutures, there is an approximately 50% chance of nerve branch strangulation. Because of this, they proposed a longitudinal open incision on the ulnar wrist to identify the DSBUN before suture application. Bednar and Osterman[40] recommend a 1-cm incision radial to the ECU tendon for safe suture retrieval and tying the suture at the level of the capsule, as opposed to the use of a suture button. As previously mentioned, the arborization pattern of the DSBUN is quite variable, and nerve injury is possible even with correct portal placement. This places the utmost importance on diligent spreading with a fine-point hemostat during portal establishment and diligent soft tissue dissection techniques for instrumentation.[8,38]

Nguyen and colleagues[41] present a case report in which near complete transection of the trunk of the ulnar nerve was caused by the trocar used for drainage at the 6U portal. Complete sensorimotor paralysis of the ulnar nerve was noted on the first postoperative day. Surgical exploration was performed, and on visualization of the injury, resection to healthy tissue was carried out and an epineural coaptation was performed. Histologic analysis of the resected nerve segment suggested trauma from the bevel of the infusion trocar placed in the 6U portal for fluid drainage. The 6U portal has been implicated with an increased risk of injury to the DSBUN due to its variable position and winding between the pisiform and ulnar styloid.[8] This report is unique for injury to the ulnar nerve proper. It is important to consider the anatomic and positional variation of the ulnar nerve with pronation/supination movements of the forearm. The ulnar nerve is more susceptible to injury from trocar shearing movements in forced pronation due to increased tension. To ensure safe application of a drainage portal, the investigators advocate to set up by mini-open access of the 6U portal after meticulous identification of anatomic structures, use of a small-diameter trocar (>20 gauge), and avoidance of arthro-pump for water intake.[41] We currently do not use drainage portals and we avoid the routine use of the 6U portal for these reasons.

SUMMARY

This article aimed to summarize the current literature regarding complications of wrist arthroscopy. The 2016 multicenter trial[6] reported a complication rate of 5.9%, greater than the previously documented systematic review of 4.7%.[4,8,15,16] Although, if further scrutinized, 110 of those complications were "failure to achieve the procedure." Extracting these numbers yields a complication rate of 4.8%, in accordance with the prior literature.

A variety of complications have been cited; including nerve injuries, tendon injuries, tendon sheath fistulae, arterial injury, development of cysts, development of CTS, de Quervain tenosynovitis, cartilage injury, chronic loss of mobility, hematoma development, equipment-related burns, and local infections. Although a clear distinction is not made, many of the complications may be classified as minor, as they resolve with little or no intervention, whereas others are more severe and subject patients to revision procedures to alleviate the deleterious consequences.

A variety of safety precautions can minimize the incidence of iatrogenic injury. These precautions include the use of a hypodermic needle to confirm portal placement; insufflation of the joint with saline before portal placement; a longitudinal incision that penetrates only the dermis; spreading of the soft tissue with a blunt, fine-tip hemostat to allow for important structures to retract; insertion of trocar with minimal resistance; and continuous monitoring of traction.[8,15,16] Avoidance of the 6U portal and appropriate placement of percutaneous needles used in ligament repairs is important to avoid nerve entrapment.

Arthroscopy of the wrist remains a valuable and safe surgical procedure for experienced surgeons and provides a broadly applicable minimally invasive approach. The likelihood of associated injuries during wrist arthroscopy is dependent on the surgeon's mastery of the anatomy coupled with correct operative technique and a thorough understanding of the equipment.[8] The literature suggests that a learning curve exists for the execution of wrist arthroscopy. Case volume and duration of experience are variables that correlate with mitigating iatrogenic injury and optimizing patient outcomes. The rate of complications decreases when a surgeon performs more than 25 cases per year and also decreases significantly after more than 5 years of operative experience.[6]

REFERENCES

1. Chen YC. Arthroscopy of the wrist and finger joints. Orthop Clin North Am 1979;10(3):723–33.
2. Roth JH, Poehling GG, Whipple TL. Arthroscopic surgery of the wrist. Instr Course Lect 1988;37:183–94.
3. Roth JH, Poehling GG, Whipple TL. Hand instrumentation for small joint arthroscopy. Arthroscopy 1988;4(2):126–8.
4. Ahsan ZS, Yao J. Complications of wrist arthroscopy. Arthroscopy 2012;29(3):406–11.
5. Shyamalan G, Jordan RW, Kimani PK, et al. Assessment of the structures at risk during wrist arthroscopy: a cadaveric study and systematic review. J Hand Surg Eur Vol 2016;41(8):852–8.
6. Leclercq C, Mathoulin C, Members of EWAS. Complications of wrist arthroscopy: a multicenter study based on 10,107 arthroscopies. J Wrist Surg 2016;5(4):320–6.
7. Beredjiklian PK, Bozentka DJ, Leung YL, et al. Complications of wrist arthroscopy. J Hand Surg Am 2004;29(3):406–11.
8. Culp RW. Complications of wrist arthroscopy. Hand Clin 1999;15(3):529–35, x.
9. De Smet L, Dauwe D, Fortems Y, et al. The value of wrist arthroscopy. An evaluation of 129 cases. J Hand Surg Br 1996;21(2):210–2.
10. Hofmeister EP, Dao KD, Glowacki KA, et al. The role of midcarpal arthroscopy in the diagnosis of disorders of the wrist. J Hand Surg Am 2001;26(3):407–14.
11. Nagle DJ, Benson LS. Wrist arthroscopy: indications and results. Arthroscopy 1992;8(2):198–203.
12. Slutsky DJ. Current innovations in wrist arthroscopy. J Hand Surg 2012;37(9):1932–41.
13. Luchetti R, Atzei A, Rocchi L. Incidence and causes of failures in wrist arthroscopic techniques. Chir Main 2006;25(1):48–53 [in French].
14. Slutsky DJ, Nagle DJ. Wrist arthroscopy: current concepts. J Hand Surg 2008;33(7):1228–44.

15. Warhold LG, Ruth RM. Complications of wrist arthroscopy and how to prevent them. Hand Clin 1995;11(1):81–9.

16. De Smet L. Pitfalls in wrist arthroscopy. Acta Orthop Belg 2002;68(4):325–9.

17. Whipple TL, Marotta JJ, Powell JH. Techniques of wrist arthroscopy. Arthroscopy 1986;2(4):244–52.

18. El-Gazzar Y, Baker CL. Complications of elbow and wrist arthroscopy. Sports Med Arthrosc 2013;21(2): 80–8.

19. Tryfonidis M, Charalambous CP, Jass GK, et al. Anatomic relation of dorsal wrist arthroscopy portals and superficial nerves: a cadaveric study. Arthroscopy 2009;25(12):1387–90.

20. Lourie GM, King J, Kleinman WB. The transverse radioulnar branch from the dorsal sensory ulnar nerve: its clinical and anatomical significance further defined. J Hand Surg Am 1994;19(2):241–5.

21. Kiliç A, Kale A, Usta A, et al. Anatomic course of the superficial branch of the radial nerve in the wrist and its location in relation to wrist arthroscopy portals: a cadaveric study. Arthroscopy 2009;25(11):1261–4.

22. Abrams RA, Petersen M, Botte MJ. Arthroscopic portals of the wrist: an anatomic study. J Hand Surg Am 1994;19(6):940–4.

23. Auerbach DM, Collins ED, Kunkle KL, et al. The radial sensory nerve. An anatomic study. Clin Orthop Relat Res 1994;308:241–9.

24. Slutsky DJ. The use of a volar ulnar portal in wrist arthroscopy. Arthroscopy 2004;20(2):158–63.

25. Ehlinger M, Rapp E, Cognet J-M, et al. Transverse radioulnar branch of the dorsal ulnar nerve: anatomic description and arthroscopic implications from 45 cadaveric dissections. Rev Chir Orthop Reparatrice Appar Mot 2005;91(3):208–14 [in French].

26. Tindall A, Patel M, Frost A, et al. The anatomy of the dorsal cutaneous branch of the ulnar nerve—a safe zone for positioning of the 6R portal in wrist arthroscopy. J Hand Surg Br 2006;31(2):203–5.

27. Pell RF IV, Uhl RL. Complications of thermal ablation in wrist arthroscopy. Arthroscopy 2004;20:84–6.

28. Shellock FG, Shields CL. Temperature changes associated with radiofrequency energy-induced heating of bovine capsular tissue: evaluation of bipolar RF electrodes. Arthroscopy 2000;16(4): 348–58.

29. Arnoczky SP, Aksan A. Thermal modification of connective tissues: basic science considerations and clinical implications. J Am Acad Orthop Surg 2000; 8(5):305–13.

30. Darlis NA, Weiser RW, Sotereanos DG. Partial scapholunate ligament injuries treated with arthroscopic debridement and thermal shrinkage. J Hand Surg Am 2005;30(5):908–14.

31. Rocchi L, Canal A, Fanfani F, et al. Articular ganglia of the volar aspect of the wrist: arthroscopic resection compared with open excision. A prospective randomised study. Scand J Plast Reconstr Surg Hand Surg 2008;42(5):253–9.

32. Gallego S, Mathoulin C. Arthroscopic resection of dorsal wrist ganglia: 114 cases with minimum follow-up of 2 years. Arthroscopy 2010;26(12): 1675–82.

33. Chen ACY, Lee WC, Hsu KY, et al. Arthroscopic ganglionectomy through an intrafocal cystic portal for wrist ganglia. Arthroscopy 2010;26(5):617–22.

34. del Piñal F, Herrero F, Cruz-Camara A, et al. Complete avulsion of the distal posterior interosseous nerve during wrist arthroscopy: a possible cause of persistent pain after arthroscopy. J Hand Surg Am 1999;24(2):240–2.

35. Geissler WB. Arthroscopic excision of dorsal wrist ganglia. Tech Hand Up Extrem Surg 1998;2(3): 196–201.

36. Weiss AP, Sachar K, Glowacki KA. Arthroscopic debridement alone for intercarpal ligament tears. J Hand Surg Am 1997;22(2):344–9.

37. Shirley DSL, Mullet H, Stanley JK. Extensor tendon sheath fistula formation as a complication of wrist arthroscopy. Arthroscopy 2008;24(11): 1311–2.

38. Tsu-Hsin Chen E, Wei J-D, Huang VWS. Injury of the dorsal sensory branch of the ulnar nerve as a complication of arthroscopic repair of the triangular fibrocartilage. J Hand Surg Br 2006;31(5):530–2.

39. McAdams TR, Hentz VR. Injury to the dorsal sensory branch of the ulnar nerve in the arthroscopic repair of ulnar-sided triangular fibrocartilage tears using an inside-out technique: a cadaver study. J Hand Surg Am 2002;27(5):840–4.

40. Bednar JM, Osterman AL. The role of arthroscopy in the treatment of traumatic triangular fibrocartilage injuries. Hand Clin 1994;10(4):605–14.

41. Nguyen MK, Bourgouin S, Gaillard C, et al. Accidental section of the ulnar nerve in the wrist during arthroscopy. Arthroscopy 2011;27(9):1308–11.

42. Doi K, Hattori Y, Otsuka K, et al. Intra-articular fractures of the distal aspect of the radius: arthroscopically assisted reduction compared with open reduction and internal fixation. J Bone Joint Surg Am 1999;81(8):1093–110.

UNITED STATES POSTAL SERVICE ®

Statement of Ownership, Management, and Circulation (All Periodicals Publications Except Requester Publications)

1. Publication Title	2. Publication Number	3. Filing Date
HAND CLINICS	000 – 709	9/18/2017

4. Issue Frequency	5. Number of Issues Published Annually	6. Annual Subscription Price
FEB, MAY, AUG, NOV	4	$398.00

7. Complete Mailing Address of Known Office of Publication (Not printer) (Street, city, county, state, and ZIP+4®)

ELSEVIER INC.
230 Park Avenue, Suite 800
New York, NY 10169

Contact Person
STEPHEN R. BUSHING
Telephone (Include area code)
215-239-3688

8. Complete Mailing Address of Headquarters or General Business Office of Publisher (Not printer)

ELSEVIER INC.
230 Park Avenue, Suite 800
New York, NY 10169

9. Full Names and Complete Mailing Addresses of Publisher, Editor, and Managing Editor (Do not leave blank)

Publisher (Name and complete mailing address)

ADRIANNE BRIGIDO, ELSEVIER INC.
1600 JOHN F KENNEDY BLVD. SUITE 1800
PHILADELPHIA, PA 19103-2899

Editor (Name and complete mailing address)

LAUREN BOYLE, ELSEVIER INC.
1600 JOHN F KENNEDY BLVD. SUITE 1800
PHILADELPHIA, PA 19103-2899

Managing Editor (Name and complete mailing address)

PATRICK MANLEY, ELSEVIER INC.
1600 JOHN F KENNEDY BLVD. SUITE 1800
PHILADELPHIA, PA 19103-2899

10. Owner (Do not leave blank. If the publication is owned by a corporation, give the name and address of the corporation immediately followed by the names and addresses of all stockholders owning or holding 1 percent or more of the total amount of stock. If not owned by a corporation, give the names and addresses of the individual owners. If owned by a partnership or other unincorporated firm, give its name and address as well as those of each individual owner. If the publication is published by a nonprofit organization, give its name and address.)

Full Name	Complete Mailing Address
WHOLLY OWNED SUBSIDIARY OF REED/ELSEVIER, US HOLDINGS	1600 JOHN F KENNEDY BLVD. SUITE 1800 PHILADELPHIA, PA 19103-2899

11. Known Bondholders, Mortgagees, and Other Security Holders Owning or Holding 1 Percent or More of Total Amount of Bonds, Mortgages, or Other Securities. If none, check box. ▶ ☐ None

Full Name	Complete Mailing Address
N/A	

12. Tax Status (For completion by nonprofit organizations authorized to mail at nonprofit rates) (Check one)
The purpose, function, and nonprofit status of this organization and the exempt status for federal income tax purposes:
☒ Has Not Changed During Preceding 12 Months
☐ Has Changed During Preceding 12 Months (Publisher must submit explanation of change with this statement)

13. Publication Title	14. Issue Date for Circulation Data Below
HAND CLINICS	AUGUST 2017

PS Form 3526, July 2014 [Page 1 of 4 (see instructions page 4)] PSN: 7530-01-000-9931 PRIVACY NOTICE: See our privacy policy on www.usps.com.

---

15. Extent and Nature of Circulation			Average No. Copies Each Issue During Preceding 12 Months	No. Copies of Single Issue Published Nearest to Filing Date
a. Total Number of Copies (Net press run)			543	467
b. Paid Circulation (By Mail and Outside the Mail)	(1)	Mailed Outside-County Paid Subscriptions Stated on PS Form 3541 (Include paid distribution above nominal rate, advertiser's proof copies, and exchange copies)	327	296
	(2)	Mailed In-County Paid Subscriptions Stated on PS Form 3541 (Include paid distribution above nominal rate, advertiser's proof copies, and exchange copies)	0	0
	(3)	Paid Distribution Outside the Mails Including Sales Through Dealers and Carriers, Street Vendors, Counter Sales, and Other Paid Distribution Outside USPS®	129	116
	(4)	Paid Distribution by Other Classes of Mail Through the USPS (e.g. First-Class Mail®)	0	0
c. Total Paid Distribution (Sum of 15b (1), (2), (3), and (4))		▶	456	412
d. Free or Nominal Rate Distribution (By Mail and Outside the Mail)	(1)	Free or Nominal Rate Outside-County Copies Included on PS Form 3541	30	55
	(2)	Free or Nominal Rate In-County Copies Included on PS Form 3541	0	0
	(3)	Free or Nominal Rate Copies Mailed at Other Classes Through the USPS (e.g. First-Class Mail)	0	0
	(4)	Free or Nominal Rate Distribution Outside the Mail (Carriers or other means)	0	0
e. Total Free or Nominal Rate Distribution (Sum of 15d (1), (2), (3) and (4))		▶	30	55
f. Total Distribution (Sum of 15c and 15e)		▶	486	467
g. Copies not Distributed (See instructions to Publishers #4 (page #3))		▶	57	0
h. Total (Sum of 15f and g)		▶	543	467
i. Percent Paid (15c divided by 15f times 100)		▶	93.83%	88.22%

* If you are claiming electronic copies, go to line 16 on page 3. If you are not claiming electronic copies, skip to line 17 on page 3.

16. Electronic Copy Circulation		Average No. Copies Each Issue During Preceding 12 Months	No. Copies of Single Issue Published Nearest to Filing Date
a. Paid Electronic Copies	▶	0	0
b. Total Paid Print Copies (Line 15c) + Paid Electronic Copies (Line 16a)	▶	456	412
c. Total Print Distribution (Line 15f) + Paid Electronic Copies (Line 16a)	▶	486	467
d. Percent Paid (Both Print & Electronic Copies) (16b divided by 16c × 100)	▶	93.83%	88.22%

☒ I certify that 60% of all my distributed copies (electronic and print) are paid above a nominal price.

17. Publication of Statement of Ownership

☒ If the publication is a general publication, publication of this statement is required. Will be printed in the NOV 2017 issue of this publication. ☐ Publication not required.

18. Signature and Title of Editor, Publisher, Business Manager, or Owner	Date
Stephen R. Bushing STEPHEN R. BUSHING - INVENTORY DISTRIBUTION CONTROL MANAGER	9/18/2017

I certify that all information furnished on this form is true and complete. I understand that anyone who furnishes false or misleading information on this form or who omits material or information requested on the form may be subject to criminal sanctions (including fines and imprisonment) and/or civil sanctions (including civil penalties).

PS Form 3526, July 2014 (Page 3 of 4) PRIVACY NOTICE: See our privacy policy on www.usps.com.

Moving?

Make sure your subscription moves with you!

To notify us of your new address, find your **Clinics Account Number** (located on your mailing label above your name), and contact customer service at:

Email: journalscustomerservice-usa@elsevier.com

800-654-2452 (subscribers in the U.S. & Canada)
314-447-8871 (subscribers outside of the U.S. & Canada)

Fax number: 314-447-8029

Elsevier Health Sciences Division
Subscription Customer Service
3251 Riverport Lane
Maryland Heights, MO 63043

*To ensure uninterrupted delivery of your subscription, please notify us at least 4 weeks in advance of move.

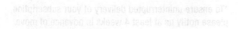

Printed and bound by CPI Group (UK) Ltd, Croydon, CR0 4YY

03/10/2024

01040304-0002